DATE DUE

DE 2 1 01			

DEMCO 38-296

ANNALS OF THE NEW YORK ACADEMY OF SCIENCES

Volume 889

EDITORIAL STAFF

Executive Editor
BARBARA M. GOLDMAN

Managing Editor
JUSTINE CULLINAN

Associate Editor
STEVEN E. BOHALL

The New York Academy of Sciences
2 East 63rd Street
New York, New York 10021

CANCER PREVENTION
NOVEL NUTRIENT AND PHARMACEUTICAL DEVELOPMENTS

ANNALS OF THE NEW YORK ACADEMY OF SCIENCES
Volume 889

CANCER PREVENTION
NOVEL NUTRIENT AND
PHARMACEUTICAL DEVELOPMENTS

Edited by H. Leon Bradlow, Jack Fishman, and Michael P. Osborne

The New York Academy of Sciences
New York, New York
1999

Library of Congress Cataloging-in-Publication Data

Cancer prevention: novel nutrient and pharmaceutical developments /edited by H. Leon Bradlow, Jack Fishman, and Michael P. Osborne
    p.   cm. — (Annals of the New York Academy of Sciences ; v. 889)
    Includes bibliographical references and index.
    ISBN 1-57331-198-7 (cloth alk. paper). — ISBN 1-57331-199-5 (paper : alk. paper)
    1. Cancer—Chemoprevention—Congresses. 2. Cancer—Prevention—Congresses. 3. Cancer—Nutritional aspects—Congresses. I. Bradlow, H. Leon. II. Fishman, Jack, 1930– III. Osborne, Michael P. IV. Series.

Q11.N5 vol. 889
[RC268.15]
500 s—dc21
[616.99'4052]   99-051355

GYAT / B-M
Printed in the United States of America
ISBN 1-57331-198-7 (cloth)
ISBN 1-57331-199-5 (paper)
ISSN 0077-8923

ANNALS OF THE NEW YORK ACADEMY OF SCIENCES
Volume 889

CANCER PREVENTION
NOVEL NUTRIENT AND
PHARMACEUTICAL DEVELOPMENTS[a]

Editors
H. LEON BRADLOW, JACK FISHMAN, AND MICHAEL P. OSBORNE

Conference Organizers
ANDREW J. DANNENBERG, MARTIN LIPKIN, ANTHONY BROWN,
AND MICHAEL P. OSBORNE

CONTENTS

[a]This volume is the result of a conference, entitled **Cancer Prevention: Novel Nutrient
and Pharmaceutical Developments,** held in New York City on November 13–14, 1998 by the
Strang Cancer Prevention Center, Cornell University Medical College, and the International
Society for Cancer Chemoprevention.

Part II. Cyclooxygenase-2 and Cancer Prevention

Part III. Calcium and Vitamin D in Cancer Prevention

Part IV. Cancer Prevention Updates

Part V. Poster Papers

Financial assistance was received from:

- **AMERICAN CANCER SOCIETY**
- **AMERICAN-ITALIAN CANCER FOUNDATION**
- **AMERICAN MEDIA, INC.**
- **DONALD BELDOCK**
- **MERCK & CO., INC.**
- **ORTHO BIOTECH, INC.**
- **WEILL MEDICAL COLLEGE OF CORNELL UNIVERSITY**
- **THE IRVING WEINSTEIN FOUNDATION**

Introduction

This volume summarizes presentations made at the Strang International Cancer Prevention Conference held on November 13 and 14, 1998, sponsored by the Strang Cancer Prevention Center and the International Society of Cancer Chemoprevention (ISCaC). The title of the meeting was Cancer Prevention: Novel Nutrient and Pharmaceutical Developments.

The educational objectives of this conference were to provide recent information to improve the participants' knowledge of several classes of nutrients and pharmaceutical agents currently believed to be important for tumor inhibition; to review novel preclinical models that facilitate analyzing chemopreventive agent efficacy and mechanisms of gene–nutrient interaction; and to provide current information on recent clinical trials under way studying chemopreventive regimens in the United States, Europe, and Asia.

The conference agenda focused on a limited number of presentations that could best fulfill these objectives and did not attempt to cover all developments emerging in this field. The main sections of the program included a review of many varieties of nutrients and pharmaceutical compounds with tumor-inhibitory properties; current strategies, including preclinical genetic models, for studying chemopreventive agents; recent studies of cyclooxygenase-2 and tumor inhibition; calcium and vitamin D in cancer prevention; an update on breast cancer prevention; and updates from Europe and Asia on cancer chemoprevention studies currently under way.

We would like to acknowledge the contribution of Dr. Michael P. Osborne in developing this program; Ms. Lorraine Bell, with the assistance of Ms. Theresa Di Meola in organizing the conference; and Dr. H. Leon Bradlow in the preparation and editing of this volume for the *Annals of the New York Academy of Sciences*. We are also grateful to the Editorial Department of the Academy, and particularly to Steven Bohall, who shepherded this volume through the press with grace and professionalism, and Stephanie J. Bludau who oversaw production.

MARTIN LIPKIN
ANDREW J. DANNENBERG

Progress in Cancer Chemoprevention

GARY J. KELLOFF,[a,c] JAMES A. CROWELL,[a] VERNON E. STEELE,[a]
RONALD A. LUBET,[a] CHARLES W. BOONE,[a] WINFRED A. MALONE,[a]
ERNEST T. HAWK,[a] RONALD LIEBERMAN,[a] JULIA A. LAWRENCE,[a]
LEVY KOPELOVICH,[a] IQBAL ALI,[a] JAYE L.VINER,[a] AND CAROLINE C. SIGMAN[b]

[a]National Cancer Institute, Division of Cancer Prevention,
Bethesda, Maryland 20892, USA

[b]CCS Associates, 1965 Landings Drive, Mountain View, California 94043, USA

ABSTRACT: More than 40 promising agents and agent combinations are being
evaluated clinically as chemopreventive drugs for major cancer targets. A few
have been in vanguard, large-scale intervention trials—for example, the studies
of tamoxifen and fenretinide in breast, 13-*cis*-retinoic acid in head and neck, vitamin E and selenium in prostate, and calcium in colon. These and other agents
are currently in phase II chemoprevention trials to establish the scope of their
chemopreventive efficacy and to develop intermediate biomarkers as surrogate
end points for cancer incidence in future studies. In this group are fenretinide,
2-difluoromethylornithine, and oltipraz. Nonsteroidal anti-inflammatories
(NSAID) are also in this group because of their colon cancer chemopreventive
effects in clinical intervention, epidemiological, and animal studies. New agents
are continually considered for development as chemopreventive drugs. Preventive strategies with antiandrogens are evolving for prostate cancer. Antiinflammatories that selectively inhibit inducible cyclooxygenase (COX)-2 are
being investigated in colon as alternatives to the NSAID, which inhibit both
COX-1 and COX-2 and derive their toxicity from COX-1 inhibition. Newer retinoids with reduced toxicity, increased efficacy, or both (e.g., 9-*cis*-retinoic acid) are being investigated. Promising chemopreventive drugs are also being
developed from dietary substances (e.g., green and black tea polyphenols, soy
isoflavones, curcumin, phenethyl isothiocyanate, sulforaphane, lycopene, in-
dole-3-carbinol, perillyl alcohol). Basic and translational research necessary to
progress in chemopreventive agent development includes, for example, (1) molecular and genomic biomarkers that can be used for risk assessment and as
surrogate end points in clinical studies, (2) animal carcinogenesis models that
mimic human disease (including transgenic and gene knockout mice), and (3)
novel agent treatment regimens (e.g., local delivery to cancer targets, agent
combinations, and pharmacodynamically guided dosing).

Cancer chemoprevention is defined as the use of specific chemical compounds to
prevent, inhibit, or reverse carcinogenesis.[1,2] In many major cancer targets, human
cancer development requires 20–40 years or more,[1] and the scope of chemopreven-

[c]Address for correspondence: National Cancer Institute, Chemoprevention Branch, Division
of Cancer Prevention, 6130 Executive Boulevard, EPN 201, Rockville, MD 20852. Voice: 301-
496-8563; fax: 301-402-0553.
  e-mail: kelloffg@dcpcepn.nci.nih.gov

tion encompasses cohorts at all phases of this process—from healthy subjects at normal risk; to populations at intermediate risk from environmental and life style factors, genetic predisposition, and precancerous lesions; and then to previous cancer patients at high risk for second primaries. The identification of efficacious and safe agents, biomarkers of efficacy and risk, and suitable cohorts for clinical intervention are critical to progress in chemoprevention.

PROMISING CHEMOPREVENTIVE AGENTS

Basic research in carcinogenesis has identified many genetic lesions and other cellular constituents associated with the initiation and progression of precancers to invasive disease. Possible mechanisms for chemoprevention involve interfering with the expression and/or activity of these molecules; examples of the mechanisms, their possible molecular targets, and agents that act at these targets are listed in TABLE 1.[1,3,4]

Systematic evaluation of classes of agents acting at molecular targets, such as those listed in TABLE 1, is an important strategy for identifying and characterizing new potential chemopreventive agents.[5] However, many promising agents have multiple chemoprevention-associated molecular activities, some of which are interrelated. Also, a single activity, even if it is the agent's predominant pharmacological activity, may not be the most important or the only one required for chemoprevention. Such may be the case for inhibition of prostaglandin synthase (particularly, cyclooxygenase (COX) activity) by nonsteroidal anti-inflammatory drugs (NSAID). These observations imply that molecular targeting should not be the only approach used to identify potential chemopreventive drugs.[6]

Experimental and epidemiological carcinogenesis studies showing that >90% of cancers are associated with mutagens and mitogens[1,6] suggest a complementary empirical approach—searching for agents that inhibit or reverse cellular processes derived from mutagenesis and mitogenesis: (1) decreased programmed cell death (from senescence; or in response to damage, environmental conditions, such as overpopulation, or hormone withdrawal), (2) decreased maturation or differentiation, and (3) increased proliferation.

Using both approaches, several thousand agents have been reported in the literature to have chemopreventive activity.[7] Since 1987 in the NCI chemoprevention testing program, more than 1,000 agents and agent combinations have been selected and evaluated in preclinical studies of chemopreventive activity, ranging from *in vitro* mechanistic assays[8] and cell-based transformation assays to carcinogen-induced[9] and transgenic animal models. More than 40 promising agents and agent combinations are being evaluated clinically as chemopreventive drugs for major cancer targets (TABLES 2 and 3). A few have been in vanguard, large-scale intervention trials—for example, the studies of tamoxifen[10] and fenretinide in breast,[11] 13-*cis*-retinoic acid in head and neck,[12] vitamin E[13] and selenium in prostate,[14] and calcium [15] in colon. These and other agents are currently in phase II chemoprevention trials to establish the scope of their chemopreventive efficacy and to develop intermediate biomarkers as surrogate end points for cancer incidence in future studies. In this group are fenretinide (bladder, cervix, lung, prostate, oral cavity, and combined with tamoxifen in breast), DFMO (breast, bladder, cervix, oral cavity, prostate, esopha-

TABLE 1. Mechanisms for chemoprevention with possible molecular targets[1]

Mechanism	Possible Molecular Targets	Representative Agents
Antimutagenesis		
Inhibit carcinogen uptake	Bile acids (bind)	Calcium
Inhibit formation/activation of carcinogen	Cytochromes P450 (inhibit)	PEITC, tea, indole-3-carbinol, soy isoflavones
	PG synthase hydroperoxidase, 5-lipoxygenase (inhibit)	NSAID, COX-2 inhibitors, lipoxygenase inhibitors, iNOS[a] inhibitors
	Bile acids (inhibit)	Ursodiol
Deactivate/detoxify carcinogen	GSH/GST (enhance)	Oltipraz, NAC
Prevent carcinogen-DNA binding	Cytochromes P450 (Inhibit)	Tea
Increase level or fidelity of DNA repair	Poly(ADP-ribosyl)transferase (enhance)	NAC, protease inhibitors (Bowman-Birk)
Antiproliferation/Antiprogression		
Modulate hormone/growth factor activity	Estrogen receptor (antagonize)	SERMs, soy isoflavones
	Androgen receptor (antagonize)	Bicalutamide, flutamide
	Steroid aromatase (Inhibit)	Exemestane, vorozole, Arimidex
	Steroid 5α-reductase (inhibit)	Finasteride, epristeride
	IGF-I (inhibit)	SERMs, retinoids
Inhibit oncogene activity	Farnesyl protein transferase (inhibit)	Perillyl alcohol, limonene, DHEA, FTI-276
Inhibit polyamine metabolism	ODC activity (inhibit)	DFMO
	ODC induction (inhibit)	Retinoids, NSAID
Induce terminal differentiation	TGF-β (induce)	Retinoids, vitamin D, SERMs
Restore immune response	COX (inhibit)	NSAID, tea, curcumin
	T, NK lymphocytes (enhance)	Selenium, tea
	Langherans' cells (enhance)	Vitamin E, NSAID
Increase intercellular communication	Connexin 43 (enhance)	Carotenoids (lycopene), Retinoids
Restore tumor suppressor function	p53 (inhibit HPV E6 protein)	—
Induce apoptosis	TGFβ (induce)	Retinoids, SERMs, vitamin D
	RAS Farnesylation (inhibit)	Perillyl alcohol, limonene, DHEA, FTI-276
	Telomerase (inhibit)	Retinoic acid
	Arachidonic acid (enhance)	NSAID, COX-2 inhibitors, lipoxygenase inhibitors
	Caspase (activate)	Retinoids
Inhibit angiogenesis	FGF receptor (inhibit tyrosine kinase)	Soy isoflavones, COX-2 inhibitors
	Thrombomodulin (inhibit)	Retinoids
Correct DNA methylation imbalances	CpG island Methylation (enhance)	Folic acid
Inhibit basement membrane degradation	Type IV collagenase (inhibit)	Protease inhibitors
Inhibit DNA synthesis	Glucose 6-phosphate dehydrogenase (inhibit)	DHEA, fluasterone

[a]Inducible nitric oxide synthase.

TABLE 2. NCI chemoprevention program: promising cancer chemopreventive agents in phase I clinical trials and preclinical toxicology

Agent	Toxicology/Phase I	Target
S-Allyl-L-cysteine	Tox	lung
Curcumin	I	colon, breast
Fluasterone	Tox	breast, colon
Genistein (soy isoflavones)	Tox	breast, prostate, colon
Ibuprofen	I	colon, bladder
Indole-3-carbinol	I	breast
Lycopene	I	prostate
Perillyl alcohol	I	breast, colon
PEITC	I	lung
9-*cis*-Retinoic acid	I	breast, cervix, prostate
Sulindac sulfone	I	colon, breast, prostate
Tea/EGCG[a]	Tox	colon, head and neck, skin
Ursodiol	I	colon
Vitamin D_3 analogues	Tox	breast, colon, prostate
L-Selenomethionine + vitamin E	I	prostate, lung, colon
NAC + DFMO	Tox	breast
DFMO + fenretinide	Tox	breast
DFMO + oltipraz	Tox	bladder, colon
Fenretinide + oltipraz	Tox	breast, bladder
NAC + oltipraz	I	lung

[a]Epigallocatechin gallate.

gus, and colon in combination with Sulindac), and oltipraz (lung, both alone and combined with NAC; liver;[16] skin). NSAID are also in this group because of their colon cancer chemopreventive effects in clinical intervention (aspirin, Sulindac), epidemiological (aspirin), and animal studies (e.g., piroxicam, Sulindac, aspirin).[3] They have also shown high activity against animal bladder cancers.

New agents are continually considered for development as chemopreventive drugs, with selection based on preliminary efficacy data, mechanistic considerations, and potential for improved chemopreventive (therapeutic) index. For example, androgen deprivation has been associated with reduced risk for prostate cancer and therapeutic benefit in treatment of the disease. Preventive strategies with antiandrogens (e.g., flutamide and 5α-reductase inhibitors[17]) are evolving. The selective estrogen receptor modulator (SERM), tamoxifen, has clinically demonstrated chemopreventive potential, but research continues to look for other SERMs that maintain tamoxifen's chemopreventive and bone and heart protective activities, without its side effects (particularly its associated increased risk for uterine cancer). Raloxifene and SERM-3 are examples.[2] Anti-inflammatory agents that selectively inhibit inducible COX-2 are being investigated in colon as alternatives to the NSAID that inhibit both COX-1 and COX-2 and derive their toxicity from COX-1 inhibition.[2,3] Retinoids have shown significant chemopreventive activity with multiple potential mechanisms of action and varied tissue specificity. Mechanisms and efficacy of new generations of retinoids with reduced toxicity, increased efficacy, or both (e.g., 9-*cis*-retinoic acid, which activates both RAR and RXR retinoid receptors, and

TABLE 3. NCI Chemoprevention Program: promising cancer chemopreventive agents in Phase II/III clinical trials

Agent	Phase	Target(s)
Retinoids		
Vitamin A	III	lung
all-*trans*-Retinoic acid	II	cervix
13-*cis*-Retinoic acid	II/III	head and neck, lung, oral cavity
9-*cis*-Retinoic acid	II	cervix
Fenretinide	II/III	bladder, breast, ovary, cervix, lung, oral cavity, prostate
Antiestrogens/antiandrogens		
Tamoxifen	II/III	breast
Fenretinide + tamoxifen	II	breast
Raloxifene	III	breast
Toremifene	II	prostate
Other SERM	II	breast
Exemestane	II	breast
Finasteride	II/III	prostate
Flutamide	II	prostate
DFMO	II	bladder, breast, cervix, colon, Barrett's esophagus, oral cavity, prostate
NSAID		
Aspirin	II/III	colon
Aspirin + calcium	II/III	colon
Aspirin + folic acid	III	colon
Piroxicam	II	colon
Sulindac	II/III	colon, multiple myeloma
DFMO + Sulindac	II	colon
COX-2 Inhibitor	II/III	colon, skin, bladder, Barrett's esophagus
Budesonide	II	lung
Oltipraz	II	liver (DNA adducts), lung
DHEA	II	multiple myeloma
Calcium	II/III	colon
Vitamin D_3	II	colon
Vitamin E	II/III	colon, lung, prostate
L-Selenomethionine	II/III	prostate, skin, colon, esophagus
Folic acid	II/III	cervix, colon
Curcumin	II	oral cavity
Soy isoflavones	II	prostate
Tea	II	skin

Targretin, which selectively activates RXR receptors)[2] are being investigated. A promising and important group of potential cancer chemopreventive drugs, because of their low toxicity and apparent benefit in other chronic diseases (e.g., protection from heart disease), are those derived from natural products, particularly dietary substances—green and black tea polyphenols,[18] lycopene,[19] soy isoflavones,[20] curcumin,[21] phenethyl isothiocyanate (PEITC),[22] indole-3-carbinol,[23] and perillyl alcohol.[24] Important aspects of developing such agents are careful characterization of the active substance(s) and the technology to ensure reproducible preparations.

The potential of single chemopreventives is limited by potency and, more importantly, toxicity at efficacious doses. Simultaneous or sequential administration of multiple agents can increase efficacy and reduce toxicity. For example, differences in the chemopreventive mechanisms among the agents can provide additive or synergistic efficacy; thus, adequate efficacy may be observed at lower and presumably less toxic doses of the individual agents. Several agent combinations are under development based on their synergistic activity in animal efficacy studies—for example, retinoids (fenretinide, 9-cis-retinoic acid) with antiestrogens (tamoxifen, raloxifene, SERM-3) in breast,[2] and 2-difluoromethylornithine (DFMO) and NSAID (piroxicam, Sulindac) in colon.[4] Also, mechanistic data may suggest the potential synergy of two agents; an example is the enhancement of electrophile-trapping activity (hence, carcinogen detoxifying activity) that might be achieved by combination of an agent, such as N-acetyl-L-cysteine (NAC), which provides substrate for glutathione (GSH) synthesis, with an agent, such as oltipraz, which enhances GSH S-transferases (GST). Another possibility is administration of second agents to counter toxicity of potent chemopreventives. Such a strategy has been proposed for NSAID, as a combination of the NSAID with a drug that inhibits associated gastrointestinal toxicity (e.g., misoprostol).[3]

CHEMOPREVENTIVE DRUG DEVELOPMENT STRATEGIES USING INTERMEDIATE BIOMARKERS OF CARCINOGENESIS

NCI's multidisciplinary approach to chemopreventive drug development and collaboration with the Food and Drug Administration to provide consensus guidance for applying this approach have been described previously.[1,3,25] Briefly the approach is an applied drug development science effort that begins with the identification of candidate agents for development and the characterization of these agents in *in vitro* and animal chemopreventive efficacy screens. Promising agents are then further evaluated in animal models to design regimens for clinical testing and use. Agents judged to have potential as human chemopreventives are subjected to preclinical toxicity and pharmacokinetic studies, and then phase I clinical safety and pharmacokinetic trials. The most successful agents then progress to clinical chemoprevention trials.

The impracticality of cancer incidence reduction as an end point is a major challenge in designing chemoprevention efficacy trials. Increased understanding of the molecular and phenotypic progression in carcinogenesis has provided a means of overcoming this obstacle, namely, with intermediate biomarkers that can be validated as surrogate end points for cancer. Primary intermediate biomarkers and targets of chemoprevention are intraepithelial neoplasia (IEN), which are almost always cancer precursors. In the NCI chemopreventive drug development program, phase II and small phase III clinical chemoprevention trials are conducted in patients with current or previous IEN. A primary goal of these studies is characterization and standardization of quantitative measurements of chemopreventive agent-induced morphometric and cytometric changes in these lesions. Results showing reversion, slowed progression, or inhibition of recurrence of the target lesions can be obtained within 3–24 months in these studies.

Further, an important component of clinical (and preclinical) studies in chemoprevention is identification of earlier intermediate biomarkers in IEN that reflect carcinogenesis/chemopreventive mechanisms—proliferation (e.g., proliferating cell nuclear antigen, MIB-1), differentiation signals (e.g., actins, vimentin, blood group antigens), and genetic/regulatory changes (e.g., apoptosis, DNA methylation, oncogene, and tumor suppressor expression).[26] The early intermediate biomarkers can be very distant developmentally from the cancer; therefore, standardized methods for sampling and measuring them and their validation against IEN are critical. Also, it is anticipated that the reliability of early biomarkers as end points for clinical trials may be improved by using them in batteries that model carcinogenesis.

CONSIDERATIONS IN DEVELOPMENT OF CHEMOPREVENTIVE DRUGS AT FOUR MAJOR CANCER TARGETS: BREAST, COLON, PROSTATE, AND LUNG

For each of four major cancer sites, the following discussion reviews promising agents and specific considerations in the development of chemoprevention strategies in these targets. In breast, the high importance of estrogen modulation is reviewed. In colon, the rationale for using adenomas as a surrogate end point in chemoprevention trials is presented, and the selection and development of antiinflammatories is described. The discussion on prostate reviews new agents under development and looks at the difficulties associated with measuring modulation of prostatic intraepithelial neoplasia (PIN) as a surrogate end point. In lung, the selection of suitable cohorts and the design of a novel local agent delivery system are described.

Breast: Estrogen Modulators as Chemopreventives[2]

Control of estrogen exposure is a key factor in breast cancer chemoprevention strategies. Many of the risk factors for breast carcinogenesis are associated with prolonged cyclical or high levels of estrogen exposure (e.g., early menarche, late menopause, or nulliparity). It is expected that estrogen exposure would couple with genetic predisposition (e.g., BRCA or Li-Fraumeni mutations) and other factors in determining an individual's risk.[6] One strategy for reducing estrogen effects is by treatment with SERMs—agents that modulate estrogen activation estrogen receptors. As noted above, the promise of the antiestrogen, tamoxifen, is widely known based on its success in reducing the risk of breast cancer in women at high risk.[10] Of equal interest is the potential protection SERMs offer against other chronic diseases; depending on the estrogen receptor response elements they affect, protection against cardiovascular disease, bone loss, and brain function are also seen. Newer generation SERMs, which also avoid estrogen agonist toxicity in sites other than breast (e.g., enhanced risk for endometrial cancer) are particularly promising. The second generation SERM, raloxifene, already approved in prevention of osteoporosis and without apparent endometrial toxicity, will be compared with tamoxifen as a breast cancer chemopreventive in postmenopausal women. A third generation SERM, related to raloxifene, but with greater efficacy in animal studies, will be evaluated in a phase II study in patients scheduled for breast surgery and in subjects at high risk with multiple biomarker abnormalities. As discussed above, synergistic activity in animal studies indicates that the combination of antiestrogen (e.g., tamoxifen, raloxifene, or SERM-3) with retinoid (e.g., fenretinide or 9-*cis*-retinoic acid) has chemopreventive potential. Phase II studies on the combination of fenretinide with tamoxifen are now ongoing. In one study, patients scheduled for breast surgery based on mammographically detected lesions are being treated for 14–21 days between diagnosis and surgery; intermediate biomarkers, primarily measures of antiproliferation, are being followed. In the second study, low-dose (5 mg/day) tamoxifen is being evaluated; the primary end point is modulation of serum insulin-like growth factor I (IGF-I). Soy isoflavones,[20] which have some direct antiestrogenic activity in the premenopausal setting, and are inhibitors of growth factor–stimulated signal transduction, are also being evaluated in clinical chemoprevention studies.

Steroid aromatase inhibitors, by preventing estrogen biosynthesis, and hence estrogen exposure, may be chemopreventive in breast, particularly in postmenopausal subjects, where estrogen biosynthesis is primarily extragonadal, and may be locally affected in breast tissue, and where the effects of inhibition are not complicated by cyclical proliferative responses.[28] Epidemiological studies have shown that consumption of cruciferous vegetables, such as broccoli, cauliflower, cabbage, and brussels sprouts is associated with decreased risk for cancer in humans.[23] Indole-3-carbinol, an autolysis product of glucobrassicin, is one component of cruciferous vegetables that may reduce breast cancer incidence through modulation of cytochrome P450-dependent estradiol metabolism, enhancing 2-hydroxyestrone (estrogen receptor antagonist) at the expense of 16α–hydroxylation (estrogen receptor agonist).[23] Also, induction of phase II enzymes by indole-3-carbinol may increase estrogen conjugation and excretion, and indole-3-carbinol metabolites, such as indolo[3,2-b]carbazole (ICZ), may exhibit direct antiestrogenic activity by downregulation of the estrogen receptor.[23]

Prostate: Considerations in Evaluating the Effect of Chemopreventive Agents on PIN[17]

Promising chemopreventive agents in prostate include antiandrogens and antiestrogens (e.g., flutamide, toremifene, raloxifene, SERM-3, and steroid aromatase inhibitors), retinoids (e.g., fenretinide and 9-*cis*-retinoic acid), RAMBA (retinoic acid metabolic blocking agents), vitamin E, organoselenium (and the combination of selenium and vitamin E), lycopene, soy isoflavones (e.g., genistein), DFMO, steroid 5α-reductase inhibitors (e.g., finasteride, dual type 1 and 2 inhibitors), apoptosis inducers (e.g., perillyl alcohol), differentiation agents (e.g., vitamin D analogues), and antiinflammatories (e.g., lipoxygenase inhibitors and selective COX-2 inhibitors). One particularly interesting finding is the epidemiologic studies suggesting that increased serum levels of lycopene, the most abundant serum carotenoid, is associated with a decreased relative risk of prostate cancer.[17] Lycopene is now in preclinical toxicity and pharmacodynamics studies to determine its distribution to prostate, and it will soon be in phase I clinical studies.

Prostate-specific antigen (PSA) and PIN are considered to be primary intermediate biomarkers for evaluating cancer risk and, potentially, chemopreventive efficacy; however, there are issues in their use. Serum PSA is well-established as a biomarker of prostate cancer, but it is not specific to neoplasia, and the data do not suggest that the level is directly related to degree of neoplastic progression. Many studies indicate that other measurements of PSA, especially density and velocity of PSA rise, may correlate better to progression than serum level alone. The validation of PSA as an intermediate biomarker awaits further data, some of which may be obtained in the large prostate, lung, colorectal, and ovary cancer screening trial in which PSA is being monitored over several years in more than 30,000 men. Even without further refinement, PSA may prove useful in identifying clinical cohorts at risk as subjects for chemoprevention studies.

There is abundant evidence that PIN is a precursor of prostatic adenocarcinoma, suggesting subjects with PIN as cohorts for chemoprevention studies. One such cohort is individuals with high-grade PIN, but without demonstrable prostatic carcinoma. These subjects are treated with a chemopreventive agent for approximately two years and then evaluated by transrectal ultrasound (TRUS)-directed biopsy every 3–6 months to determine the modulation of PIN, changes in proliferation indices, and nuclear abnormalities. Because PIN is nearly always also observed in conjunction with prostatic adenocarcinomas, patients with newly diagnosed early stage prostate cancers form a cohort for biomarker studies using PIN. Such patients are usually not scheduled for prostatectomy until 3–8 weeks after diagnosis. Chemopreventive intervention can be made in the period between diagnosis and prostatectomy. The removed prostate gland is analyzed for PIN modulation and other potential biomarkers.

PIN demonstrates the difficulty in tissue sampling that must be addressed in chemoprevention studies using surrogate end points. In men aged ≥50 years, HGPIN incidence is 50 percent. However, of all sextant prostate biopsies taken in this subpopulation for any reason, when no cancer is present, only 5% HGPIN incidence is detected (i.e., only 10% of the expected cases). In the general population, <1% HGPIN incidence is detected in sextant prostate biopsies. These discrepancies are most probably due to inability to adequately visualize the prostate for ensuring detection of suspect tissue, and, at the least, call for standardization of measurement methods (e.g., number and location of biopsies). The situation is improved when the whole gland is available after prostatectomy. Even in this case, the number and location of samples from invasive cancer, HGPIN, and adjacent normal-appearing tissue, as well as the thickness/number of histologic sections processed and scored are important parameters that will affect variability, accuracy, and reproducibility.

Colon: Colorectal Adenomas and the Development Path for Anti-inflammatory Drugs

The developmental path for most colorectal cancer is well-documented. Histopathologically, it starts with hyperproliferation in colon mucosa, formation of adenomas (IEN) with varying degrees of malignant potential, and finally adenocarcinoma.[29,30] This well-documented histopathology along with the accessibility of all stages of colon carcinogenesis facilitates the evaluation of chemopreventive activity in colon.[3]

Patients with a history of adenomatous polyps provide a feasible cohort for clinical chemoprevention studies, because their risk of developing new adenomas is high. In several studies, new adenomas were seen at rates ranging from 37–60% within 1–4 years following polypectomy.[31] In the National Polyp Study, a recurrence rate of 29–35% was seen in patients after removal of all synchronous adenomas. Patients with FAP are a special subset of this high-risk group, because they develop many adenomas, some of which inevitably progress to adenocarcinoma. Several chemoprevention trials with colorectal adenoma recurrence and regression as the end point are currently in progress in this cohort; the agents being evaluated are Sulindac; Sulindac sulfone; and the combination of β-carotene, vitamin C, and vitamin E; as well as a selective COX-2 inhibitor (see below). The high incidence of adenomas in the general population suggests that adequate accrual for such studies is possible.

Antiinflammatories that show potent chemopreventive activity in animal colorectal carcinogenesis models (primarily against AOM or DMH-induced cancers in rats and mice) include the NSAID Sulindac, piroxicam, aspirin, and ibuprofen, as well as curcumin, tea polyphenols, and the selective COX-2 inhibitor, celecoxib.[9,32] As noted above, the agent combination of DFMO and Sulindac is being evaluated in colon based on the synergism of DFMO and piroxicam observed in animal efficacy screens.

Use of such COX inhibitors as the NSAID, sulindac and aspirin, has a particularly strong association with prevention of gastrointestinal cancers.[3] In case studies and limited intervention studies (patients with FAP or Gardner's syndrome), Sulindac consistently caused regression of existing colonic polyps and prevented formation of new polyps. Epidemiology studies of aspirin use provide evidence of an association with reduced risk for gastrointestinal (esophagus, stomach, colon, and rectum) cancer and colon cancer mortality. In fact, one complicating factor in estimating sample size required for adenoma prevention trials is the widespread use of aspirin as a cardioprotective in the target population.

Despite NSAID's potent chemopreventive activity, their promise for extended chronic use is limited by toxicity. The most common side effects of the NSAID, which inhibit both COX-1 and COX-2, are gastrointestinal effects, such as bleeding and ulcers (occurring in $\geq 30\%$ of treated patients).[33] These effects have been attributed to reduced PGE_2 leading to less protective mucus secretion in the gut. Several strategies have been proposed to limit the impact of these side effects, including combinations with other agents (e.g., DFMO). Another is administering a second drug that inhibits associated gastrointestinal toxicity (e.g., the PGE_2 analogue, misoprostol). A third is the development of chemical structural or pharmacological derivatives of NSAID that retain chemopreventive activity while minimizing the side effects. Examples are the sulfone metabolite of Sulindac and selective inhibitors of COX-2.

COX-2, the inducible form of COX, predominates at inflammation sites and in macrophages and synoviocytes. By contrast, constitutive COX-1 predominates in the stomach, gastrointestinal tract, platelets, and kidney.[34] The traditional NSAID inhibit both forms of the enzyme, but other compounds (e.g., NS-398, MF tricyclic, celecoxib) inhibit COX-2 selectively at therapeutic doses and do not interfere with COX-1–mediated synthesis of PGE_2 in the gastric mucosa. Both celecoxib and MF tricyclic inhibit colorectal adenomas in the Min mouse (a transgenic mouse with a mutation in the APC gene, analogous to mutations in FAP patients);[35] celecoxib is also a potent inhibitor of colorectal adenocarcinomas in rats.[32] A clinical chemoprevention study of celecoxib is in progress in FAP patients.

Lung: Smokers and Local Agent Delivery

Tobacco use is by far the greatest risk factor for lung cancer, and chronic smokers are a primary target for chemopreventive strategies in lung.[36] Potential lung chemopreventives—NAC, oltipraz, and PEITC—have pronounced antimutagenic activity against tobacco carcinogens. PEITC is an analogue and potent inhibitor of the metabolic activation of NNK. Mutated p53 is observed in >50% of lung cancers; the tobacco carcinogens B(*a*)P and nitrosamines, such as NNK, which mutate p53, are inhibited by oltipraz. Based on animal studies, other antioxidant/anti-inflammatory agents, such as lipoxygenase inhibitors, also have potential as lung cancer chemopreventives.

One strategy in lung is local, topical administration of agent by aerosol delivery, which minimizes systemic toxicity and circumvents bioavailability problems. Wattenberg has demonstrated chemopreventive activity of aerosolized corticosteroids (budesonide) in B(a)P-induced mouse lung,[37] and budesonide is now being evaluated for prevention and regression of bronchial dysplasia in chronic smokers. The concept of local delivery of chemopreventive agents is also likely to find application in such other target tissues as colon and upper aerodigestive tract, and, of course, topical application of sunscreens has long set the precedent for local delivery of chemopreventives to skin. In fact, a study of topical tea polyphenols in prevention of actinic keratosis has recently begun.

FUTURE PROGRESS IN CHEMOPREVENTION

Our understanding of carcinogenesis continues to grow, accelerated by advances in functional genomics and proteomics such as are being produced by the Cancer Genome Anatomy Project. Basic and translational research capitalizing on this new technology are necessary to progress in chemopreventive agent development. A major contribution of this research will be characterization of molecular and genomic biomarkers that can be used to identify and quantify risk in prospective cohorts as well as finding use as surrogate end points in clinical studies. Another will be leads to new animal models of carcinogenesis that mimic human disease (including transgenic and gene knockout mice) and that can be used to validate surrogate end points. New treatment regimens to improve the therapeutic ratio of chemopreventives will also be important. As suggested by the discussion above on topical delivery of aerosolized steroids, the development of systems allowing local delivery to cancer targets is one possibility. Others include agent combinations and pharmacodynamically guided dosing regimens. Use of foods and dietary supplements present another important safe chemopreventive strategy. Besides epidemiological studies, basic science research to detect mechanisms and evaluate the chemopreventive potential of food components is necessary. Talalay's research on phase II enzyme induction by molecular components of broccoli sprouts is the prototype of what is required to demonstrate chemopreventive potential of foods.[38] The results of epidemiological[19] and molecular studies of lycopene are another example.

REFERENCES

1. KELLOFF, G.J. *et al.* 1997. Progress in clinical chemoprevention. Semin. Oncol. **24:** 241–252.
2. HONG, W.K. & M.B. SPORN. 1997. Recent advances in chemoprevention of cancer. Science **278:** 1073–1077.
3. KELLOFF, G.J. *et al.* 1996. Strategies for identification and clinical evaluation of promising chemopreventive agents. Oncology **10:** 1471–1484.
4. KELLOFF, G.J. *et al.* 1994. Mechanistic considerations in chemopreventive drug development. J. Cell. Biochem. Suppl. **20:** 1–24.
5. KELLOFF, G.J. *et al.* 1996. Mechanistic considerations in the evaluation of chemopreventive data. Principles of Chemoprevention, IARC Scientific Publication No. 139, Lyon, France: International Agency for Research on Cancer. 203–221.
6. KELLOFF, G.J. *et al.* 1997. Risk biomarkers and current strategies for cancer chemoprevention. J. Cell. Biochem. Suppl. **25:** 1–14, 1996.
7. BAGHERI, D. *et al.* 1989. Database of inhibitors of carcinogenesis. J. Environ. Sci. Health **6:** 261–414.
8. STEELE, V.E. *et al.* 1996. Use of *in vitro* assays to predict the efficacy of chemopreventive agents in whole animals. J. Cell. Biochem. Suppl. **26:** 29–53.
9. STEELE, V.E. *et al.* 1994. Preclinical efficacy evaluation of potential chemopreventive agents in animal carcinogenesis models: methods and results from the NCI chemoprevention testing program. J. Cell. Biochem. Suppl. **20:** 32–54.
10. FISHER, B. *et al.* 1998. Tamoxifen for prevention of breast cancer: Report of the National Surgical Adjuvant Breast and Bowel Project P1 Study. J. Natl. Cancer Inst. **90:** 1371–1388.
11. DE PALO, G. *et al.* 1996. Ongoing clinical chemoprevention study of breast cancer with fenretinide. Int. Congr. Ser. **1120:** 249–254.
12. HONG, W.K. *et al.* 1990. Prevention of second primary tumors with isotretinoin in squamous-cell carcinoma of the head and neck. N. Engl. J. Med. **323:**795–801.
13. Heinonen, O.P. *et al.* 1998. Prostate cancer and supplementation with α–tocopherol and β–carotene: Incidence and mortality in a controlled trial. J. Natl. Cancer Inst. **90:** 440–446.
14. CLARK, L. C. *et al.* 1998. Decreased incidence of prostate cancer with selenium supplementation: Results of a doubleblind cancer prevention trial. Br. J. Urol. **81:** 730–734.
15. BARON, J.A. *et al.* 1999. Calcium supplements for the prevention of colorectal adenomas. Calcium polyp prevention study group. N. Engl. J. Med. **340:** 101–107.
16. KENSLER, T.W. *et al.* 1998. Oltipraz chemoprevention trial in Qidong, People's Republic of China: Modulation of serum aflatoxin albumin adduct biomarkers. Cancer Epidemiol. Biomarkers Prev. **7:** 127–134.
17. KELLOFF, G.J., *et al.* 1999. Chemoprevention of prostate cancer: Concepts and strategies. Eur. J. Urol. **35:** 342–350.
18. KELLOFF, G.J. *et al.* 1996. Clinical development plan: Tea extracts, green tea polyphenols, epigallocatechin gallate. J. Cell. Biochem. Suppl. **26:** 236–257.
19. GIOVANNUCCI, E.G. *et al.* 1995. Intake of carotenoids and retinol in relation to risk of prostate cancer. J. Natl. Cancer Inst. **87:**1767–1776.
20. KELLOFF, G.J. *et al.* 1996. Clinical development plan: Genistein. J. Cell. Biochem. Suppl. **26:** 114–126.
21. KELLOFF, G.J. *et al.* 1996. Clinical development plan: Curcumin. J. Cell. Biochem. Suppl. **26:** 72–85.

22. KELLOFF, G.J. *et al.* 1996. Clinical development plan: Phenethyl isothiocyanate (PEITC). J. Cell. Biochem. Suppl. **26:** 149–157.
23. KELLOFF, G.J. *et al.* 1996. Clinical development plan: Indole-3-carbinol. J. Cell. Biochem. Suppl. **26:** 127–136.
24. KELLOFF, G.J. *et al.* 1996. Clinical development plan: Perillyl alcohol. J. Cell. Biochem. Suppl. **26:** 137–148.
25. KELLOFF, G.J. *et al.* 1995. Approaches to the development and marketing approval of drugs that prevent cancer. Cancer Epidemiol. Biomarkers Prev. **4:** 1–10.
26. KELLOFF, G.J. *et al.* 1994. Surrogate endpoint biomarkers for Phase II cancer chemoprevention trials. J. Cell. Biochem. Suppl. **19:** 1–9.
27. LAWRENCE, J.A. *et al.* 1999. The clinical development of estrogen modulators for breast cancer chemoprevention in premenopausal *vs.* postmenopausal women. J. Cell. Biochem. Suppl. In press.
28. KELLOFF, G.J. *et al.* 1998. Aromatase inhibitors as potential cancer chemopreventives. Cancer Epidemiol. Biomarkers Prev. **7:** 65–78.
29. HAMILTON, S.R. 1992. The adenoma-adenocarcinoma sequence in the large bowel: Variations on a theme. J. Cell. Biochem. **16** (Suppl. **G**): 41–46.
30. LIPKIN, M. 1992. Prototypic applications of intermediate endpoints in chemoprevention. J. Cell. Biochem. **16** (Suppl. **G**): 1–13.
31. WINAWER, S.J. *et al.* 1990. Risk and surveillance of individuals with colorectal polyps. Bull. W.H.O. **68:** 789–795.
32. KAWAMORI, T. *et al.* 1998. Chemopreventive activity of celecoxib, a specific cyclooxygenase-2 inhibitor, against colon carcinogenesis. Cancer Res. **58:** 409–412.
33. SINGH, G. *et al.* 1994. Comparative toxicity of non-steroidal anti-inflammatory agents. Pharm. Ther. **62:** 175–191.
34. MITCHELL, J.A. *et al.* 1993. Selectivity of nonsteroidal antiinflammatory drugs as inhibitors of constitutive and inducible cyclooxygenase. Proc. Natl. Acad. Sci. USA **90:**11693–11697.
35. OSHIMA, M. *et al.* 1996. Suppression of intestinal polyposis in Apc delta716 knockout mice by inhibition of cyclooxygenase 2 (COX-2). Cell **87:** 803–809.
36. KELLOFF, G.J. *et al.* 1994. Progress in cancer chemoprevention: Perspectives on agent selection and short-term clinical intervention trials. Cancer Res. **54:** 2015s–2024s.
37. WATTENBERG, L.W. *et al.* 1997. Chemoprevention of pulmonary carcinogenesis by aerosolized budesonide in female A/J mice. Cancer Res. **57:** 5489–5492.
38. FAHEY, J.W., Y.-S. ZHANG & P. TALALAY. Broccoli sprouts: an exceptionally rich source of inducers of enzymes that protect against chemical carcinogens. Proc. Natl. Acad. Sci. USA **94:** 10367–10372.

Preclinical Mouse Models for Cancer Chemoprevention Studies

MARTIN LIPKIN,[a,f] KAN YANG,[a] WINFRIED EDELMANN,[b] LEXUN XUE,[c] KUNHUA FAN,[a] MAURO RISIO,[d] HAROLD NEWMARK,[a,e] AND RAJU KUCHERLAPATI[b]

[a]Strang Cancer Research Laboratory at The Rockefeller University, New York, New York 10021, USA

[b]Albert Einstein College of Medicine, Bronx, New York 19161, USA

[c]Henan Medical University, Henan, People's Republic of China 450052

[d]Istituto per La Ricerca e La Cura del Cancro, 10060 Candiolo, Torino, Italy

[e]Rutgers University Laboratory for Cancer Research, Piscataway, New Jersey 08854-8020, USA

ABSTRACT: To aid in identifying the ability of chemopreventive agents to inhibit tumor development, new preclinical *in vivo* rodent models have recently been developed. Some of the models contain targeted mutations capable of increasing the incidence and progression of neoplastic lesions, whereas in other models dietary nutrients induce preneoplastic lesions in normal mice. These new preclinical models are assisting the analysis of genetic and environmental factors leading to neoplasia, and clinical studies to evaluate the chemopreventive efficacy of specific nutrients and pharmacological agents.

GASTROINTESTINAL NEOPLASMS IN MICE INDUCED BY A TARGETED Apc1638 MUTATION

Preclinical models have previously used chemical carcinogens to test the possible efficacy of chemopreventive agents. Recently, however, new rodent models have been developed that produce preneoplastic and neoplastic lesions in the gastrointestinal tract without chemical carcinogens. The adenomatous polyposis coli (*Apc*) gene is important in the development of human gastrointestinal tumors. Mice carrying a truncated *Apc* allele with a nonsense mutation at amino acid position 1638 of exon 15 were generated by gene targeting and embryonic stem cell technology and were designated *Apc1638* mice.[1] Numerous gastrointestinal neoplasms consisting of adenomas and adenocarcinomas develop in mice carrying the truncated *Apc* allele. Adenomas and carcinomas were located in the stomach, duodenum, jejunum, ileum, and colon, occurring mostly in the small intestine. Adenomas were tubular, tubulovillous and villous, and a majority had severe dysplasias. The adenocarcinomas invaded the muscularis mucosa, submucosa, or inner layer of propria muscularis. Polypoid hyperplasias with dysplasias also were found in the colons of young mice; adenomas, focal areas of dysplasias, and polypoid hyperplasias were found in older

[f]Address for correspondence: Voice: 212-734-0567 ext. 208; fax: 212-570-6995.
e-mail: lipkin@rockvax.rockefeller.edu

mice. These findings revealed a new rodent model based on a specific *Apc* gene mutation for studies of tumor development in the gastrointestinal tract and tumor prevention.[1,2]

NEOPLASMS IN *Apc1638* MICE ARE INCREASED BY A WESTERN-STYLE DIET

The development of the colonic lesions in these *Apc1638* mice was recently modified with dietary intervention. Young *Apc1638* mice developed colonic polypoid hyperplasias containing dysplasias; older mice developed carcinomas throughout the gastrointestinal tract. Both benign and malignant lesions were significantly increased by feeding a Western-style diet containing reduced calcium and vitamin D and increased fat content compared with AIN-76A diet; and lesions were decreased by decreasing fat content and increasing dietary calcium and vitamin D. This was the first animal model, rapidly producing intestinal and colonic lesions without a chemical carcinogen, that rapidly responded to dietary modulation of developing colonic lesions.[3]

During the development of these tumors, further studies revealed apoptotic cell distribution to be modified in flat mucosa of the colon, with fewer apoptotic cells present on the mucosal surface of colonic crypts. After feeding the Western-style diet, Bcl-2 expression increased, bax decreased, and cyclin D1 expression increased. Computer-assisted cell image analysis revealed significant increases in nuclear Feulgen staining and nuclear area in *Apc1638* colonic epithelial cells after Western-style diet feeding. These findings further quantitated Western-style diet modulation of growth characteristics of *Apc1638* cells for application to studies of mechanisms contributing to tumor progression, and for studies of the effects of chemopreventive agents.[4]

INCREASED TUMOR INCIDENCE IN MICE HAVING BOTH *Mlh1* AND *Apc* TARGETED MUTATIONS

Germline mutations in DNA mismatch repair genes, including *Mlh1*, cause hereditary nonpolyposis colon cancer in humans. We have now studied tumor development in mice having mutations both in *Mlh1* and *Apc* genes.[5] Mice with four different genotypes were evaluated, and differences were found between genotypes in the following measurements: tumors developed in 38% of *Mlh1* ± mice; in 69% of *Mlh1*−/− mice; in 82% of *Mlh1* ± *Apc1638* ± mice; and in 100% of *Mlh1*−/− *Apc1638* ± mice. Gastrointestinal tumors were adenomas and adenocarcinomas with the same histopathology in mice having single or multiple mutations. The number of gastrointestinal tumors per mouse also increased markedly in *Mlh1* −/− *Apc1638* ± mice. Tumors outside the gastrointestinal tract occurred more frequently in mice with single mutations and included non-Hodgkin's lymphomas, and cancers of the skin, cervix, and lung.[5]

COMPUTER-ASSISTED QUANTITATIVE IMAGE ANALYSIS OF EPITHELIAL CELL IN *Apc1638* AND NORMAL MICE

Nuclear morphometry has been further evaluated in *Apc*1638[*Apc*±] mouse colonic epithelial cells and compared to normal C57Bl/6J[*Apc*+/+] nuclei, using a Samba 4000 computer-assisted cell image analyzer. Twenty features were studied: five related to nuclear-integrated optical density (IOD), reflecting DNA content; six related to size and shape of nuclei; and nine related to nuclear texture. Significant findings in the colonic mucosa of [*Apc*±] mice compared to corresponding nuclei in [*Apc*+/+] were as follows: (1) In the flat mucosa, epithelial cell nuclei exhibited decreased IOD, chromatin condensation, and frequency of chromatin clumps; (2) focal areas of dysplasia (FAD) showed intralesional increase in nuclear size, IOD, and chromatin condensation; (3) adenomas and carcinomas in *Apc*± mice showed further intralesional increase in nuclear size compared to nuclei of focal areas of dysplasia. These findings documented and quantified progressive increases in nuclear size, shape, DNA content, and alteration of chromatin texture in *Apc*± mice for application to studies of tumor development and progression, and for preclinical chemoprevention studies.[6]

NORMAL MICE: COLONIC WHOLE CRYPT DYSPLASIAS INDUCED BY A WESTERN-STYLE DIET

We have carried out long-term studies of Western-style diet feeding to normal mice. Our previous short-term studies of neoplasm development in normal mouse colon showed that Western-style diets induced colonic epithelial cell hyperproliferation and hyperplasia.[7,8] In a more recent study, two Western-style diets with increased fat content and low calcium and vitamin D were fed to normal C57BL/6J mice for two years, essentially throughout their entire life span; the Western-style diets contained either American blend fat or corn oil. Hyperproliferation and hyperplasia developed and were followed by other changes in the colon, including dysplasias, similar to those seen in the human colon in diseases that increase risk of colon cancer; they occurred without administering any chemical carcinogen. The Western-style diets induced the development of atypical mitosis and the eventual development of colonic whole-crypt dysplasias in the normal rodent colon. The quantitation of these findings throughout the entire life span of the rodents[9] has been carried out to facilitate analyses of tumor development and progression and for chemoprevention studies. These further observations revealed modifications in differentiation-associated properties of the colonic epithelial cells: lectin SBA binding significantly increased after Western-style diet feeding, together with increased expression of cytokeratins AE1 and RPN 1160, and total acidic mucins.[10]

NORMAL MICE: CELL PROLIFERATION AND HYPERPLASIA IN MAMMARY GLAND INCREASED BY A WESTERN-STYLE DIET

In related studies,[11,12] mammary glands of female C57BL/6J mice were analyzed after feeding a Western-style diet or control AIN-76A diet for short-durations up to

20 weeks; mammary glands were removed for morphometric and radiographic measurements. The number of terminal ducts in the mammary glands of mice on the Western-style diet significantly increased compared to the control group; this is the region in mammary gland where precancerous lesions and carcinomas characteristically develop in rodent models and in humans. Moreover, there was a significant increase in [^{3}H]dThd and bromodeoxyuridine (BrdU) labeling indices of mammary terminal ductal epithelial cells in mice fed the Western-style diet. Thus, the Western-style diet induced both increased epithelial cell proliferation and increased number of terminal ducts in female mice when fed during young adult growth and development. The findings raise the possibility that the ingestion of a diet low in calcium and vitamin D might induce similar changes during the early development of mammary gland in adolescent young women whose calcium and vitamin D intakes are characteristically low, for example, cell hyperproliferation that could facilitate the later evolution of neoplastic lesions.

NORMAL MICE: CELL PROLIFERATION IN EXOCRINE PANCREAS AND PROSTATE OF MICE INCREASED BY A WESTERN-STYLE DIET

The effects of a Western-style diet with increased fat and low calcium and vitamin D on epithelial cell proliferation in pancreas, prostate, and bladder of C57BL/6J mice also have been studied.[13,14] After feeding a Western-style diet for short durations up to 16 weeks, mice were infused with BrdU for 72 hours using subcutaneous Alzet pumps. In the pancreas, the number of pancreatic ducts or acini was unchanged in mice on Western-style diet or AIN-76A control diets; however, BrdU-labeling indices of epithelial cells lining pancreatic inter- and intralobular ducts and centroacinar cells significantly increased in the Western-style diet group compared to control diet groups. These corresponded to regions in the pancreas where carcinomas develop in rodent models and in humans. In the prostate, BrdU-labeling indices significantly increased in anterior and dorsal, but not in ventral lobes after feeding Western-style diet for 16 weeks compared to feeding control diet. This also corresponded to the regions in the prostate gland where carcinomas develop in humans and in rodent models. In the bladder, epithelial cell BrdU-labeling indices were not significantly modified in Western-style diet and control groups. Western-style diet effects are thus similar in the colon, mammary gland, and pancreas, suggesting a role of Western diets in human carcinogenesis in these organs and additional strategies that can be considered for the chemoprevention of cancer.

INFLUENCE OF ADDED DIETARY CALCIUM AND VITAMIN D ON WESTERN-STYLE DIET-INDUCED EPITHELIAL CELL HYPERPROLIFERATION IN MICE

Previous epidemiologic and laboratory studies, including some from our own laboratory, have suggested that a high-fat diet increases the risk of cancer development in the pancreas, prostate, colon, and breast and that carcinogenesis in some of these organs may be influenced by alterations in dietary calcium and vitamin D. A study of the effect of added dietary calcium or vitamin D investigated the development of the above-noted epithelial cell hyperproliferation induced by a Western-style diet in the exocrine pancreas, prostate, and mammary gland of mice. Four-week-old C57BL/6J mice were given either a control AIN-76A diet, a Western-style diet, or a putative chemopreventive diet (a Western-style high-fat diet with the addition of dietary calcium and vitamin D). Nine weeks after dietary intervention, osmotic pumps were subcutaneously implanted in the mice to provide three days of the BrdU infusion. Mice on the Western-style diet had statistically significant increases in BrdU-labeling indices of epithelial cells in the interlobular and intralobular ducts and centroacinar cells of the pancreatic duct system, the dorsal lobe of the prostate, and the terminal ducts of the mammary gland, compared to mice in the respective control diet groups. Adding dietary calcium and vitamin D significantly suppressed the Western-style diet-induced hyperproliferation of epithelial cells in those tissues. This study further confirmed previous findings that a Western-style diet produces hyperproliferation of epithelial cells in several organs and that the changes can be prevented by increasing dietary calcium and vitamin D alone.[15]

REFERENCES

1. FODDE, R., W. EDELMANN, K.YANG, C. VAN LEEUWEN, C. CARLSON, B. RENAULT, C. BREUKEL, E. ALT, M. LIPKIN, P. KHAN & R. KUCHERLAPATI. 1994. A targeted chain-termination mutation in the mouse *Apc* gene results in multiple intestinal tumors. Proc. Natl. Acad. Sci. USA **91:** 8969–8973.

2. YANG, K., W. EDELMANN, K. FAN, K. LAU, V.R. KOLLI, R. FODDE, M. KHAN, R. KUCHERLAPATI & M. LIPKIN. 1997. A mouse model of human familial adenomatous polyposis. J. Exp. Zool. **277:** 245–254.

3. YANG, K., W. EDELMANN, K. FAN, K. LAU, D. LEUNG, H. NEWMARK, R. KUCHERLAPATI & M. LIPKIN. 1998. Dietary modulation of carcinoma development in a mouse model for human familial adenomatous polyposis. Cancer Res. **58:** 5713–5717.

4. YANG, K., K.H. FAN, H. SHINOZAKI, Y. LIU, W. YANG, L. AUGENLICHT, H. NEWMARK, W. EDELMANN, R. KUCHERLAPTI & M. LIPKIN. 1999. Western-style diet modifies growth characteristics of colonic epithelial cells of mice with an *Apc* mutation. Proc. Am. Assoc. Cancer Res. **40:** 58.

5. YANG, K., K.H. FAN, W. EDELMANN, R. KUCHERLAPATI & M. LIPKIN. 1998. Increased tumor incidence in mice having both Mlh1 and Apc targeted mutations. Proc. Am. Assoc. Cancer Res. **39:** 114.

6. FAN, K.H., K. YANG, C. BOONE, W. EDELMANN, R. KUCHERLAPATI & M. LIPKIN. 1998. Computer-assisted quantitative image analysis of epithelial cell in *Apc1638* and normal mice. Proc. Am. Assoc. Cancer Res. **39:** 116.

7. NEWMARK, H.L., M. LIPKIN & N. MAHESWARI. 1990. Colonic hyperplasia and hyperproliferation induced by a nutritional stress diet with four components of Western-style diet. J. Natl. Cancer Inst. **82:** 491–496.

8. NEWMARK, H.L., M. LIPKIN & N. MAHESWARI. 1991. Colonic hyperproliferation induced in rats and mice by nutritional stress diets containing four components of a human Western-style diet (series 2). Am. J. Clin. Nutr. **54:** 209–214s.

9. RISIO, M., M. LIPKIN, H. NEWMARK, K. YANG, F. ROSSINI, V. STEELE, C. BOONE & G. KELLOFF. 1996. Apoptosis, cell replication, and Western-style diet-induced tumorigenesis in mouse colon. Cancer Res. **56:** 4910–4916.

10. YANG, K., K. FAN, H. NEWMARK, D. LEUNG, M. LIPKIN, V. STEELE & G. KELLOFF. 1996. Cytokeratin, lectin, and acidic mucin modulation in differentiating colonic epithelial cells of mice after feeding Western-style diets. Cancer Res. **56:** 4644–4648.

11. KHAN, N., K. YANG, H. NEWMARK, G. WONG, N. TELANG, R. RIVLIN & M. LIPKIN. 1994. Mammary ductal epithelial cell hyperproliferation and hyperplasia induced by a nutritional stress diet containing four components of a Western-style diet. Carcinogenesis **15:** 2645–2648.
12. XUE, L., H. NEWMARK, K. YANG & M. LIPKIN. 1996. Model of mouse mammary gland hyperproliferation and hyperplasia induced by a Western-style diet. Nutr. Cancer **26:** 281–287.
13. XUE, L., K. YANG, H. NEWMARK, D. LEUNG & M. LIPKIN. 1996. Epithelial cell hyperproliferation induced in the exocrine pancreas of mice by a Western-style diet. J. Natl. Cancer Inst. **88:** 1586–1590.
14. XUE, L., K. YANG, H. NEWMARK & M. LIPKIN. 1997. Induced hyperproliferation in epithelial cells of mouse prostate by a Western-style diet. Carcinogenesis **18:** 995–999.
15. XUE, L., M. LIPKIN, H. NEWMARK & J. WANG. 1999. Influence of dietary calcium and vitamin D on diet-induced epithelial cell hyperproliferation in mice. J. Natl. Cancer Inst. **91:** 176–181.

Cellular Mechanisms of Risk and Transformation

LEONARD H. AUGENLICHT,[a] MICHAEL BORDONARO,[b]
BARBARA G. HEERDT, JOHN MARIADASON, AND ANNA VELCICH

*Department of Oncology, Albert Einstein Cancer Center, Montefiore Medical Center,
Bronx, New York 10467, USA*

ABSTRACT: Our early work using the first array and imaging methods for the
quantitative analysis of the expression of 4000 cDNA sequences suggested that
modulation of mitochondrial gene expression was a factor in determining
whether colonic epithelial cells displayed a differentiated or transformed phenotype. We have since dissected a pathway in which mitochondrial function is
a key element in determining the probability of cells undergoing cell-cycle arrest, lineage-specific differentiation, and cell death. Moreover, this pathway is
linked to signaling through β-catenin-Tcf, but in a manner that is independent
of effects of the APC gene on β-catenin-Tcf activity. Utilization of unique
mouse genetic models of intestinal tumorigenesis has confirmed that mitochondrial function is an important element in generation of apoptotic cells in the colon *in vivo* and has demonstrated that modulation of cell death may be involved
in intestinal tumor progression rather than initiation. Normal spatial and temporal patterns of cell proliferation, differentiation, and apoptosis in the colonic
mucosa are determined by developmentally programmed genetic signals and
external signals generated by homo- and heterotypic cell interactions, humoral
agents, and lumenal contents. Mitochondrial function may play a pivotal role
in integrating these signals and in determining probability of cells entering different maturation pathways. How this is accomplished is under investigation
using high-density cDNA microarrays.

INTRODUCTION

A principal focus in chemoprevention research is based on the assumption that
the initiation of transformation can be minimized by limiting exposure to mutagens,
or by increasing the rate at which mutagenic agents are inactivated or the mutations
that they induce are repaired. There are, however, more complex mechanisms that
may play a role in minimizing the probability of tumor formation. For example, Laboisse and associates have isolated clonal variants of the HT29 colon carcinoma cell
line that are highly undifferentiated and phenotypically transformed when the cells
are rapidly growing but upon confluence form a monolayer of well-differentiated absorptive or goblet cells that are nontumorigeneic in nude mice.[1] Upon reseeding the

[a]Address correspondence to: Leonard H. Augenlicht, Department of Oncology, Albert Einstein Cancer Center, Montefiore Medical Center, 111 East 210th Street, Bronx, NY 10467.
Voice: 718-920-4663; fax: 718-882-4464
  e-mail: augen@aecom.yu.edu
  [b]Current address: Department of Pharmacology, Yale University School of Medicine, New
Haven, CT 06520.

cells at lower density, they reacquire their undifferentiated, transformed phenotype. The cells have been cycled through these phenotypes for over a decade. Because the cells are clonally derived, such genetic alterations as *APC* and p53 mutations, c-*myc* amplification, and hundreds of other deletions, point mutations, and amplifications are identical in the two different phenotypes. Clearly, therefore, there are pathways that can be activated or repressed *even in the presence of structural alterations in critical growth regulatory genes*, which can circumvent these defects, and which can then lead to normal cell growth and differentiation. A second area of research in chemoprevention is, therefore, the identification of these important "modulatable" pathways and how they are regulated, interact, and can be recruited into minimizing the probability of progression of a potentially transformed cell to tumor formation.

Candidates for important pathways that may contribute to tissue homeostasis in the colon come from knowledge of the histology and of cell turnover in the normal colonic crypt. Epithelial cells synthesize DNA and divide in the lower two thirds of the crypt. As they migrate up, they undergo maturation, differentiating along a number of lineages—the most prominent being the absorptive cell lineage and the goblet, or secretory cell, lineage. Cells also undergo apoptosis. However, the number of apoptotic cells in the colonic crypt is actually very low, amounting to 2–3% of the total epithelial cells determined by either morphological criteria or by TUNEL assay of cells with fragmented DNA.[2] Therefore, most cells undergo maturation without entering, or completing, an apoptotic pathway, before they are sloughed into the lumen.

The importance of proper temporal and spatial regulation of these cellular events—proliferation, differentiation, and apoptosis—is intuitive: imbalances between cell production and maturation would lead to lack of mucosal homeostasis and disrupted tissue architecture, the hallmark of tumor pathology. In addition, investigation of several genes that are critical in colon tumor development has shown that they are regulated in expression during the migration of cells from the lower portions of the crypt to the regions of differentiation. This includes *APC*[3] and p21[WAF1/cip1],[4] both of which are upregulated after cells leave the proliferative compartment, and c-*myc*, which is expressed more highly in proliferating cells than in differentiated cells.[5,6]

EXPERIMENTAL APPROACH

To identify genes and pathways important in both normal growth and maturation of colonic cells or in transformation, we developed the first scanning and image analysis systems using arrayed, cloned, cDNA sequences capable of quantifying level of expression of each of thousands of corresponding genes in small biopsies or cell samples.[7] Using this approach for analysis of mucosal biopsies from patients with familial adenomatous polyposis (FAP) and hereditary nonpolyposis colon cancer (HNPCC), we identified a panel of 30 sequences whose pattern of expression distinguished the colonic mucosa of these patients at elevated risk for development of colon cancer from the mucosa of patients at low risk.[8] It was important that the pattern of expression of these 30 clones was the same in the high risk mucosa from FAP and HNPCC patients, implying that although the genetic etiology of risk is very different in these two high-risk populations, common pathways were initiated in the mucosa.

A number of the sequences that all decreased in expression in association with risk for tumor development were mitochondrial genes.[9] That these sequences were coordinately downregulated with risk was consistent with the fact that polycistronic mRNA molecules are transcribed from a single promoter common to the heavy and light strands of the mitochondrial genome, which are then processed by cleavage into individual mRNA species. Thus, coordinate regulation of transcription of mitochondrial genes is to be expected.

To investigate further the mechanistic role of altered mitochondrial gene expression and, hence, potentially, altered mitochondrial function in colon tumorigenesis, we turned to more simple cell culture systems, reasoning that changes in key genes and pathways seen upon risk and transformation might be modulated in a complementary way when colon carcinoma cells were induced to develop a more normal, differentiated phenotype in culture. To pursue this line of work, we investigated the induction of differentiation of colon carcinoma cell lines with short-chain fatty acids (SCFAs), especially the 4 carbon unbranched SCFA butyrate. This was chosen for a number of reasons. First, butyrate had been well documented to induce differentiation along the absorptive cell lineage. In particular, butyrate induces growth arrest of colonic carcinoma cells and expression of differentiation markers of the absorptive cell lineage, including alkaline phosphatase.[10–12] Second, SCFAs, such as butyrate, are physiological modulators of differentiation in the colon. High levels of SCFAs in the colonic lumen are present from microbial fermentation of fiber and also from significant levels of SCFAs found in dairy products.[13] Moreover, in diversion colitis, in which the colonic mucosa does not make contact with the fecal stream, differentiation of the mucosa can be promoted by instillation of SCFAs by enema.[14] Finally, SCFAs serve as the principal energy source for colonic epithelial cells,[15] and in this role their metabolism by β-oxidation in the mitochondria provided a potential link (and experimental tool) to understand induction of growth arrest and differentiation pathways by SCFAs and our observation of decreased mitochondrial gene expression in risk for, and development of, colonic cancer.

In a series of studies, we confirmed that butyrate elevated alkaline phosphatase mRNA levels and enzymatic activity, and also elevated depressed levels of mitochondrial gene expression back to levels more characteristic of the normal colonic mucosa of individuals at low risk for development of colon cancer.[9,16] Mitochondrial cytochrome oxidase activity was also elevated, suggesting that synthesis of mitochondrially encoded subunits of this enzyme was rate limiting in assembling active enzyme. Moreover, we showed that structural analogues of SCFAs that were inefficiently metabolized in the mitochondria—the branched 4 carbon SCFA isobutyric acid (isoC4) and the fluorine-substituted SCFA heptafluorobutyric acid (fluoroC4)—stimulated neither alkaline phosphatase activity nor mitochondrial gene expression. These observations were then extended to demonstrate that butyrate stimulated apoptosis of colonic epithelial cells in culture,[17] an observation also made by others,[18] and that the stimulation of apoptosis was not induced by iso- and fluoroC4. Moreover, DMSO and DMF, both of which had been reported to normalize the phenotype of colonic carcinoma cell lines, induced mitochondrial gene expression and apoptosis. By contrast, forskolin, an inducer of the human *MUC2* gene, which encodes the peptide backbone of the principal colonic mucin characteristic of the goblet cell lineage, did not induce mitochondrial gene expression or apoptosis. Thus, there was a tight link between the ability of agents to elevate mitochondrial gene expression and their ability to induce apoptosis of colonic carcinoma cells in culture.[19]

The pathway induced by butyrate was investigated further and shown to be characterized by an early and sustained induction of the cyclin-dependent kinase inhibitor, p21[WAF1/cip1], and growth arrest in G_0/G_1 beginning approximately 12 hours after induction, and coincident with a dissipation of the mitochondrial membrane potential ($\Delta\Psi_m$). This was followed closely by activation of caspase-3 and, finally, an increase in cells in the end stages of apoptosis measured by either the extent of DNA fragmentation or the number of cells with a subdiploid DNA content.[20,21]

To understand the role of mitochondrial function in this sequence of events initiated by butyrate, we used a number of inhibitors of mitochondrial function that either blocked various complexes, and hence steps, in electron transport, or that collapsed the mitochondrial membrane potential. Each was shown to inhibit DNA fragmentation when given simultaneously with butyrate, or within 8 hours following butyrate treatment. However, when the cells were exposed to butyrate for 16 hours or longer before treatment with the inhibitors, they became refractory to the effects of the inhibitors. Thus, there was an early period of commitment, lasting approximately until cell cycle arrest, dissipation of the $\Delta\Psi_m$ and caspase-3 activation, during which mitochondrial electron transport and the presence of an intact $\Delta\Psi_m$ was essential for entry into the pathway culminating in apoptosis. We subsequently demonstrated that the maintenance of a $\Delta\Psi_m$ was also necessary for caspase activation.[20,21]

The work of others made it clear that mitochondria were critically involved in the generation of apoptotic cascades, at least in part by the release of cytochrome c, which is mechanistically involved in caspase activation (reviewed in ref. 22). Other factors are also released from mitochondria in some apoptotic cascades.[23,24] Thus, it was possible to envision why mitochondrial functions play a role in stimulation of events temporally downstream of the dissipation of the $\Delta\Psi_m$, that is, caspase activation and DNA fragmentation. However, our data showed that collapse of the $\Delta\Psi_m$ also prevented the early induction, within 2 hours of butyrate treatment, of p21[WAF1/cip1], as well as the arrest of cells in G_0/G_1. Thus, we concluded that mitochondrial function may play a critical role in coordinating the pathways of cell growth and apoptosis in the colonic mucosa, and that SCFAs, by modulating mitochondrial function, influence the balance of cell renewal and death critical for homeostasis of the mucosa.[21]

Moreover, recent data have raised the possibility that SCFAs also modulate lineage-specific differentiation in the colonic mucosa. Butyrate, which does not induce expression of the *MUC2* gene, in fact, inhibits the expression of this gene in two cell systems used to study the development of the goblet, or secretory cell, lineage (Velcich, unpublished). Thus, three important features contributing to colonic mucosal homeostasis—rates of cell proliferation, cell death, and the balance of differentiation along two major cell lineages—may all be modulated, at least in part, by SCFAs in the colon.

The question arises as to how these pathways of cell proliferation, cell death, and lineage-specific differentiation interact with pathways known to be important in colonic epithelial cell transformation. To address this, we turned our attention to the β-catenin-Tcf pathway, inasmuch as this is an important signaling pathway that is altered by mutation of the *APC* gene, the initiating event in development of most human colon cancers. Wild-type *APC* protein binds β-catenin in a complex with GSK and targets β-catenin for degradation.[25–27] However, mutant *APC* does not target β-catenin for degradation. β-catenin levels rise, and a complex of β-catenin with Tcf, a transcriptional modulator, similarly increases in the nucleus, constitutively activating a gene program that brings about transformation.[28–31]

We have found that butyrate treatment of colonic carcinoma cells increases β-catenin-Tcf complex formation and Tcf activity, independent of decreases brought about by expression of a wild-type *APC* cDNA in these cells.[32] Moreover, other inducers of apoptosis of these cells, trichostatin A (TSA), like butyrate, an inhibitor of histone deacetylase, and Sulindac, an NSAID, which also induces a G_0/G_1 cell cycle arrest and a dissipation of the $\Delta\Psi_m$, also elevate Tcf activity. By contrast, isoC4 and fluoroC4, structural analogues of butyrate that do not induce an apoptotic cascade, and curcumin, a chemopreventive agent found in tumeric, which induces an S and G_2/M arrest without inducing apoptosis, do not increase Tcf activity.[32] Therefore, increases in this signaling pathway are associated with the induction of an apoptotic cascade, similar to the upregulation of a homologous pathway in *Drosophila* stimulated by a mutant *APC* gene that leads to retinal cell apoptosis.[33]

It has been suggested that wild-type *APC* normally triggers apoptosis of colonic epithelial cells[34] and that, consequently, the upregulation of signaling through the β-catenin-Tcf pathway brought about by mutant *APC* decreases apoptosis in the colonic mucosa, which is the cellular mechanism that initiates tumorigenesis due to the mutation. This, however, is in contrast to the link between elevated apoptosis and upregulation of the pathway that we have found for butyrate, TSA, and Sulindac,[32] as well as the upregulation in *Drosophila* retinal degeneration.[33] How can these observations be reconciled with the model proposed to link mutant *APC*, β-catenin-Tcf signaling, and apoptosis in the colonic mucosa?

First, it is possible that the mechanisms that regulate an apoptotic cascade in *Drosophila*, and in colonic cells in response to chemopreventive agents, differ significantly from the mechanisms induced by mutation in *APC*, and that the regulation of entry into an apoptotic cascade is much more complex than we understand. For example, it has recently been reported that there is a functional Tcf binding site in the c-*myc* gene, and hence that c-*myc* is a critical target for the transformation of colonic epithelial cells by *APC*.[35] This is consistent with earlier reports that c-*myc* is overexpressed in colonic tumors, sometimes in conjunction with its amplification;[36–40] c-*myc* expression has also been shown to be decreased in butyrate-induced apoptosis, probably related to the cell cycle arrest that is characteristic of the response to butyrate.[41–45] However, the decrease in c-*myc* expression has been attributed to a transcriptional pause mechanism in exon 2 of the gene,[44] therefore bypassing any effect of butyrate on Tcf activity, and hence on initiation of transcription of the gene. Further, alterations in c-*myc* and cell cycling are only one aspect of entry into an apoptotic cascade. We have found that events downstream of butyrate treatment, including induction of p21[WAF1/cip1], cell cycle arrest, caspase activation, elevation of Tcf activity, and DNA fragmentation are all dependent upon the presence of an intact $\Delta\Psi_m$,[20,21] thus suggesting that a mitochondrial function may be a critical determinant of the probability of a cell entering and completing the apoptotic cascade. There is reason, therefore, to believe that further research may reconcile the suggestion that apoptosis is associated with decreased Tcf activity induced by wild-type *APC* and the increases in Tcf activity we see in induced apoptosis in colonic carcinoma cells, which is similar to the observation in *Drosophila* retina. However, careful consideration of some of the assumptions that underlie the model of colonic cell transformation induced by mutant *APC* is also informative. First, the observation that *APC* regulates a pathway leading to apoptosis may not be correct. Although it has been reported that transfection of a wild-type *APC* can induce apoptosis in colonic carcinoma cell lines,[34] this is not true of all cell lines.[46] Moreover, we have recently found that spontaneous differentiation of the Caco-2 cell line, which takes place in the absence of apoptosis, is characterized by a downregulation of Tcf activity similar to that seen with *APC* (Mariadason, unpublished). Thus, expression of *APC*, and attendant downregulation of β-catenin-Tcf signaling, may be associated with aspects of colonic cell maturation other than apoptosis, which is consistent with the observations that although most colonic epithelial cells express *APC* as they migrate up the crypt, most do not, in fact, undergo, or at least complete, an apoptotic pathway before being sloughed into the lumen. Second, although it has been reported that FAP patients,[47] and mice with a targeted inactivation of the *APC* gene,[48] exhibit decreases in apoptosis in the colonic mucosa, these observations need to be carefully scrutinized. Colonic tumorigenesis is associated with homozygous inactivation of both *APC* alleles, and there is no evidence of a dominant affect of the loss of a single allele on apoptosis. Further, in both the human and mouse studies in which inheritance of a mutant *APC* was reported to decrease apoptosis in the flat mucosa, the control patients and mice exhibited very high levels of apoptosis, exceeding 25%.[47,48] As pointed out earlier, rates of apoptosis in the colonic mucosa determined either by morphology or TUNEL assay are an order of magnitude lower; extensive numbers of apoptotic cells are not seen in the upper third of the crypt, where cells exhibit their differentiated properties; and the higher rates would seem to be incompatible with normal development and growth.

Finally, we have recently found that alterations in apoptosis are neither necessary nor sufficient for tumorigenesis in mice that develop intestinal tumors in response to an inherited, targeted inactivation of the *Apc* gene.[2] Like other mouse models in which there is an inherited mutation of the *Apc* gene, the *Apc*1638 mouse develops gastrointestinal tumors, principally in the duodenum. We have demonstrated that there is no alteration in levels of apoptosis, or the ratio of apoptotic to proliferating cells, in the duodenum, proximal or distal colon of these animals. Moreover, we have introduced a homozygous deletion of the gene for short-chain acyl dehydrogenase into these mice, which encodes the first enzyme in the β-oxidation of SCFAs in the mitochondria. This is associated with a decrease of approximately 50% in apoptotic cells in the duodenum and distal colon, and a complete elimination of apoptotic cells in the proximal colon, presumably due to the dependence of apoptosis in these cells on the mitochondrial metabolism of SCFAs that we described above. However, these alterations in frequency of apoptosis did not change the tumor incidence (percent of mice with tumors) or number (tumors per mouse), or site distribution of tumors in the gastrointestinal tract. Thus, alterations in apoptosis are neither necessary nor sufficient for apoptosis in response to a mutant *Apc* gene.[2]

Does this absence of a role for altered apoptosis in the flat mucosa in tumor initiation by an *Apc* mutation mean that apoptosis is unimportant in colon tumorigenesis? The answer clearly is no. First, we have recently found that a stress diet, which increases tumor formation in the *Apc*1638 mice, increases proliferation and decreases apoptosis in the flat mucosa of these animals (Augenlicht, unpublished). Because the stress diet has been suggested to influence tumor progression, rather than initiation, alterations in the ratio of apoptotic to proliferating cells may be more important in progression of tumors than in earlier events. Second, in colon tumors, there is inactivation (or deletion) of both alleles of the *Apc* gene. Moreover, several chemopreventive agents, including NSAIDs, have been shown to induce apoptosis in causing regression of these lesions, although it is not certain if this is the sole, or most important, mechanism by which they act. Thus, although loss of a single *Apc* allele may not affect apoptosis in the intestinal mucosa, other agents that both promote and inhibit tumor formation and progression may indeed act by altering the balance between rates of apoptosis and proliferation either in the mucosa or in early tumors.

FUTURE DIRECTION

There are three particular areas that we will pursue using the cell and mouse models discussed above: mechanisms that distinguish tumor initiation from tumor progression; mechanisms that determine site specificity of tumor formation in the gastrointestinal tract; and coordination of pathways that determine probability of tumor formation, behavior, and response to agents that promote or inhibit tumorigenesis.

Initiation versus Progression

The distinction between genetic and other effects on tumor initiation and progression is an important one, and the *Apc*1638 model is an excellent opportunity to explore the biochemistry and molecular biology that underlie this distinction. We have recently documented the formation of aberrant crypt foci (ACF) in the colon of this mouse model (Augenlicht and Pretlow, unpublished). ACF are morphological lesions found in mice treated with colon-specific chemical carcinogens and in the colons of patients at high risk for development of colon cancer.[49] ACF show alterations in proliferation and gene mutation, as well as pathology, which indicate that at least some ACF have the potential to progress to carcinoma. Interestingly, although the number of ACF increase in the *Apc*1638 mouse between 9 and 25 weeks of age, their size (i.e., number of colonic crypts per aberrant focus) does not change. Thus, the *Apc* mutation may be involved in ACF initiation. Studies are underway to determine if dietary constituents that increase tumorigenesis in this mouse model also cause an expansion in size, and progression (i.e., pathology), of these early ACF. Another intriguing aspect of ACF is that they exhibit a depletion in goblet cells in this genetic model, as well as in ACF of mice treated with chemical carcinogens and in patients at high risk. Investigation of whether there is a block in differentiation of this lineage in ACF, and identification of the genetic and dietary influences that underlie such a block, are important areas of research. In this regard, we have analyzed the structure and mechanisms of regulation of both the human and mouse *MUC2* genes and continue to investigate mechanisms that determine lineage-specific expression of these sequences.[50–52] Moreover, our recent development of a mouse with a targeted inactivation of the *MUC2* gene should be a valuable tool in determining whether loss of the ability to synthesize mucin is a key step in promoting expansion of ACF to colon tumors and on to frankly malignant cancers (Velcich, unpublished).

Site Specificity of Tumor Formation

Epidemiological data, especially on changes in tumor incidence and tissue specificity in migrant populations, makes it clear how important environment—and especially diet—is in colon tumorigenesis. A particularly interesting observation that illustrates the important relationship between diet and genetics comes from the work of Warthin and Lynch in defining the HNPCC syndrome. Warthin initially identified family "G" as exhibiting a high incidence of uterine and gastric cancer.[53] Of note, at the turn of the century, gastric cancer was the principal GI cancer in the United States. By the time Lynch reinvestigated family G in his studies of hereditary cancer, the family exhibited high incidence of colon cancer, which had become the principal GI cancer in the United States.[54] We now know that such HNPCC families have a defect in DNA mismatch repair, due to an inherited mutation in any one of a number of different genes involved in a DNA mismatch repair (reviewed in ref. 55). Thus, the high incidence of cancer in family G is due to this genetic defect, but the site specificity appears to be determined by an environmental factor that also manifests itself in the site specificity of sporadic cancer.

This has important implications for genetic models of colon cancer. All three mouse models that have been reported, in which there is inheritance of a mutation in the *Apc* gene, develop small intestinal tumors, principally in the duodenum, rather than large intestinal tumors, as in the analogous FAP syndrome.[56–59] The reason for this is not understood. However, we have found that a combination of dietary factors and introduction of additional gene mutations cannot only increase the incidence of tumors in the *Apc*1638 model, but can also shift the tumors to more distal regions of the small intestine, and into the colon as well (Augenlicht, unpublished). We are investigating whether this is associated with a shift in patterns of cell proliferation and apoptosis in the GI tract, and the underlying molecular alterations in different regions of the intestine that may influence tumor formation initiated by inheritance of a mutant *Apc* allele.

Coordination of Pathways in Tumor Initiation, Promotion, and Chemoprevention

Finally, the development of colon tumors, and the influence of dietary constituents on their progression or regression, are complex events regulated by intersecting and interregulated biochemical pathways. Identification of genes that have undergone mutation in tumorigenesis has given us insight into some of the pathways involved, but our knowledge is clearly incomplete, and the coordination of these pathways is still obscure. However, new technology makes it possible to probe the pathways involved in normal and abnormal development in great detail. Using microarrays of cloned sequences, we are now able to analyze patterns of gene expression with far greater accuracy and sensitivity, and at a more complex level, than when we first approached these questions in the mid-1980s.[7,8] We are applying this methodology to colon cell lines in culture, to unique mouse genetic models, and to mucosal tissue from patients, to develop multiple data bases that can reveal pathways important in lineage-specific colon cell differentiation, colon cell apoptotic cascades, and colon cell transformation.

REFERENCES

1. AUGERON, C. & C.L. LABOISSE. 1984. Emergence of permanently differentiated cell clones in a human colonic cancer cell line in culture after treatment with sodium butyrate. Cancer Res. **44:** 3961–3969.
2. AUGENLICHT, L.H., G.M. ANTHONY, T.L. CHRUCH, W. EDELMANN, R. KUCHERLAPATI, K.Y. YANG, M. LIPKIN & B.G. HEERDT. Short chain fatty acid metabolism, apoptosis and Apc initiated tumorigenesis in the mouse gastrointestinal mucosa. Submitted.
3. SMITH, K.J., K.A. JOHNSON, T.M. BRYAN, D.E. HILL, S. MARKOWITZ, J.K.V. WILLSON, C. PARASKEVA, G.M. PETERSEN, S.R. HAMILTON, B. VOGELSTEIN & K.W. KINZLER. 1993. The APC gene product in normal and tumor cells. Proc. Natl. Acad. Sci. USA **90:**2846–2850.
4. EL-DEIRY, W.S., T. TOKINO, T. WALDMAN, J.D. OLINER, V.E. VELCULESCU, M. BURRELL, D.E. HILL, E. HEALY, J.L. REES, S. R. HAMILTON, K.W. KINZLER & B. VOGELSTEIN. 1995. Topological control of p21 waf1/cip1 expression in normal and neoplastic tissues. Cancer Res. **55:** 2910–2919.
5. MELHEM, M.F., A.I. MEISLER, G.G. FINLEY, W.H. BRYCE, M.O. JONES, I.I. TRIBBY, J.M. PIPAS & R.A. KOSKI. 1992. Distribution of cells expressing myc proteins in human colorectal epithelium, polyps, and malignant tumors. Cancer Res. **52:** 5853–5864.
6. CHIN, L., N. SCHREIBER-AGUS, I. PELLICER, K. CHEN, H.-W. LEE, M. DUDAST, C. CORDON-CARDO & R.A. DEPINHO. 1995. Contrasting roles for myc and mad proteins in cellular growth and differentiation. Proc. Natl. Acad. Sci. USA **92:** 8488–8492.
7. AUGENLICHT, L.H., M.Z. WAHRMAN, H. HALSEY, L. ANDERSON, J. TAYLOR & M. LIPKIN. 1987. Expression of cloned sequences in biopsies of human colonic tissue and in colonic carcinoma cells induced to differentiate *in vitro*. Cancer Res. **47:** 6017–6021.
8. AUGENLICHT, L.H., J. TAYLOR, L. ANDERSON & M. LIPKIN. 1991. Patterns of gene expression that characterize the colonic mucosa in patients at genetic risk for colonic cancer. Proc. Natl. Acad. Sci. USA **88:** 3286–3289.
9. HEERDT, B.G., H.K. HALSEY, M. LIPKIN & L.H. AUGENLICHT. 1990. Expression of mitochondrial cytochrome c oxidase in human colonic cell differentiation, transformation, and risk for colonic cancer. Cancer Res. **50:** 1596–1600.
10. KIM, Y.S., D. TSAO, B. SIDDIQUI, J.S. WHITEHEAD, P. ARNSTEIN, J. BENNETT & J. HICKS. 1980. Effects of sodium butyrate and dimethylsulfoxide on biochemical properties of human colon cancer cells. Cancer **45:**1185–1192.
11. MORITA, A., D. TSAO & Y.S. KIM. 1982. Effect of sodium butyrate on alkaline phosphatase in HRT-18, a human rectal cancer cell line. Cancer Res. **42:** 4540–4545.
12. TSAO, D., Z.-R. SHI, A. WONG & Y.S. KIM. 1983. Effect of sodium butyrate on carcinoembryonic antigen production by human colonic adenocarcinoma cells in culture. Cancer Res. **43:** 1217–1222.
13. CUMMINGS, J.H., E.W. POMARE, W.J. BRANCH, C.P.E. NAYLOR & G.T. MACFARLANE. 1987. Short chain fatty acids in human large intestine, portal, hepatic and venous blood. Gut **28:** 1221–1227.
14. HARIG, J.M., K.H. SOERGEL, R.A. KOMOROWSKI & C.M. WOOD. 1989. Treatment of diversion colitis with short-chain-fatty acid irrigation. N. Engl. J. Med. **320:** 23–28.
15. ROEDIGER, W.E. 1980. Role of anaerobic bacteria in the metabolic welfare of the colonic mucosa in man. Gut **21:** 793–798.
16. HEERDT, B.G. & L.H. AUGENLICHT. 1991. Effects of fatty acids on expression of genes encoding subunits of cytochrome c oxidase and cytochrome c oxidase activity in HT29 human colonic adenocarcinoma cells. J. Biol. Chem. **266:** 19120–19126.

17. HEERDT, B.G., M.A. HOUSTON & L.H. AUGENLICHT. 1994. Potentiation by specific short-chain fatty acids of differentiation and apoptosis in human colonic carcinoma cell lines. Cancer Res. **54:** 3288–3294.
18. HAGUE, A., A.M. MANNING, K.A. HANLON, L.I. HUSCHTSCHA, D. HART & C. PARASKEVA. 1993. Sodium butyrate induces apoptosis in human colonic tumor cell lines in a p53-independent pathway: Implications for the possible role of dietary fibre in the prevention of large-bowel cancer. Int. J. Cancer **55:** 498–505.
19. HEERDT, B.G., M.A. HOUSTON, J.J. REDISKE & L.H. AUGENLICHT. 1996. Steady-state levels of mitochondrial messenger RNA species characterize a predominant pathway culminating in apoptosis and shedding of HT29 human colonic carcinoma cells. Cell Growth & Differen. **7:** 101–106.
20. HEERDT, B. G., M.A. HOUSTON & L.H. AUGENLICHT. 1997. Short chain fatty acid-initiated cell cycle arrest and apoptosis of colonic epithelial cells is linked to mitochondrial function. Cell Growth & Differen. **8:** 523–532.
21. HEERDT, B.G., M.A. HOUSTON, G.M. ANTHONY & L.H. AUGENLICHT. 1998. Mitochondrial membrane potential in the coordination of p53-independent proliferation and apoptosis pathways in human colonic carcinoma cells. Cancer Res. **58:** 2869–2875.
22. REED, J. C. 1997. Cytochrome c: Can't live with it—Can't live without it. Cell **91:** 559–562.
23. MARCHETTI, P., S.A. SUSIN, D. DECAUDIN, S. GAMEN, M. CASTEDO, T. HIRSCH, N. ZAMZAMI, J. NAVAL, A. SENIK & G. KROEMER. 1996. Apoptosis-associated derangement of mitochondrial function in cells lacking mitochondrial DNA. Cancer Res. **56:** 2033–2038.
24. ZAMZAMI, N., S.A. SUSIN, P. MARCHETTI, T. HIRSCH, I. GOMEZ-MONTERREY, M. CASTEDO, & G. KROEMER. 1996. Mitochondrial control of nuclear apoptosis. J. Exp. Med. **183:** 1533–1544.
25. RUBINFELD, B., B. SOUZA, I. ALBERT, O. MULLER, S.H. CHAMBERLAIN, F.R. MASIARZ, S. MUNEMITSU, P. POLAKIS. 1993. Association of the APC gene product with β-catenin. Science **262:** 1731–1734.
26. SU, L.-K., B. VOGELSTEIN & K. KINZLER. 1993. Association of the APC tumor suppressor protein with catenins. Science **262:** 1734–1737.
27. MUNEMITSU, S., I. ALBERT, B. SOUZA, B. RUBINFELD & P. POLAKIS. 1995. Regulation of intracellular β-catenin levels by the adenomatous polyposis coli (APC) tumor-suppressor protein. Proc. Nalt. Acad. Sci. USA **92:** 3046–3050.
28. MOLENAAR, M., M. VAN DE WETERING, M. OSTERWEGEL, J. PETERSON-MADURO, S. GODSAVE, V. KORINEK, J. ROOSE, O. DESTREE & H. CLEVERS. 1996. XTcf-3 transcription factor mediates β-catenin-induced axis formation in Xenopus embryos. Cell **86:** 391–399.
29. BEHRENS, J., J.P. VON KRIES, M. KUHL, L. BRUHN, D. WEDLICH, R. GROSSCHEDL & W. BIRCHMEIER. 1996. Functional interaction of β-catenin with the transcription factor LEF-1. Nature **382:** 638–642.
30. KORINEK, V., N. BARKER, P.J. MORIN, D. VAN WICHEN, R. DE WEGER, K.W. KINZLER, B. VOGELSTEIN & H. CLEVERS. 1997. Constitutive transcriptional activation by a β-catenin-Tcf complex in APC−/− colon carcinoma. Science **275:** 1784–1787.
31. MORIN, P.J., A.B. SPARKS, V. KORINEK, N. BARKER, H. CLEVERS, B. VOGELSTEIN & K.W. KINZLER. 1997. Activation of β-catenin-Tcf signaling in colon cancer by mutations in β-catenin or APC. Science **275:** 787–1790.
32. BORDONARO, M., J.M. MARIADASON, B.G. HEERDT & L.H. AUGENLICHT. 1999. Butyrate induced cell cycle arrest and apoptotic cascade in colonic carcinoma cells: Modulation of the β-catenin-Tcf pathway, and concordance with effects of Sulindac and trichostatin, but not curcumin. Cell Growth & Differen. In press.

33. AHMED, Y., S. HAYASHI, A. LEVINE & E. WIESCHAUS. 1998. Regulation of Armadillo by a *Drosophila* APC inhibits neuronal apoptosis during retinal development. Cell **93:** 1171–1182.
34. MORIN, P.J., B. VOGELSTEIN & K.W. KINZLER. 1996. Apoptosis and APC in colorectal tumorigenesis. Proc. Natl. Acad. Sci. USA **93:** 7950–7954.
35. HE, T.-C., A.B. SPARKS, C. RAGO, H. HERMEKING, L. ZAWEL, L.T. DA COSTA, P.J. MORIN, B. VOGELSTEIN & K.W. KINZLER. 1998. Identification of c-*myc* as a target of the APC pathway. Science **281:** 1509–1512.
36. YANDER, G., H. HALSEY, M. KENNA & L.H. AUGENLICHT. 1985. Amplification and elevated expression of c-*myc* in a chemically induced mouse colon tumor. Cancer Res. **45:** 4433–4438.
37. HEERDT, B.G., S. MOLINAS, D. DEITCH & L.H. AUGENLICHT. 1991. Aggressive subtypes of human colorectal tumors frequently exhibit amplification of the c-*myc* gene. Oncogene **6:** 125–129.
38. AUGENLICHT, L.H., S.WADLER, G. CORNER, C. RICHARDS, L. RYAN, A.S. MULTANI, S. PATHAK, A. BENSON, D. HALLER & B.G. HEERDT. 1997. Low-level c-*myc* amplification in human colonic carcinoma cell lines and tumors: A frequent, p53-independent mutation associated with improved outcome in a randomized multi-institutional trial. Cancer Res. **57:** 1769–1775.
39. ERISMAN, M.D., J.K. SCOTT, R.A. WATT & S.M. ASTRIN. 1988. The c-*myc* protein is constitutively expressed at elevated levels in colorectal carcinoma cell lines. Oncogene **2:** 367–378.
40. ERISMAN, M.D., P.G. ROTHBERG, R.E. DIEHL, C.C. MORSE, J.M. SPANDORFER & S.M. ASTRIN. 1985. Deregulation of c-*myc* gene expression in human colon carcinoma is not accompanied by amplification or rearrangement of the gene. Mol. Cell. Biol. **5:** 1969–1976.
41. HEROLD, K.M. & P.G. ROTHBERG. 1988. Evidence for a labile intermediate in the butyrate induced reduction of the level of c-*myc* RNA in SW837 rectal carcinoma cells. Oncogene **3:** 423–428.
42. TAYLOR, C.W., Y.S. KIM, K.E. CHILDRESS-FIELDS & L.C. YEOMAN. 1992. Sensitivity of nuclear c-myc levels and induction to differentiation-inducing agents in human colon tumor cell lines. Cancer Lett. **62:** 95–105.
43. COLLINS, J.F., P. HERMAN, C. SCHUCH & G.C. BAGBY. 1992. c-myc antisense oligonucleotides inhibit the colony-forming capacity of Colo 320 colonic carcinoma cells. J. Clin. Invest. **89:** 1523–1527.
44. HERUTH, D.P., G.W. ZIRNSTEIN, J.F. BRADLEY & P.G. ROTHBERG. 1993. Sodium butyrate causes an increase in the block to transcriptional elongation in the c-myc gene in SW837 rectal carcinoma cells. J. Biol. Chem. **268:** 20466–20472.
45. BARNARD, J.A. & G. WARWICK. 1993. Butyrate rapidly induces growth inhibition and differentiation in HT-29 cells. Cell Growth & Differen. **4:** 495–501.
46. GRODEN, J., G. JOSLYN, W. SAMOWITZ, D. JONES, N. BHATTACHARYYA, L. SPIRIO, A. THLIVERIS, M. ROBERTSON, S. EGAN, M. MEUTH & R. WHITE. 1995. Response of colon cancer cell lines to the introduction of APC, a colon-specific tumor suppressor gene. Cancer Res. **55:** 1531–1539.
47. BEDI, A., P.J. PASRICHA, A.J. AKHTAR, J.P. BARBER, G.C. BEDI, F.M. GIARDIELLO, B.A. ZEHNBAUER, S.R. HAMILTON & R.J. JONES. 1995. Inhibition of apoptosis during development of colorectal cancer. Cancer Res. **55:** 1811–1816.
48. BOOLBOL, S.K., A.J. DANNENBERG, A. CHADBURN, C. MARTUCCI, X.J. GUO, J.T. RAMONETTI, M. ABREU-GORIS, H.L. NEWMARK, M. LIPKIN, J.J. DECOSSE & M.M. BERTAGNOLLI. 1996. Cyclooxygenase-2 overexpression and tumor formation are blocked by sulindac in a murine model of familial adenomatous polyposis. Cancer Res. **56:** 2556–2560.

49. PRETLOW, T.P., B. SIDDIKI, L.H. AUGENLICHT, T.G. PRETLOW & Y.S. KIM. 1999. Aberrant crypt foci (ACF)—earliest recognized players or innocent bystanders in colon carcinogenesis. *In* Colorectal Cancer: Molecular Mechanisms, Premalignant State, and its Prevention. W. Schmiegel, Ed.: Kluwer Academic Publishers. Lancaster, England.
50. VELCICH, A. & L.H. AUGENLICHT. 1993. Regulated expression of an intestinal mucin gene in HT29 colonic carcinoma cells. J. Biol. Chem. **268:** 13956–13961.
51. VELCICH, A., L. PALUMBO, A. JARRY, C. LABOISSE, J. RACEVSKIS & L. AUGENLICHT. 1995. Patterns of expression of lineage specific markers during the *in vitro* differentiation of HT29 colon carcinoma cells. Cell Growth & Differen. **6:** 749–757.
52. VELCICH, A., L. PALUMBO, L. SELLERI, G. EVANS & L. AUGENLICHT. 1997. Organization and regulatory aspects of the human intestinal mucin gene (MUC2) locus. J. Biol. Chem. **272:** 7968–7976.
53. WARTHIN, A.S. 1913. Heredity with reference to carcinoma. Arch. Intern. Med. **12:** 546–555.
54. LYNCH, H.T. & A.J. KRUSH. 1971. Cancer family G revisited: 1895–1970. Cancer **27:** 1505–1511.
55. MARRA, G. & C.R. BOLAND. 1995. Hereditary nonpolyposis colorectal cancer: The syndrome, the genes, and historical perspectives. J. Natl. Cancer Inst. **87:** 1114–1125.
56. FODDE, R., W. EDELMANN, K. YANG, C. VAN LEEUWEN, C. CARLSON, B. RENAULT, C. BREUKEL, E. ALT, M. LIPKIN, P.M. KHAN & R. KUCHERLAPATI. 1994. A targeted chain-termination mutation in the mouse Apc gene results in multiple intestinal tumors. Proc. Natl. Acad. Sci. USA **91:** 8969–8973.
57. YANG, K., W. EDELMANN, K. FAN, K. LAU, V.R. KOLLI, R. FODDE, P.M. KHAN, R. KUCHERLAPATI & M. LIPKIN. 1997. A mouse model of human familial adenomatous polyposis. J. Exp. Zool. **277:** 245–254.
58. SU, L.-K., K.W. KINZLER, B. VOGELSTEIN, A.C. PREISINGER, A.R. MOSER, C. LUONGO, K.A. GOULD & W.F. DOVE. 1992. Multiple intestinal neoplasia caused by a mutation in the murine homolog of the APC gene. Science **256:** 668–670.
59. OSHIMA, M., H. OSHIMA, K. KITAGAWA, M. KOBAYASHI, C. ITAKURA & M. TAKETO. 1995. Loss of Apc heterozygosity and abnormal tissue building in nascent intestinal polyps in mice carrying a truncated Apc gene. Proc. Natl. Acad. Sci. USA **92:** 4482–4486.

APC and Intestinal Carcinogenesis

Insights from Animal Models

MONICA M. BERTAGNOLLI[a]

The New York Hospital-Cornell Medical Center and Strang Cancer Prevention Center, New York, New York 10021, USA

ABSTRACT: The APC protein is a crucial regulator of intestinal cell growth, and mutations in the *APC* gene are a common initial event in the process of human colorectal carcinogenesis. Animals bearing germline mutations in *Apc* are therefore important models for human colorectal cancer. These animals have been used both to understand the biology of human colorectal cancer and to screen for agents able to prevent malignant transformation of susceptible intestinal cells.

FAMILIAL ADENOMATOUS POLYPOSIS, THE *APC* GENE, AND SPORADIC COLORECTAL CANCER

The *APC* (adenomatous polyposis coli) gene was recognized as an important safeguard against colon cancer when germline mutations were linked to a syndrome of colon cancer predisposition, familial adenomatous polyposis (FAP).[1–4] FAP is characterized by multiple intestinal adenomas and, if untreated, eventual progression to colorectal cancer in the third to fourth decade of life. The phenotype of FAP is variable. In addition to colorectal tumors, it includes many other abnormalities of cellular proliferation, such as periampullary neoplasms, mandibular osteomas, desmoid tumors of the abdomen, congenital hypertrophy of the retinal pigmented epithelium, gastric fundic gland polyps, and medulloblastomas.[5] FAP is a very rare disorder, affecting only 1/8,000 individuals in the United States.[6] Somatic mutations of the *APC* gene, however, are very common and are associated with 80–85% of sporadic colorectal cancers.[7] Genetic analyses of the adenoma-carcinoma sequence for colorectal cancer suggest that mutation of *APC* is not only common, it is an initiating factor in the disease.[8,9] Because of this, understanding the rare syndrome of FAP provides the key to preventing most of the 60,000 deaths that occur annually as a result of colorectal cancer.[10]

The *APC* gene, located at 5q21, encodes a protein of 2843 amino acids in length. *APC* is a tumor suppressor gene, because single allele mutations result in defective APC protein function and precede the loss of heterozygosity evident in tumors.[8,9] APC forms one component of an intracellular complex that includes GSK-3β, a serine-

[a]Address for correspondence: The New York Hospital-Cornell Medical Center, 525 East 68th Street, Suite F-1913, New York, NY 10021. Voice: 212-746-2195; fax: 212-746-8765.
e-mail: mbertagn@mail.med.cornell.edu

threonine kinase, and the intracellular proteins, conductin and β-catenin.[11,12] This complex facilitates the phosphorylation of β-catenin, which, in turn, targets β-catenin for degradation via ubiquitination.[13,14] Deficient APC function results in the intracellular accumulation of β-catenin. β-Catenin is a protein associated with the adherens junction and actin cytoskeleton of epithelial cells. β-Catenin is also present in the nucleus, where it binds to the transcription factor, Tcf, and induces transcription of a number of genes, including *c-myc*.[15–17] These observations suggest that β-catenin plays a role in signaling changes in the arrangement of actin filaments and cell-cell adhesion. These critical signaling pathways, in turn, may control epithelial cell growth.

The APC protein contains several functional domains, including an oligomerization domain at the amino terminus, and a central β-catenin binding domain that includes both constitutive and inducible binding sites.[4,18] The carboxy terminus of APC binds microtubules, as well as the human homologue of *Drosophila* discs large (DLG) and EB1, a protein of unknown function. Most of the mutations associated with FAP and sporadic colorectal cancer occur in the central portion of the molecule, producing loss of some or all of the β-catenin binding regions.[13,14,19] Most clinically relevant mutations in *APC* create premature termination codons that yield truncations of the protein product. Several important genotype-phenotype correlations have been noted in patients with FAP. For instance, truncations in the extreme 5′ end of the coding sequence (prior to codon 169) produce an attenuated form of FAP, with fewer intestinal tumors and later progression to colorectal cancer.[20–23] The great majority of mutations found in patients with FAP result in stable truncated proteins of greater than 80 kDa.[24–26] The "profuse" FAP phenotype, characterized by extremely numerous lower intestinal adenomas, is associated with mutations from codon 1250 to codon 1464.[23] Germline mutations after codon 1700 are few,[25] suggesting that mutations in the 3' end of the coding sequence produce little or no phenotype.

ANIMAL MODELS OF *APC*-ASSOCIATED CANCER

For *APC*, as for other genes implicated in human cancer, animal models provide important insight into the nature of the disease and the means by which tumor formation may be prevented or disease progression delayed. At the present time, there are three animal models for FAP, each bearing germline mutations in *Apc*: (1) C57BL/6J-Min/+ (Min/+ mouse);[27,28] (2) APC$^{\Delta716}$;[29] and (3) *Apc*1638N.[30] Intestinal tumor formation in these animals differs significantly from that of humans, in that the mice have many tumors in the small intestine, but few in the colon. It is possible that this discrepancy arises from differences in the microenvironment of the murine intestine, which has a different distribution of bacterial content and a faster rate of cell turnover than that of humans. In spite of this difference, clinically relevant methods to decrease *Apc*-associated tumor formation have been identified by studying these animals. In addition to their use as a screen for chemopreventive agents, these animal models exhibit important phenotypic differences produced by *Apc* mutations. These distinct phenotypes provide additional insight into the mechanism of *Apc*-associated carcinogenesis.

MODULATION OF *APC*-ASSOCIATED CARCINOGENESIS
BY CHEMOPREVENTIVE AGENTS

Studies of FAP patients suggest that it is possible to decrease APC-associated intestinal tumors by drugs or dietary modification. The nonsteroidal antiinflammatory drug (NSAID), sulindac, decreased both the size and number of intestinal polyps in patients with FAP.[31–33] In addition, dietary modification by increasing intake of fiber and vitamin C decreased rectal tumors in a randomized trial of patients with FAP.[34] These promising results in humans suggested that effective chemoprevention of colonic tumors is an achievable goal and that the search should begin with NSAIDs and antioxidants.

Due to its wide availability and relatively severe phenotype, the Min/+ mouse has been the animal model chosen for most tumor modulation studies to date. Early work showed that Min/+ intestinal tumor number increased as a result of a high fat diet,[28] confirming an association implicated in human sporadic colorectal cancer. Administration of bile acids in the diet enhanced tumor formation in the duodenum of Min/+ mice, supporting another widely held theory of intestinal tumor promotion.[35] The modulation of bile acid effect by increased dietary fiber may be the reason for the clinical response to fiber in FAP patients.[34] Other known modulators of tumorigenesis in Min/+ mice include the Bowman-Birk protease inhibitor,[36] NSAIDs,[37–40] and phenolic antioxidants. The last two categories have been the focus of work in our laboratory.

A number of different NSAIDs prevent tumor formation in Min/+ mice (TABLE 1). Animals treated for 2.5 months with a dose of sulindac equivalent to an effective regimen in FAP patients exhibited a >90% reduction in tumor number.[38] In a tumor regression study, dietary sulindac administration decreased tumor size and number after only 4 days of administration, with maximal effect at 20 days after initiation of treatment.[41] Sulindac treatment lowered mucosal prostaglandin-E_2 (PGE_2) levels, confirming an effect of this dose on cyclooxygenase activity.[38] Tumor formation was not affected by treatment of Min/+ mice with the sulfone metabolite of sulindac, an agent that does not decrease prostaglandin activity.[42] Aspirin, in a dose equivalent to 100 mg per day in humans, decreased tumor formation in Min/+ mice by 44%.[39,40] Finally, administration of the selective cyclooxygenase-2 (Cox-2) inhibitor, SC58635, inhibited Min/+ intestinal tumors by more than 90% (R. Jacoby, personal communication). The antitumor effects of NSAIDs in Min/+ mice, therefore, parallel those in humans with FAP and suggest that NSAID use will also prevent sporadic human colorectal cancer.

Phenolic antioxidants are plant-derived compounds with chemopreventive activity in cell culture systems. These compounds have antiinflammatory activity and, like NSAIDs, are able to inhibit cyclooxygenase activity *in vitro*.[43] In animal bioassays, such as carcinogen-induced rodent models, some phenolic antioxidants inhibit tumor formation at both the initiation and promotional phases. Two phenolic antioxidants, caffeic acid phenethyl ester (CAPE) and curcumin, were administered in the diet to Min/+ mice. At doses previously shown to inhibit azoxymethane-induced intestinal tumors in rats, both of these agents significantly decreased Min/+ adenoma formation (TABLE 1).

TABLE 1. NSAIDs and phenolic antioxidants decrease tumors in Min/+ mice

Agent	Dose	Tumor reduction	Reference
Sulindac	0.016%	>90%	38,41
Sulindac sulfide	0.016%	>90%	42
Aspirin	0.02–0.05%	44–51%	39,40
SC58635	0.15%	>90%	R. Jacoby, personal communication
CAPE	0.15%	63.1%	M. Bertagnolli, manuscript in preparation
Curcumin	2%	63.7%	M. Bertagnolli, manuscript in preparation

In addition to supporting the use of prostaglandin-inhibiting agents in colon cancer prevention, studies of chemopreventive agents in Min/+ mice have identified some tissue-specific correlates of antitumor efficacy. Humans with FAP treated with sulindac exhibited increased apoptosis in the nonadenomatous tissue of the rectum.[44] A similar effect was observed in the Min/+ mouse, where treatment with tumor-inhibiting doses of sulindac, aspirin, CAPE, or curcumin produced a significant increase in apoptosis in the enterocytes of the small intestine (FIG. 1). In conjunction with this increase in apoptosis, a compensatory increase in enterocyte proliferation, as measured by PCNA expression, was observed (FIG. 2). Taken together, these results suggest that chemopreventive agents increase the turnover rate of cells in the

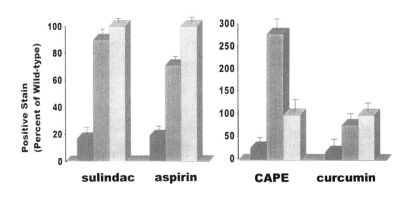

Min/+   **Min/+ drug**   **+/+**

FIGURE 1. Enterocyte apoptosis is increased by chemopreventive drugs. Specimens of small intestine from animals at 16 weeks of age were formalin fixed, embedded in paraffin, and sectioned at 5 μm. Where indicated, animals were treated for 10 weeks with sulindac (0.016%), aspirin (0.02%), CAPE (0.15%), or curcumin (2%) mixed in an AIN76A diet. Sections of small intestine were analyzed by TUNEL. The percent staining of enterocytes in these crypt-villus units was measured by an observer blinded to the animal's genetic status using the Cell Analysis System 200 (CAS 200). Values expressed are % ± SEM of total cells positive relative to enterocytes in the wild-type animals.[38,39,41]

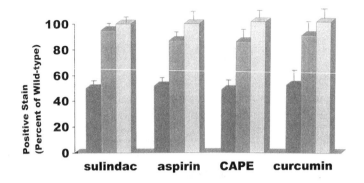

■ Min/+ ■ Min/+ drug □ +/+

FIGURE 2. Enterocyte proliferation is increased by chemopreventive drugs. Where indicated, animals were treated for 10 weeks with sulindac (0.016%), aspirin (0.02%), CAPE (0.15%), or curcumin (2%) mixed in an AIN76A diet. Specimens of small intestine were harvested and formalin fixed, embedded in paraffin, and sectioned at 5 μm. Sections of small intestine were stained with antibody to PCNA, and the percent staining of enterocytes in these crypt-villus units was measured by an observer blinded to the animal's genetic status using the CAS 200. Values expressed are % ± SEM of total cells positive relative to enterocytes in the wild-type animals.[39,41]

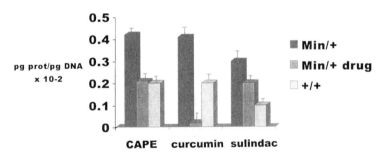

FIGURE 3. Modulation of tissue β-catenin expression by chemopreventive drugs. Specimens of small intestine from animals at 16 weeks of age were formalin fixed, embedded in paraffin, and sectioned at 5 μm. Where indicated, animals were treated with CAPE (0.15%), curcumin (2%), or sulindac (0.016%) mixed in an AIN76A diet. Sections were stained with antibody to β-catenin. The percent staining of enterocytes in these crypt-villus units was measured by an observer blinded to the animal's genetic or treatment status using the CAS 200. Values represented are ± SEM.[38,45]

intestinal mucosa. In addition to altering enterocyte growth, chemopreventive agents modulated the expression of β-catenin in murine small intestine enterocytes (FIG. 3). When the enterocytes of wild-type animals lacking the mutant *Apc* allele were compared to those of the untreated Min/+ mice, a 2- to 4-fold increase in tissue β-catenin expression was observed. Treatment with chemopreventive agents lowered β-catenin expression in the small intestine, thereby "normalizing" the effect of the mutation.[45]

These experiments suggest that administration of NSAIDs and phenolic antioxidants can partially reverse the deleterious effects of an *APC* mutation. The doses administered in these studies, in human equivalents, are relatively nontoxic, suggesting that these agents alone or in combination may be effective in reducing sporadic colorectal cancer in humans.

GENETIC MODULATION OF *APC*-ASSOCIATED CARCINOGENESIS

Carcinogenesis in the gastrointestinal epithelium is the result of successive accumulation of numerous mutations in cellular oncogenes and tumor suppressors, resulting in a transformed phenotype and eventual progression of the enterocyte to invasive cancer. In 1988, Vogelstein *et al.*[46] published a report describing specific mutations in human colorectal cancer and defined their relationship to the adenoma-carcinoma sequence. Through the use of transgenic technology to induce tumor-associated mutations in study animals, a more precise understanding of the correlation between specific mutations and the different stages of carcinogenesis is emerging.

As mentioned previously, mutations in *APC* are among the earliest events in intestinal carcinogenesis.[8,9] Additional mutations associated with human colorectal cancer include those of *hMLH-1, hMSH-2, K-ras, DCC, Dpc-4,* and *p53.*[46] Transgenic animals bearing inactivating mutations in these genes, when crossed with *Apc*-mutant mice, provide insight into the relative contribution of the various genes implicated in the adenoma-carcinoma sequence (TABLE 2). In some cases, the results have confirmed a role for suspected cancer-associated genes in intestinal tumorigenesis.

The *Apc*1638N mouse bears a germline mutation in *Apc* that produces a minimal phenotype, with few intestinal tumors and an increased lifespan relative to that of Min/+ mice.[30] When these animals were crossed with a mouse lacking in mismatch repair capability, such as the *Mlh-1* knock-out mouse, the number of tumors in the intestine were greatly increased, leading to much earlier death of the animal (R. Kucherlapati, unpublished data). The same result was obtained by crossing the Min/+ mouse with an animal lacking the *Msh-2* gene.[47] These data indicate that lack

TABLE 2. Genetic modulation of *Apc*-deficient animals

Genotype	Result	Reference
Min/+ × Cox-1$^{-/-}$	Decreased tumor number and size	54
Min/+ × Cox-2$^{-/-}$	Decreased tumor number and size	54
APC$^{\Delta 176}$ × Cox-2$^{-/-}$	Decreased tumor number	53
Min/+ × Mom-1$^{-/-}$	Decreased tumor number	49
Min/+ × MMP-7$^{-/-}$	Decreased tumor number and size	51
Min/+ × *Dpc-4*$^{-/-}$	Increased tumor invasiveness	48
Min/+ × *Msh-2*$^{-/-}$	Increased tumor number	47
*Apc*1638N × *Mlh*-1$^{-/-}$	Increased tumor number	R. Kucherlapati, unpublished data
Min/+ × *p53*$^{-/-}$	No change in tumor number or progression	52

of mismatch repair capability accelerates intestinal carcinogenesis. The mismatch repair pathway corrects postreplication errors and allows repair via homologous recombination. Deficiencies in mismatch repair function increase the spontaneous rate of mutation, a consequence that is consistent with the requirement for multiple mutations for tumor progression. Similarly, when the $APC^{\Delta716}$ mouse was crossed with an animal lacking the function of *Dpc4*, a gene regulating signaling by the growth factor, TGF-β, increased tumor invasiveness was observed.[48] This latter result supports a large body of data linking defects in TGF-β signaling to intestinal tumor formation.

Some of the knockout experiments in *Apc*-deficient animals yielded surprising results. In early studies of the Min/+ mice, a mutation at the Mom-1 (modifier of min-1) locus was identified as producing an attenuated phenotype.[49] Mom-1 was later discovered to be a gene encoding secretory phospholipase-A, and the Mom-1/ Min/+ result is consistent with dietary studies implicating phospholipid metabolism in intestinal carcinogenesis.[50] In a fascinating study, the cross of the Min/+ mouse with an animal lacking p53 function (p53−/−) showed no change in tumor incidence or rate of progression, and no difference in tumor cell apoptosis.[51] The influence of p53 in early intestinal carcinogenesis is therefore unclear.

In addition to clarifying the role of cancer-associated genes, knockout studies in *Apc*-deficient mice provided insight into the role of key enzymes in intestinal tumorigenesis. When the $APC^{\Delta716}$ mouse was crossed with an animal lacking murine Cox-2 activity, a 90% decrease in tumor number was observed.[52] Similar results were obtained when Cox-2 activity was eliminated in the Min/+ mouse.[53] In addition, eliminating Cox-1 activity in the Min/+ mouse also produced an 80–90% reduction in tumor number, suggesting that both cyclooxygenase isoforms are important in intestinal tumorigenesis.[53] Finally, when matrix metalloproteinase activity was decreased in Min/+ mice by loss of the MMP-7 (matrilysin) gene, tumors were reduced in number and size. This result suggests that enzymes mediating invasion and metastasis by destruction of the basement membrane and connective tissue may also play a role in early carcinogenesis.[54]

GENOTYPE-PHENOTYPE CORRELATION IN ANIMAL MODELS OF FAP

The *Apc* gene product mediates coordinated cell growth in the intestinal mucosa. In humans with FAP, the severity of tumor formation in the intestine varies depending upon the length of the protein expressed by the mutant allele. Truncations producing very small APC fragments result in the attenuated APC phenotype, with fewer intestinal tumors and later progression to colorectal cancer.[20–23] The classic FAP phenotype, characterized by abundant colorectal tumors, is associated with stable truncated proteins of greater than 80 kDa.[24–26] To study the relationship between APC protein size and tumor formation, we compared the intestinal mucosa from Min/+ mice, an animal model of classic FAP, and the *Apc*1638N mouse, a model of attenuated FAP.[55] Because earlier work suggested that Min/+ mice exhibit increased

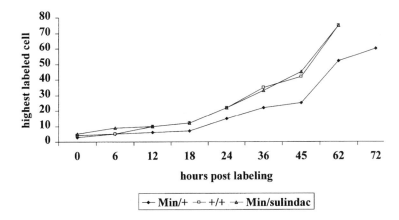

FIGURE 4. Enterocyte migration in Min/+ mice. Ten mice from each experimental group (Min/+, +/+, and Min/+ treated with sulindac, 0.016%) were injected with 0.3 µg/kg of BrdU (Sigma, St. Louis, MO). Small intestine from each group was examined at the indicated intervals postinjection by staining with anti-BrdU antibody. Eight intact histologically normal crypt-villus units from each animal were examined by an observer blinded to the animal's genetic status or treatment group. Decreased enterocyte migration was observed in Min/+ small intestine. By ANOVA, a significant group-time interaction ($p < 0.0001$) was observed. Further pairwise analysis showed that the cell height-by-time curves for +/+ and Min/sulindac were not different from one another.[45]

enterocyte turnover rates when compared to wild-type littermates, we compared the rates of crypt-villus migration for enterocytes in the small intestine of Min/+ and Apc1638N mice. Following labeling of actively dividing enterocytes with BrdU, their movement was tracked by harvesting and examining intestinal tissue at successive postlabeling intervals. For Min/+ mice, a 20% delay in enterocyte migration was observed at all time points (Fig. 4). This delay was eliminated by treatment of the mice with sulindac, an observation predicted by the previous observation that sulindac increased enterocyte apoptosis and proliferation (Figures 1 and 2). In comparison, no migration delay was found in the Apc1638N animals, and sulindac administration did not alter the enterocyte migration rate (Fig. 5). A comparison of enterocyte β-catenin expression for Min/+ and Apc1638N mice also indicated the absence of tumor-associated changes in the enterocytes of animals displaying the attenuated phenotype (Fig. 6). Whereas β-catenin expression was elevated in the enterocytes of Min/+ mice and reduced by sulindac administration, there was no difference between β-catenin levels in tissues from Apc1638N mice, wild-type littermates, or Apc1638N mice treated with sulindac. These observations suggest that a dominant negative effect producing altered cell migration may be exerted by the truncated APC protein present in the Min/+ mouse, perhaps explaining the difference in tumor phenotype.[45,55] These data also suggest that the effectiveness of chemopreventive agents in preventing Apc-related tumor formation may depend upon which type of mutation is present.

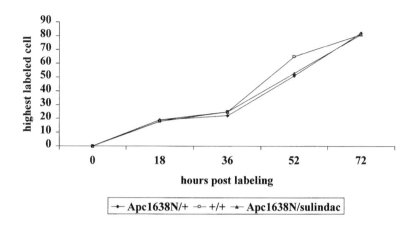

FIGURE 5. Enterocyte migration in *Apc*1638N mice. Ten mice from each experimental group (+/+, *Apc*1638N, and *Apc*1638N treated with sulindac, 0.016%) were injected with 0.3 µg/kg of BrdU (Sigma, St. Louis, MO). Small intestine from each group was examined at the indicated intervals postinjection by staining with anti-BrdU antibody. Eight intact histologically normal crypt-villus units from each animal were examined by an observer blinded to the animal's genetic status or treatment group. No significant difference in enterocyte migration rate was observed among wild-type (+/+), *Apc*1638N, or *Apc*1638N mice treated with sulindac. Analysis of variance (ANOVA) with time as a covariate was used to assess differences between group and time, $p > 0.05$.[55]

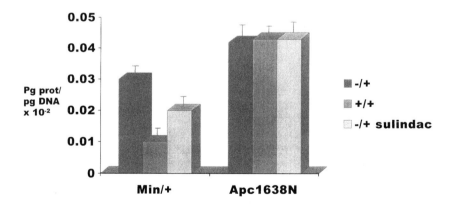

FIGURE 6. Differences in tissue β-catenin expression in Min/+ versus *Apc*1638N mice. Specimens of small intestine from animals at 65 days of age were formalin fixed, embedded in paraffin, and sectioned at 5 µm. Where indicated, animals were treated with sulindac (0.016%). Sections were stained with antibody to β-catenin. The percent staining of enterocytes in these crypt-villus units was measured by an observer blinded to the animal's genetic or treatment status using the CAS 200. Values represented are ± SEM.

SUMMARY: IMPLICATIONS FOR DESIGNING HUMAN CHEMOPREVENTION STRATEGIES

Studies of *Apc*-deficient mice support several observations related to human colorectal cancer, such as the importance of dietary fats, the acceleration of carcinogenesis by mismatch repair defects, and the role of bile acids in tumor promotion. The relationship between cyclooxygenase expression and tumor formation in these animals strongly supports the use of NSAIDs to prevent sporadic colorectal tumors in humans. If proven to have low toxicity in humans, phenolic antioxidants or related compounds may increase cancer prevention activity when used in combination with NSAIDs. Studies of the *Apc*-deficient mice also illustrate the importance of tumor genotype to the progression of intestinal cancer and may even suggest that the efficacy of chemopreventive agents depends upon the genotype. These models will undoubtedly continue to be useful tests of new potential chemopreventive agents, and particularly of combination chemoprevention regimens.

REFERENCES

1. NISHISHO, I., Y. NAKAMURA, Y. MIYOSHI, Y. MIKI, H. ANDO, A. HORII, K. KOYAMA, J. UTSUNOMIYA, S. BABA & P. HEDGE. 1991. Mutations of chromosome 5q21 genes in FAP and colorectal cancer patients. Science **253**: 665–669.
2. KINZLER, K.W., M.C. NILBERT, L.K. SU, B. VOGELSTEIN, T.M. BRYAN, D.B. LEVY, K.J. SMITH, A.C. PREISINGER, P. HEDGE, D. MCKETCHNIE *et al.* 1991. Identification of FAP locus genes from chromosome 5q21. Science **253**: 661–665.
3. GRODEN, J., A. THLIVERIS, W. SAMOWITZ, M. CARLSON, L. GELBERT, H. ALBERTSEN, G. JOSLYN, J. STEVENS, L. SPIRIO, M. ROBERTSON, L. SARGEANT, K. KRAPCHO, E. WOLFF, R. BURT, J.P. HUGHES, J. WARRINGTON, J. MCPHERSON, J. WASMUTH, D. LE PASLIER, H. ADBERRAHIM, D. COHEN, M. LEPPERT & R. WHITE. 1991. Identification and characterization of the familial adenomatous polyposis coli gene. Cell **66**: 589–600.
4. JOSLYN, G., M. CARLSON, A. THLIVERIS, H. ALBERTSEN, L. GELBERT, W. SAMOWITZ, J. GRODEN, J. STEVENS, L. SPIRIO, M. ROBERTSON, K. KRAPCHO, L. SARGENT, E. WOLFF, R. BURT, J.P. HUGHES, J. WARRINGTON, J. MCPHERSON, J. WASMUTH, D. LE PASLIER, H. ABDERRAHIM, D. COHEN, M. LEPPERT & R. WHITE. 1991. Identification of deletion mutations and three new genes at the familial polyposis locus. Cell **66**: 601–613.
5. RHODES, M. & D.M. BRADBURN. 1993. Overview of screening and management of familial adenomatous polyposis. Gut **33**:125–131.
6. ALM, T. & G. LICZNERSKI. 1973. The intestinal polyposis. Clin. Gastroenterol. **2**: 577–602.
7. JEN, J., S. POWELL, N. PAPADOPOULOS, K.J. SMITH, S.R. HAMILTON, B. VOGELSTEIN & K.W. KINZLER. 1994. Molecular determinants of dysplasia in colorectal lesions. Cancer Res. **54**: 5523–5526.
8. LEVY, D.B., K.J. SMITH, Y. BEAZER-BARCLAY, S.R. HAMILTON, B. VOGELSTEIN & K.W. KINZLER. 1994. Inactivation of both APC alleles in human and mouse tumors. Cancer Res. **54**: 5953–5958.
9. LOUNGO, C., A.R. MOSER, S. GLEDHILL & W.F. DOVE. 1994. Loss of Apc+ in intestinal adenomas from Min mice. Cancer Res. **54**: 5947–5952.
10. AMERICAN CANCER SOCIETY. 1997. Cancer Facts and Figures.
11. BEHRENS, J., B.-A. JERCHOW, M. WURTELE, J. GRIMM, C. ASBRAND, R. WIRTZ, M. KUHL, D. WEDLICH & W. BIRCHMEIER. 1998. Functional interaction of an axin homolog, conduction, with β-catenin, APC & GSK3β. Science **280**: 596–599.

12. RUBINFELD, B., I. ALBERT, E. PORFIRI, C. FIOL, S. MUNEMITSU & P. POLAKIS. 1996. Binding of GSK3β to the APC-β-catenin complex and regulation of complex assembly. Science **272:** 1023–1026.
13. RUBINFELD, B., B. SOUZA, I. ALBERT, O. MULLER, S. CHAMBERLAIN, F.R. MASIARZ, S. MUNEMITSU & P. POLAKIS. 1993. Association of the APC gene product with beta-catenin. Science **262:** 1731–1734.
14. SU, L.-K., B. VOGELSTEIN & K.W. KINZLER. 1993. Association of the APC tumor suppressor protein with catenins. Science **262:** 1734–1737.
15. MORIN, P.J., A.B. SPARKS, V. KORINEK, N. BARKER, H. CLEVERS, B. VOGELSTEIN & K.W. KINZLER. 1997. Activation of β-catenin-Tcf signaling in colon cancer by mutations in β-catenin or APC. Science **275:** 1787–1790.
16. ERISMAN, M.D., J.K. SCOTT & S.M. ASTRIN. 1989. Evidence that the familial adenomatous polyposis gene is involved in a subset of colon cancers with a complementable defect in *c-myc* regulation. Proc. Natl. Acad. Sci. USA **86:** 4264–4268.
17. HE, T.-C,, A.B. SPARKS, C. RAGO, H. HERMEKING, L. ZAWEL, L.T. DA COSTA, P.J. MORIN, B. VOGELSTEIN & K.W. KINZLER. 1998. Identification of c-MYC as a target of the APC pathway. Science **281:** 1509–1512.
18. JOSLYN, G., D.S. RICHARDSON, R. WHITE & T. ALBER. 1993. Dimer formation by an N-coiled coil in the APC protein. Proc. Natl. Acad. Sci. USA **90:** 11109–11113.
19. MUNEMITSU, A., I. ALBERT, B. SOUZA, B. RUBINFELD & P. POLAKIS. 1995. Regulation of intracellular β-catenin levels by the adenomatous polyposis coli (APC) tumor-suppressor protein. Proc. Natl. Acad. Sci. USA **92:** 3046–3050.
20. LYNCH, H.T., T. SMYRK, T. MCGINN, S. LANSPA, J. CAVALIERI, J. LYNCH, S. SLOMINSKI-CASTOR, M.C. CAYOUETTE, I. PRILUCK & M.C. LUCE. 1995. Attenuated familial adenomatous polyposis (AFAP). Cancer **76:** 2427–2433.
21. SPIRIO, L., S. OLSCHWANG, J. GRODEN, M. ROBERTSON, W. SAMOWITZ, G. JOSLYN, L. GELBERT, A. THLIVERIS, M. CARLSON, B. OTTERUD, H. LYNCH, P. WATSON, J.P. HUGHES, G. THOMAS, M. LEPPERT & R. WHITE. 1993. Alleles of the *APC* gene: An attenuated form of familial polyposis. Cell **75:** 951–957.
22. WU, J.S., P. PAUL, E,A. MCGANNON & J.M. CHURCH. 1998. *APC* genotype, polyp number, and surgical options in familial adenomatous polyposis. Ann. Surg, **227:** 57–62.
23. NAGASE, H., Y. MIYOSHI, A. HORII, T. AOKI, M. OGAWA, J. UTSUNOMIYA, S. BABA, T. SASAZUKI & Y. NAKAMURA. 1992. Correlation between the location of germ-line mutations in the *APC* gene and the number of colorectal polyps in familial adenomatous polyposis patients. Cancer Res. **52:** 4055–4057.
24. SMITH, K.J., K.A. JOHNSON, T.M. BRYAN, D.E. HILL, S. MARKOWITZ, J.V.K. WILLSON, C. PARASKEVA, G.M. PETERSEN, S.R. HAMILTON, B. VOGELSTEIN & K.W. KINZLER. 1993. The APC gene product in normal and tumor cells. Proc. Natl. Acad. Sci. USA **90:** 2846–2850.
25. MURAOKA, M., H. TAKAHASHI, Y. AMADA, M. FUKAYAMA, Y. MAEDA, T. IWAMA, Y. MISHIMA, T. MORI & M. KOIKE. 1994. Characteristics of somatic mutation of the adenomatous polyposis coli gene in colorectal tumors. Cancer Res. **54:** 3011–3020.
26. DOBBIE, Z., M. SPYCHER, J.L. MARY, M. HANER, I. GULDENSCHUH, R. HURLIMAN, R. AMMAN, J. ROTH, H. MULLER & R.J. SCOTT. 1996. Correlation between the development of extracolonic manifestations in FAP patients and mutations beyond codon 1403 in the APC gene. J. Med. Genet. **33:** 274–280.
27. SU, L.-K., K.W. KINZLER, B. VOGELSTEIN, A.C. PREISINGER, A.R. MOSER, C. LUONGO, K.A. GOULD, W.F. DOVE. 1992. Multiple intestinal neoplasia caused by a mutation in the murine homolog of the APC gene. Science **256:** 668–670.
28. MOSER, A.R., H.C. PITOT & W.F. DOVE. 1990. A dominant mutation that predisposes to multiple intestinal neoplasia in the mouse. Science **247:** 322–324.

29. OSHIMA, M., H. OSHIMA, K. KITAGAWA, M. KOBAYASHI, C. ITAKURA & M. TAKETO. 1995. Loss of Apc heterozygosity and abnormal tissue building in nascent intestinal polyps in mice carrying a truncated Apc gene. Proc. Natl. Acad. Sci. USA **92:** 4482–4486.

30. FODDE, R., W. EDELMANN, K. YANG, C. VAN LEEUWEN, C. CARLSON, B. RENAULT, C. BREUKEL, E. ALT, M. LIPKIN, P. MEERA KHAN & R. KUCHERLAPATI. 1994. A target chain termination mutation in the mouse *Apc* gene results in multiple intestinal tumors. Proc. Natl. Acad. Sci. USA **91:** 8969–8973.

31. WADDELL, W.R. & R.W. LOUGHRY. 1983. Sulindac for polyposis of the colon. J. Surg. Oncol. **24:** 83–87.

32. GIARDIELLO, F.M., S.R. HAMILTON, A.J. KRUSH *et al.* 1993. Treatment of colonic and rectal adenomas with sulindac in familial adenomatous polyposis. N. Engl. J. Med. **328:** 1313–1316.

33. LABAYLE, D., D. FISCHER, P. VIELH, F. DROUHIN, A. PARIENTE, C. BORIES, O. DUHAMEL, M. TROUSSET & P. ATTALI. 1991. Sulindac causes regression of rectal polyps in familial adenomatous polyposis. Gastroenterology **101:** 635–639.

34. DECOSSE, J.J., H.H. MILLER & M.L. LESSER. 1989. Effect of wheat fiber and vitamins C and E on rectal polyps in patients with familial adenomatous polyposis. J. Natl. Cancer Inst. **81:** 1290–1297.

35. MAHMOUD, N.N., A.J. DANNENBERG, R.T. BILINSKI, M.R. CHURCHILL, J. MESTRE, C. MARTUCCI, M.M. BERTAGNOLLI. 1999. Administration of an unconjugated bile acid increases duodenal tumors in a murine model of familial adenomatous polyposis. Carcinogenesis **20:** 299–303.

36. KENNEDY, A.R., Y. BEAZER-BARCLAY, K.W. KINZLER & P.M. NEWBERNE. 1996. Suppression of carcinogenesis in the intestines of Min mice by the soybean-derived Bowman-Birk inhibitor. Cancer Res. **56:** 679–682.

37. JACOBY, R.F., D.J. MARSHALL, M.A. NEWTON, K. NOVAKOVIC, K. TUTSCH, C.E. COLE, R.A. LUBET, G.J. KELLOFF, A. VERMA, A.R. MOSER & W.F. DOVE. 1996. Chemoprevention of spontaneous intestinal adenomas in the Apc^{Min} mouse model by the nonsteroidal anti-inflammatory drug piroxicam. Cancer Res. **56:** 710–714.

38. BOOLBOL, S.K., A.J. DANNENBERG, A. CHADBURN, C. MARTUCCI, X.-J. GUO, J.T. RAMONETTI, M. ABREU-GORIS, H.L NEWMARK, M.L. LIPKIN, J.J. DECOSSE & M.M. BERTAGNOLLI. 1996. Cyclooxygenase-2 overexpression and tumor formation are blocked by sulindac in a murine model of familial adenomatous polyposis. Cancer Res. **56**(11)**:** 2556–2560.

39. MAHMOUD, N.N., A.J. DANNENBERG, J. MESTRE, R.T. BILINSKI, M.R. CHURCHILL, C. MARTUCCI, H. NEWMARK, M.M. BERTAGNOLLI. 1998. Aspirin prevents tumors in a murine model of familial adenomatous polyposis. Surgery **124**(2)**:** 225–231.

40. BARNES, C.J. & M. LEE. 1998. Chemoprevention of spontaneous intestinal adenomas in the adenomatous polyposis coli Min mouse model with aspirin. Gastroenterology **114:** 873–877.

41. CHIU, C.-H., M.F. MCENTEE & J. WHELAN. 1997. Sulindac causes rapid regression of preexisting tumors in Min/+ mice independent of prostaglandin biosynthesis. Cancer Res. **57:** 4267–4273.

42. MAHMOUD, N.N., S.K. BOOLBOL, A.J. DANNENBERG, J.R. MESTRE, R.T. BILINSKI, H.L. NEWMARK, A. CHADBURN & M.M. BERTAGNOLLI. 1998. The sulfide metabolite of sulindac prevents tumors and restores enterocyte apoptosis in a murine model of familial adenomatous polyposis. Carcinogenesis **19:** 87–91.

43. ZHANG, F., N.K. ALTORKI, J.R. MESTRE, K. SUBBARAMAIAH & A.J. DANNENBERG. 1999. Curcumin inhibits cyclooxygenase-2 transcription in bile acid- and phorbol ester-treated human gastrointestinal epithelial cells. Carcinogenesis **20:** 445–451.

44. PASRICHA, P.J., A. BEDI, K. O'CONNOR, A. RASHID, A.J. AKHTAR, M.L. ZAHURAK, S. PIANTADOSI, S.R. HAMILTON & F.M. GIARDIELLO. 1995. The effects of sulindac on colorectal proliferation and apoptosis in familial adenomatous polyposis. Gastroenterology **109:** 994–998.

45. MAHMOUD, N.N, S.K. BOOLBOL, R.T. BILINSKI, C.M. MARTUCCI, A. CHADBURN. M.M. BERTAGNOLLI. 1997. *Apc* gene mutation is associated with a dominant negative effect upon intestinal cell migration. Cancer Res. **57**(22): 5045–5050.

46. VOGELSTEIN, B., E.R. FEARON, S. HAMILTON, S.E. KERN, A.C. PREISINGER, M. LEPPERT, Y. NAKAMURA, R. WHITE, A.M.M. SMITS & J.L. BOS. 1988. Genetic alterations during colorectal tumor development. N. Engl. J. Med. **319:** 525–532.

47. REITMAIR, A.H., J.C. CAI, M. BJERKNES, M. TEDSTON, H. CHENG, M.T. PIND, K. HAY, A. MITRI, B.V. BAPAT & S. GALLINGER. 1996. MSH2 deficiency contributes to accelerated APC-mediated intestinal tumorigenesis. Cancer Res. **56:** 2922–2926.

48. TAKAKU, K., M. OSHIMA, H. MIYOSHI, M. MATSUI, M.F. SELDIN & M.M. TAKETO. 1998. Intestinal tumorigenesis in compound mutant mice of both *Dpc4* (*Smad4*) and *Apc* genes. Cell **92:** 645–656.

49. DIETRICH, W.F., E.S. LANDER, J.S. SMITH, A.R. MOSER, K.A. GOULD, C. LUONGO, N. BORENSTEIN & W. DOVE. 1993. Genetic identification of *Mom-1*, a major modifier locus affection *Min*-induced intestinal neoplasia in the mouse. Cell 1993 **75:** 631–639.

50. MACPHEE, M., K.P. CHEPENIK, R.A. LIDDELL, K.K. NELSON, L.D. SIRACUSA & A.M. BUCHBERG. 1995. The secretory phospholipase A2 gene is a candidate for the *Mom1* locus, a major modifier of *Apc^{Min}*-induced intestinal neoplasia. Cell **81:** 957–966.

51. FAZELI, A., R.G. STEEN, S.L. DICKINSON, D. BAUTISTA, W.F. DIETRICH, R.T. BRONSON, R.S. BRESALIER, E.S. LANDER, J. COSTA & R.A. WEINBERG. 1997. Effects of *p53* mutations on apoptosis in mouse intestinal and human colonic adenomas. Proc. Natl. Acad. Sci. USA **94:** 10199–10204.

52. OSHIMA, M., J.E. DINCHUK, S.L. KARGMAN, H. OSHIMA, B. HANCOCK, E. KWONG, J.M. TRZASKOS, J.F. EVANS & M.M. TAKETO. 1996. Suppression of intestinal polyposis in Apc$^{\Delta716}$ knockout mice by inhibition of cyclooxygeanse 2 (COX-2). Cell **87:** 803–809.

53. CHULADA, P.C., C. DOYLE, B. GAUL, H. TIANO, J. MAHLER, C. LEE, S. MORHAM & R. LANGENBACH. 1998. Cyclooxygenase-1 and −2 deficiency decrease spontaneous intestinal adenomas in the *Min* mouse. Proc. Am. Assoc. Cancer Res. **39:** 1332.

54. WILSON, C.L., K.J. HEPPNER, P.A. LABOSKY, B.L.M. HOGAN & L.M. MATRISIAN. 1997. Intestinal tumorigenesis is suppressed in mice lacking the metalloproteinase matrilysin. Proc. Natl. Acad. Sci. USA **94:** 1402–1407.

55. MAHMOUD, N.N., R. KUCHERLAPATI, R.T. BILINSKI, M.R. CHURCHILL, A. CHADBURN & M.M. BERTAGNOLLI. 1999. Genotype-phenotype correlation in murine *Apc* mutation: Differences in enterocyte migration and response to sulindac. Cancer Res. **59:** 353–359.

Oncogenic Activating Mutations in the *neu/erbB-2* Oncogene Are Involved in the Induction of Mammary Tumors

RICHARD CHAN,[a,c] WILLIAM J. MULLER,[a,b,c,d] AND PETER M. SIEGEL[a,c]

[a]*Institute for Molecular Biology and Biotechnology,* [b]*Department of Pathology,*
[c]*Department of Biology, McMaster University, Hamilton, Ontario, Canada, L8S 4K1*

ABSTRACT: Amplification and overexpression of *erbB-2/neu* is an important determinant in the initiation and progression of human breast cancer. Indeed,
transgenic mice that overexpress the *neu* proto-oncogene heritably develop
mammary adenocarcinomas. Tumorigenesis in these transgenic strains is associated with activation of the intrinsic catalytic activity of Neu. In many of these
tumors, activation of Neu occurs as a result of somatic mutations located within
the transgene itself. Examination of the altered *neu* transcripts revealed the
presence of in-frame deletions that encode aberrant Neu receptors lacking 5 to
12 amino acids within the extracellular domain proximal to the transmembrane region of Neu. In addition to these deletion mutants we have also detected single point mutations within this juxtatransmembrane region. The
majority of the mutations analyzed affect the one of several conserved cysteine
residues present within this region. Introduction of these activating mutations
into the wild-type *neu* cDNA results in its oncogenic conversion. Taken together, these observations suggest that this cysteine-rich region plays an important
role in regulating the catalytic activity of Neu.

INTRODUCTION

The progression of a primary mammary epithelial cell to the malignant phenotype is thought to involve multiple genetic events, including activation of dominant-
acting oncogenes and the loss of specific tumor supressor genes. Activation of
certain tyrosine kinases have been implicated in the malignant progression of a significant proportion of human breast cancers. For example, amplification and overexpression of the *erbB-2/neu* oncogene has been implicated in the initiation and
progression of a large percentage of primary breast cancers.[1–4] The *neu* oncogene
encodes a receptor tyrosine kinase (RTK) belonging to the epidermal growth factor
receptor (EGFR) family. In addition to *neu*, the EGFR family comprises three other
closely related genes, including EGFR, *erbB-3*, and *erbB-4*.[5–7] Interestingly, mem-

[d]Address correspondence to W.J. Muller, Institute for Molecular Biology and Biotechnology,
McMaster University, 1280 Main Street West, Hamilton, Ontario, Canada, L8S 4K1. Voice:
905-525-9140, ext. 2730; fax: 905-521-2955.
e-mail: muller@mcmail.cis.mcmaster.ca

bers of the EGFR family can interact with each other. For example, Neu is a substrate for the activated EGFR, following stimulation of cells with EGF,[8–10] or activated ErbB-4, following stimulation with heregulin.[11,12] The observed tyrosine phosphorylation of Neu by EGFR is thought to be mediated by heterodimerization between Neu and EGFR family members, resulting in a high affinity receptor for these mitogenic ligands.[9,13] In addition to activation of ErbB-2/Neu by a variety of physiological ligands, overexpression or mutation of the receptor can result in its oncogenic activation.[14]

Direct evidence for the involvement of Neu in the induction of mammary tumors stems from observations made with transgenic mice expressing a constitutively activated version of Neu[15] in the mammary epithelium.[16,17] In several of these transgenic strains, high level expression of activated Neu resulted in the development of multifocal mammary adenocarcinomas that affected every female carrier.[16] Consistent with these observations, infection of the mammary epithelium of rats with a retroviral vector bearing the activated *neu* cDNA[15] also resulted in the rapid development of multifocal mammary tumors.[18] Taken together, these observations suggest that activated Neu can act as a potent oncogene in the mammary epithelium.

In human breast cancer, examination of primary breast cancer samples has thus far failed to reveal a comparable transmembrane mutation in ErbB-2.[19] These observations argue that elevated expression of the *erbB-2* proto-oncogene is the primary mechanism by which ErbB-2 induces malignant transformation. To directly test the oncogenic potential of wild-type Neu in the mammary epithelium, several independent strains of transgenic mice carrying an MMTV-driven *neu* proto-oncogene have been established.[20] In contrast to transgenic mice expressing the activated version of *neu*, mammary gland–specific expression resulted in the appearance of focal mammary tumors after a long latency period. Biochemical analyses of these mammary tumors revealed that tumorigenesis in these mice was correlated with increased Neu intrinsic tyrosine kinase activity and the appearance of several tyrosine phosphorylated proteins.[20]

Because activation of the catalytic activity of Neu can occur through the mutation of a single amino acid in the transmembrane domain,[15] we investigated whether this mutation could be detected during tumor progression in these transgenic strains. To this end, total RNA from both breast tumors and adjacent morphologically normal mammary epithelium was subjected to reverse transcription followed by the polymerase chain reaction (RT-PCR). The resulting PCR products were then hybridized to oligonucleotides corresponding to both the wild-type sequence and transmembrane point mutation in Neu. The results showed that although there was no evidence of the point mutation, many of the PCR products derived from the Neu-induced tumors possessed deletions.[21] Significantly, sequence analyses of the altered products revealed that these deletions were located in a confined region of the extracellular domain and that they encoded functional Neu proteins due to maintenance of the protein's reading frame. Furthermore, it was demonstrated that these in-frame deletions resulted in constitutive activation of the kinase activity of Neu. The observation that the identified activating mutations reside in a region of Neu not previously known to be involved in its oncogenic activation raises the intriguing possibility that comparable mutations within the ErbB-2 protein might be functionally involved in human breast cancer.

RESULTS AND DISCUSSION

Previous studies with tumors induced by the expression of *neu* revealed that 65% of the tumors analyzed displayed evidence of altered transcripts (35 samples analyzed[21]). In addition, these deletions were noted in mammary tumors arising in three independent transgenic strains expressing the MMTV/*neu* fusion gene.[21] Because the initial riboprobe used in these analyses spans both the extracellular and intracellular region, it was unclear whether these RNase protection analyses would detect single base pair mutations. To test this possibility, specific antigen riboprobes complimentary to the extracellular and transmembrane region were hybridized to RNA derived from tumors from the MMTV/neu mice and subjected to RNase protection analyses under stringent conditions. In addition to the previously described deletions, this stringent RNase protection analysis revealed additional tumor samples that had not previously demonstrated evidence of alterations (unpublished observations).

To precisely define the nature of these mutations, these altered RNA transcripts were subjected to RT-PCR and the PCR products inserted into plasmid vectors and subjected to DNA sequence analyses. For each matched pair of samples, several independent subclones were analyzed. The results of these alterations are summarized in FIGURE 1. Sequence analyses of these PCR products revealed that two types of single base pair mutations were detected. In one class of mutations, cysteine residues located at positions 635, 639, and 647 were converted to a variety of different amino acids (FIG. 1). A second class of mutations resulted in the conversion of a tryptophan residue located at position 619, a tyrosine residue at position 621 and a serine residue at 638 to cysteine residues. In both classes of mutations, the observed alterations resulted in either a net increase or net loss of a single cysteine residue. The observation that these point mutations affected the balance of cysteine residues like the previously described deletions suggested[21] that these alterations may be directly involved in the activation of the intrinsic catalytic domain of Neu. Indeed, previous observations have demonstrated that insertion of several of these deletions in an otherwise wild-type *neu* cDNA resulted in its oncogenic activation.[21] To confirm that the other deletion and insertion mutants behaved in a similar manner, three of the deletion mutants and the single insertion mutant were placed into a wild-type *neu* expression cassette and tested for their capacity to transform Rat-1 fibroblasts. Consistent with previous observations,[21] expression of these altered Neu receptors was capable of transforming Rat 1 fibroblasts whereas expression of the wild-type *neu* cDNA was not (unpublished observations).

Because the transforming activity of Neu is closely correlated with its activation of intrinsic tyrosine kinase activity,[23–25] we also measured the state of tyrosine phosphorylation of Neu in cell lines transformed by these altered cDNAs. The results showed that tyrosine-phosphorylated Neu was detected in cell lines expressing these altered *neu* cDNAs but was not detected in cell lines expressing elevated levels of wild-type Neu.[21] Thus the increase in the levels of tyrosine-phosphorylated Neu in these cell lines likely reflects the catalytic activation of these altered receptors. The above observations suggest that activation of the Neu tyrosine kinase is a pivotal step in the initiation of mammary tumorigenesis and occurs primarily through somatic mutations in this transgenic mouse model of human breast cancer. The observation

Mutant Neu Amino Acid Sequences

	628 631 635 639 647 TM
Neu(WT)	WYKPDEEGICQPCPINCTHSCVDLDERGCPAEQRASPVTF
3 BT-1	WKYPDEEGICQPCPINYTHSCVDLDERGCPAEQRASPVTF
3 BT-2	WKYPDEEGICQPCPINGTHSCVDLDERGCPAEQRASPVTF
6 BT-2 7 BT-1	CKYPDEEGICQPCPINCTHSCVDLDERGCPAEQRASPVTF
7 BT-4	WKYPDEEGICQPCPINCTHSCVDLDERGYPAEQRASPVTF
7 BT-6 11 BT-1	WKYPDEEGICQPCPINCTHSSVDLDERGCPAEQRASPVTF
11 BT-2	WKCPDEEGICQPCPINCTHSCVDLDERGCPAEQRASPVTF
11 BT-3	WKYPDEEGICQPCPINCTHCCVDLDERGCPAEQRASPVTF
16 Lg-7	WKYPDEEGICQPCPINCTHSYVDLDERGCPAEQRASPVTF

FIGURE 1. Activation of Neu can occur through single amino acid mutations in the juxtatransmembrane region. Amino acid sequence alignment of altered Neu receptors. In each case, the balance of cysteine residues is directly affected by either conversion of cysteine residue to another amino acid or conversion of unrelated amino acid to a cysteine residue.

that the identified mutations are located in a region of Neu previously not known to be involved in its oncogenic activation raises the intriguing possibility that comparable mutations might be detected in human breast cancers.

It is striking that the mutations we have detected reside in a relatively narrow region of Neu located outside the transmembrane domain (FIG. 1). In fact, this region in Neu appears to be conserved among the other members of the EGFR family, including EGFR, ErbB-3, and ErbB-4.[22] Specifically, the region of all four known family members contains five cysteine residues that are perfectly conserved.[22] Moreover, the amino acids located adjacent to these cysteine residues exhibit a high degree of similarity.[22] Interestingly, with the exception of the deletion detected in a single tumor, the alterations that have been sequenced thus far have removed or altered at least one of the conserved cysteine residues.[22] Furthermore, in the mutant Neu molecule possessing the three-amino acid insertion, one of the inserted amino acids is a cysteine residue. These data suggest that the balance of cysteine residues within this region of Neu may play an important role in activation of the receptor.

Although these observations suggest that these cysteine residues may be involved in the oncogenic activation of the Neu receptor, the precise molecular mechanism by which this occurs remains to be addressed. In this regard, it has been reported that transforming Neu mutants possessing the point mutation in the transmembrane domain demonstrate an increased propensity to homodimerize.[22,26–28] Indeed, immunoprecipitation analyses of this mutant Neu receptor under both reducing and nonreducing conditions revealed that the activated Neu species could be detected as a multimeric complex under nonreducing conditions, which was converted to a monomeric species under reducing conditions.[25] By contrast, the wild-type Neu receptor remained a monomer species under both reducing and nonreducing conditions. These observations suggest that receptor dimerization is occurring through the formation of disulfide bonds.

Given that many of the deletions and insertions mutants affect different cysteine residues, it is conceivable that, like the transmembrane point mutation, alteration of these cysteine residues in the mutants promotes receptor dimerization through the formation of cysteine disulfide bonds. Indeed we have recently demonstrated that these altered receptors dimerize in a manner dependent on the formation of disulfide bonds.[22] It is possible that these deletions and insertions of cysteine residues disrupt the normal cysteine pairing that occurs in the wild-type receptor. As a consequence this unpaired cysteine residue would be free to participate in disulfide bond formation with another altered receptor.

Consistent with this proposed model, it has recently been demonstrated that in inherited forms of endocrine neoplasia type 2A, a single mutation in a cysteine residue located in the cysteine rich juxtatransmembrane domain of the Ret RTK is responsible for its oncogenic activation. Similar to the Neu deletion mutants, the generation of this cysteine imbalance results in the constitutive dimerization of the Ret RTK in a manner dependent on the formation of disulfide bonds.[29,30] In addition to these studies, dimerization of the hematopoietic/cytokine receptor superfamily is thought to involve cysteine disulfide bonding. For example, replacement of specific amino acids with cysteine residues in the juxtatransmembrane domain of either the thrombopoietin receptor or the erythropoietin receptor results in the formation of disulfide-linked dimers that constitutively activate these receptors.[31–33] In addition, it has recently been demonstrated that disruption of disulfide bonding by the administration of reducing agents to the external media of cultured cells can interfere with signaling from the thrombopoietin receptor by preventing dimerization of the receptor.[30] Indeed, we have recently demonstrated that addition of 2-mercaptoethanol to the external media of cells can interfere with the transforming potential of these altered Neu receptors in a dose-dependent manner.[22] Taken together these observations suggest that this mode of receptor dimerization may be shared by other receptor systems.

The data generated thus far suggests that the occurrence of these deletions within Neu in this transgenic mouse model are likely directly involved in the induction of mammary tumors expressing the MMTV/wild-type *neu* fusion gene. To directly assess the significance of these activating mutations in Neu, we have recently established transgenic mice that express certain of these activated *neu* alleles under the transcriptional control of the MMTV promoter. Although we are still in the early stages of characterization of these lines, preliminary observations suggest that in contrast to the parental strains expressing the wild-type *neu* gene these mice develop multifocal mammary tumors with a relatively shorter latency period (Siegel and Muller, unpublished observations). However, unlike the transgenic mice expressing the transmembrane point mutation that exhibits rapid progression phenotype,[16] these mice possess preneoplastic lesions. One potential explanation for these observations is that in the latter strains the level of Neu-associated tyrosine kinase activity is below a certain threshold required for the rapid transformation of the mammary epithelial cell, whereas the rapid progression strains exceed this critical threshold. In addition to the elevated expression these activated *neu* alleles, we have frequently detected elevated expression of the *erbB-3* (Siegel and Muller, unpublished observations). Indeed, erbB-3 is tyrosine phosphorylated in these tumors (Siegel and Muller, unpublished observations). Given the fact that erbB-3 does not possess catalytic activity, it is likely that the observed tyrosine phosphorylation of ErbB-3 derives from transphosphorylation by these activated neu alleles. Future experiments with these various strains should allow this hypothesis to be rigorously tested.

The frequent occurrence of activating mutations in the juxtatransmembrane of Neu raises the possibility that comparable mutations in ErbB-2 might also be involved in the genesis of human breast cancer. We are currently examining human breast cancer biopsies for the occurrence of these mutations to test this hypothesis. Given that activating mutations in Ret RTK can result in the hereditary predisposition to development of endocrine neoplasias, it is conceivable that a comparable germ-line mutation in erbB-2 may, in part, be responsible the development of hereditary breast and ovarian cancers.

Finally, the observation that the region that is deleted in Neu appears to be highly conserved among the different EGFR family members raises the possibility that mutational activation of these other members may also be involved in the genesis of human breast cancer. Indeed, there is considerable evidence to suggest that these other EGFR family members are overexpressed in human breast cancer.[6,7] Although no direct evidence exists for mutational activation of these EGFR family members in human cancers, it has recently been demonstrated that the *Caenorhabditis elegans* EGFR homologue, LET-23, can be activated by mutation of a single cysteine residue in the extreme amino terminus of the protein.[34] Given the potential of the various EGFR family members to heterodimerize, it is conceivable that mutational activation of any one of the EGFR family can activate the other family members. Future studies should allow these issues to be addressed.

REFERENCES

1. KING, C.R., M.H. KRAUS & S.A. AARONSON. 1985. Science **229:** 974–976.
2. SLAMON, D.J., G.M. CLARK, S.G. WONG, W.J. LEVIN, A. ULLRICH & W.L. McGUIRE. 1987. Science **235:** 177–182.
3. SLAMON, D.J., W. GODOLPHIN, L.A. JONES, J.A. HOLT, S.G. WONG, D.E. KEITH, W.J. LEVIN, S.G. STYART, G. UDOVE, A. ULLRICH & M.F. PRESS. 1989. Science **244:** 707–712.
4. VAN DE VIJER, M., J. PEYERSE, W.J. MOOI, P. WISMAN, J. LOMANS, O. DALESIO & R. NUSSE. 1988. N. Engl. J. Med. **319:** 1239–1245.
5. ULLRICH, A., L. COUSSENS, J.S. HAYFLICK, T.J. DULL, A. GRAY, A.W. TAM, J. LEE, Y. YARDEN, T.A. LIBERMANN, J. SCHLESSINGER, J. DOWNWARD, E.L.V. MAYES, N. WHITTLE, M.D. WATERFIELD & P.H. SEEBURG. 1984. Nature **309:** 418–425.
6. KRAUS, M.H., I. ISSING, T. MIKI, N.C. POPESCU & S.A. AARONSON. 1989. Proc. Natl. Acad. Sci. USA **86:** 9193–9197.
7. PLOWMAN, G., G. WHITNEY, M. NEUBAUER, J. GREEN, V. McDONALD, G. TODARO & M. SHOYAB. 1990. Proc. Natl. Acad. Sci. USA **87:** 4905–4909.
8. STERN, D.F. & M.P. KAMPS. 1988. EMBO J. **7:** 995–1001.

9. WADA, T., X. QIAN & M.I. GREENE. 1990. Cell **61:** 1339–1347.
10. QIAN, X., S.J. DECKER & M.I. GREENE. 1992. Proc. Natl. Acad. Sci. USA **89:** 1330–1334.
11. RIESE II, D.J., T.M. VAN RAAJI, G.D. PLOWMAN, G.C. ANDREWS & D.F. STERN. 1995. Mol. Cell. Biol. **15:** 5770–5776.
12. BEERLI, R.R., D. GRAUS-PORTA, K. WOODS-COOK, X. CHEN, Y. YARDEN & N.E. HYNES. 1995. Mol. Cell. Biol. **15:** 6496–6505.
13. GOLDMAN, R., R. BEN LEVY, E. PELES & Y. YARDEN. 1990. Biochemistry **29:** 11024–11028.
14. HYNES, N.E. & D.F. STERN. 1994. Biochim. Biophys. Acta **1198:** 165–184.
15. BARGMANN, C.I., M-C. HUNG & R.A. WEINBERG. 1986. Cell **45:** 649–657.
16. MULLER, W.J., E. SINN, R. WALLACE, P.K. PATTENGALE & P. LEDER. 1988. Cell **54:** 105–115.
17. BOUCHARD, L., L. LAMARRE, P.J. TREMBLAY, P. JOLICOEUR. 1989. Cell **57:** 931–936.
18. WANG, B., W.J. KENNAN, J. YASUKAWA-BARNES, M.J. LINDSTROM & M.N. GOULD. 1991. Cancer Res. **51:** 5649–5654.
19. LEMOINE, N.R., S. STADDON, C. DICKSON, D.M. BARNES & W.J. GULLICK. 1990. Oncogene **5:** 237–239.
20. GUY, C.T., M.A. WEBSTER, M. SCHALLER, T.J. PARSONS, R.D. CARDIFF & W.J. MULLER. 1992. Proc. Natl. Acad. Sci. USA **89:** 10578–10582.
21. SIEGEL, P.M., D.L. DANKORT, W.R. HARDY & W.J. MULLER. 1994. Mol. Cell. Biol. **14:** 7068–7077.
22. SIEGEL. P.M. & W.J. MULLER. 1996. Proc. Natl. Acad. Sci. USA **93:** 8878–8883.
23. BARGMANN, C.I. & R.A. WEINBERG. 1988. Proc. Natl. Acad. Sci. USA **85:** 5394–5398.
24. STERN, D.F., M.P. KAMPS & H. CAO. 1988. Mol. Cell. Biol. **8:** 3969–3973.
25. WEINER, D.B., Y. KOKAI, T. WADA, J.A. COHEN, W.V. WILLIAMS & M.I. GREENE. 1989. Oncogene **4:** 1175–1183.
26. WEINER, D.B., J. LIU, J.A. COHEN, W.V. WILLIAMS & M.I. GREENE. 1989. Nature **339:** 230–231.
27. BRANDT-RAUF, P.W., S. RACKOVSKY & M.R. PINCUS. 1990. Proc. Natl. Acad. Sci. USA **87:** 8660–8664.
28. CAO, H., L. BANGALORE, B.J. BORMANN & D.F. STERN. 1992. EMBO J. **11:** 923–932.
29. SANTORO, M., F. CARLOMAGNO, A. ROMANO, D.P. BOTTARO, N.A. DATHAN, M. GRIECO, A. FUSCO, G. VECCHIO, B. MATOSKOVA, M.H. KRAUS & P.P. DIFIORE. 1995. Science **267:** 381–383.
30. ASAI, N., T. IWASHITA, M. MATSUYAMA & M. TAKAHASHI. 1995. Mol. Cell. Biol. **15:** 1613–1619.
31. ALEXANDER, W.S., D. METCALF & A.R. DUNN. 1995. EMBO J. **14:** 5569–5578.
32. WATOWICH, S.S., A. YOSHIMURA, G.D. LONGMORE, D.J. HILTON, Y. YOSHIMURA & H.F. LODISH. 1992. Proc. Natl. Acad. Sci. USA **89:** 2140–2144.
33. WATOWICH, S.S., D.J. HILTON & H.F. LODISH. 1994. Mol. Cell. Biol. **14:** 3535–3549.
34. KATZ, W.S., G.M. LESA, D. YANNOUKAKOS, T.R. CLANDININ, J. SCHLESSINGER & P.W. STERNBERG. 1996. Mol. Cell. Biol. **16:** 529–537.

Cyclooxygenase-deficient Mice

A Summary of Their Characteristics and Susceptibilities to Inflammation and Carcinogenesis

ROBERT LANGENBACH,[a] CHARLES D. LOFTIN, CHRISTOPHER LEE, AND HOWARD TIANO

National Institute of Environmental Health Sciences,
Research Triangle Park, North Carolina 27709, USA

ABSTRACT: Cyclooxygenase (COX)-1- and COX-2-deficient mice have unique physiological differences that have allowed investigation into the individual biological roles of the COX isoforms. In the following, the phenotypes of the two COX knockout mice are summarized, and recent studies to investigate the effects of COX deficiency on inflammatory responses and cancer susceptibility are discussed. The data suggest that both isoforms have important roles in the maintenance of physiological homeostasis and that such designations as housekeeping and/or response gene may not be entirely accurate. Furthermore, data from COX-deficient mice indicate that both isoforms can contribute to the inflammatory response and that both isoforms have significant roles in carcinogenesis.

INTRODUCTION

Two isoforms of cyclooxygenase, COX-1[1,2] and COX-2,[3–6] are known. Both enzymes catalyze the first committed step in the synthesis of prostaglandins (PGs), the conversion of arachidonic acid (AA) to PGH_2.[7] The PGH_2 produced by both isoforms can then be further metabolized to the biologically active prostaglandins, PGE_2, PGI_2, $PGF_{2\alpha}$, PGD_2, and thromboxane A_2. Since the discovery of COX-2, elucidating the physiological functions of each COX isoform has been an area of intense study.

COX-1 is considered the "housekeeping" isoform,[7] because it is constitutively expressed in at least some cells of most tissues. By contrast, COX-2 is normally not detectable in most tissues; but it can be induced by various endogenous and exogenous agents and has therefore been referred to as the "inducible" isoform.[7] However, COX-2 is now known to be constitutively expressed in some cells of several tissues.[8–10] Recent studies have indicated that the two isoforms may have different cellular localizations[11] and that the cytosolic localization of COX-1 may give rise to PGs with autocrine or paracrine activity, whereas the perinuclear localization of COX-2 may lead to PGs with intracrine activity.[7] Indeed, both cell-surface mem-

[a]Address for communication: National Institute of Environmental Health Sciences, 101 Alexander Drive, P.O. Box 12233, Research Triangle Park, NC 27709. Voice: 919-541-7558; fax: 919-541-1460.

e-mail: langenbach@niehs.nih.gov

brane and nuclear receptors for PGs have been identified.[12–14] Furthermore, it has been demonstrated in certain cell types that COX-1 and COX-2 use AA generated by different phospholipases,[15] which further supports the possibility that the isoforms are involved in different signaling pathways.

Vane[16] first reported that COX was the pharmacological target of NSAIDs (nonsteroidal anti-inflammatory drugs), and much of our current knowledge about the physiological roles of the COXs and PGs has been obtained from studies with NSAIDs. With the recent characterization of COX-2, NSAIDs with varying degrees of isoform specificity have been developed.[17–24] In addition to their potential therapeutic benefit, isoform selective inhibitors are also being used to elucidate the physiological functions of the COX isoforms. However, several studies have indicated that NSAIDs have pharmacological mechanisms in addition to, or other than, the inhibition of COX activity,[25–32] and therefore effects observed with NSAIDs may not always reflect the physiological roles of the COX isoforms.

We have used a genetic approach to develop mouse models to study the roles of the COX isoforms in normal and diseased states. Gene-targeting techniques were used to inactivate the COX genes and to produce mice genetically deficient in COX-1 or COX-2.[33,34] Dinchuk *et al.*[35] have also described the development of a COX-2-deficient mouse. One of our original goals for making the COX null mice was to investigate the individual roles of COX-1 and COX-2 in carcinogenesis. Two types of cancers, colon cancer and skin cancer, had been chosen for study. The rationales for the COXs having roles in colon cancer are based on both rodent and human epidemiologic data.[36] Reddy and colleagues[37] had conducted many studies indicating that NSAIDs reduced carcinogen-induced intestinal cancer in rodents. Furthermore, epidemiological studies indicated that aspirin reduced colon cancer mortality in humans.[38–40] Further support for a role of COX-2 in intestinal neoplasia has been presented by Oshima *et al.*[41] who observed that COX-2 deficiency reduced intestinal polyp formation by 86% in Apc knockout mice. A role for the COXs in skin carcinogenesis was also based on observations that NSAIDs could inhibit tumor formation[42–44] and that supplementation with specific PGs restored papilloma formation.[43–44] Furthermore, recent studies have indicated that COX-2, and not COX-1, was upregulated in human and rodent intestinal tumors[45–49] and in rodent skin papillomas.[44]

In the following, the general characteristics of both COX-deficient mice are described, and recent studies using the COX-1- and COX-2-knockout mice in inflammation and carcinogenesis studies are discussed.

GENERAL CHARACTERISTICS OF COX-1- AND COX-2-DEFICIENT MICE

The DNA manipulations used to disrupt the genes coding for COX-1 and COX-2 have been reported.[33–35] Both COX-1- and COX-2-deficient mice lacked the respective normal size message and protein. Mice heterozygous for COX-1 or COX-2 expressed the respective messages and proteins at about 50% of the levels observed in wild-type mice. In the tissues examined, COX-1 null mice did not compensate by upregulating the expression of COX-2, nor did COX-2-null mice appear to upregulate the expression of COX-1. Furthermore, in many biological responses to exogenous stimuli, both COX knockout mice showed gene dosage effects with heterozygous knockouts, being intermediate between null and wild-type mice. The health of mice heterozygous for COX-1 or COX-2 appeared to be normal.

COX-1-null mice were born in the expected ratios and lived normal life spans, even though their PG levels, in most tissues, were reduced by 99 percent. Indeed, the health of COX-1-deficient mice was surprising given the "housekeeping" functions attributed to COX-1. As expected, an impairment of platelet aggregation was observed in the COX-1-null mice.[33] Additionally, whereas COX-1-null female mice produced litters of normal size, they had difficulty with parturition, and most pups were born dead or died shortly after birth.[33] Other aspects of the female reproductive process in COX-1-null mice appeared normal.[50] Gross et al.[51] also observed that the onset of parturition was delayed in COX-1-null mice and that the administration of $PGF_{2\alpha}$ facilitated parturition. The upregulation of COX-1 in the uterus in wild-type females suggests this isoform to be the source of the $PGF_{2\alpha}$. Male COX-1-deficient mice exhibited normal fertility.

The lack of gastric and kidney pathologies in COX-1-null mice was especially noteworthy, as the PGs produced by COX-1 were believed to have key roles in the physiology of these tissues.[16,19,52–55] The current hypothesis about the medicinal usage of NSAIDs is that inhibition of COX-2 is responsible for their beneficial effects, whereas the inhibition of COX-1 is responsible for their adverse effects, the most common of which is gastric ulceration. Therefore it was surprising that COX-1-deficient mice did not spontaneously develop gastric ulcers.[33] Measurement of gastric PG levels in the COX-1-null mice indicated a greater than 99% reduction, and this reduction in gastric PGs was similar to that caused by an ulcerative dose of indomethacin. Compensation by upregulation of COX-2 was considered; however, gastric COX-2 message levels did not differ from wild-type mice.[33] Therefore, if compensation was occurring, it did not appear to involve PGs. Thus, the data from the COX-1-deficient mice indicated that elimination of COX-1-derived PGs alone was not sufficient to cause gastric ulcers.

In contrast to COX-1-deficient mice, mice lacking COX-2 expression manifested various pathologies. COX-2-null pups were born at the expected ratio; but only about 60% of the pups survived to weaning, and of those only about 75% survived to one year of age. The causes of death prior to three weeks of age are unknown. The deaths of mice after three weeks of age were attributed to peritonitis or kidney malfunction.[34]

Although the deficiency of COX-1 appeared to affect only parturition, COX-2-null female mice were essentially infertile.[35,50,56] Lim et al.[50] observed that few eggs were recovered from COX-2-null female mice, even after superovulation, and only about 2% were fertilized compared to wild-type females. Davis et al.[56] demonstrated that ovarian PGE_2 was upregulated by pituitary gonadotropins in wild-type and COX-1-, but not COX-2-deficient mice, indicating that COX-2 accounted for increased ovarian PG production following the luteinizing hormone surge. Furthermore, cumulus activation, stigmata formation, and ovulation were also abnormal in COX-2-null mice, but these processes could be restored by PGE_2 administration. COX-2-null male mice showed normal fertility.

Renal abnormalities were present in all adult COX-2-null mice,[34,35] and the renal pathology became more severe with age, resulting in end-stage renal disease. As the kidneys of 3-day-old wild-type and COX-2 nulls were indistinguishable, the renal pathology was ascribed to postnatal developmental causes. The kidney pathology observed in adult COX-2-null mice did not resemble the toxicity induced by NSAIDs in adult mice or humans.[53,57] However, to compare kidney pathologies between COX-2-deficient mice and NSAID-treated mice, neonatal mice treated with NSAIDs should be studied.

EFFECTS OF COX DEFICIENCY ON THE INFLAMMATORY RESPONSE

Inflammation is a complex biological response modulated by various chemical mediators with which prostaglandins have a synergistic role.[58,59] To better understand the relative contributions of the COX isoforms in the inflammatory process, we compared the inflammatory responses of wild-type and COX-1- and COX-2-null mice.

In our initial studies, AA and the potent tumor promoter, TPA (12-*O*-tetradecanoylphorbol-13-acetate), were used to induce edema in the mouse ear as the measure of inflammation.[33,34] In COX-1-, but not COX-2-deficient mice, edema induced by AA was reduced about 70% compared to wild-type mice.[33] Heterozygous COX-1 mice showed a response to AA intermediate between null and wild-type mice. The data do suggest that the initial inflammatory response could be due to COX-1, and implicates COX-1 in the inflammatory process.

TPA was equally inflammatory in the mouse ear edema assay in both COX-1- and COX-2-null mice.[33,34] This observation was unexpected, as COX-2 was induced by TPA and was thought to mediate, at least partially, the inflammatory response to TPA. Because COX-2-null mice still express COX-1, it is possible that COX-1 is contributing sufficient levels of PGs for the inflammatory process to occur. However, the induction of non-PG inflammatory mediators by TPA is probably also occurring. The results with AA and TPA indicate that COX-1, as well as COX-2, can contribute PGs during an inflammatory response. The extent to which each isoform contributes PGs may depend on the inflammatory stimuli, the time after insult, and the relative levels of each isoform in the target tissue.

We have continued to study inflammatory responses in the COX-null mice using the air pouch model.[60] By six hours after carrageenan treatment, PGE_2 production was significantly elevated in the pouch exudate of all genotypes compared to solvent-treated controls. In COX-2-null mice the increase in PGs was only about 25% of wild-type mice, whereas PG levels in COX-1-null mice were about 75% of wild type. The COX-2 inhibitor, NS-398, reduced PG production in wild-type mice to levels comparable to those seen in COX-2-null mice. Thus, both COX-2 deficiency and NSAID inhibition indicated that COX-2 is the major pathway for PG production during the early stages of inflammation in this model. However, the data indicated that COX-1 contributed about 25% of the PGs produced during this early stage. By day 3 following carrageenan treatment, PG levels had declined in all genotypes, but the number of neutrophils and macrophages in the exudates of all genotypes were elevated. However, compared to wild-type mice, macrophage infiltration into the pouch was reduced by about 50% in COX-2-null mice and was slightly reduced in COX-1-null mice. By day 7, higher levels of apoptotic neutrophils were present in the pouch fluid of COX-2-null mice, and little resolution of inflammation was apparent compared to wild-type or COX-1-null mice. These findings with the air pouch model indicate that both COX-1 and COX-2 contribute to PG production during inflammation and also that COX-2-derived PGs appear to have roles in the resolution or healing phase as well as in the early stages of the inflammatory process.

EFFECTS OF COX-1 AND COX-2 DEFICIENCY ON CARCINOGENESIS

To study the effects of COX deficiency on intestinal tumorigenesis, we have used the Min (multiple intestinal neoplasia) mouse model.[61,62] The Min mouse has a chemically induced mutation in the Apc gene, which leads to a 100% incidence of intestinal neoplasia. Using a breeding strategy, we produced COX-1- or COX-2-deficient Min mice. Our results showed that both COX deficiencies caused about an 80% decrease in the number of intestinal polyps.[63] Our findings with the COX-2-null Min mice are similar to those of Oshima et al. with COX-2 null/Apc knockout mice; however, this group had not investigated the effects of COX-1 deficiency.[41] For intestinal tumorigenesis, the observation that deficiency of COX-1, as well as COX-2,[63] decreases intestinal tumorigenesis may not be surprising, as aspirin is a more effective COX-1, than COX-2 inhibitor,[23] and aspirin has been shown to reduce intestinal tumors in rodents and in humans.[38,39,64]

Further evidence that the absence of either COX-1 or COX-2 can reduce tumorigenesis comes from studies using a mouse skin initiation/promotion model. In the mouse skin model, we observed that the number of papillomas was reduced by about 75% in mice lacking expression of either COX-1 or COX-2.[65] Additional support for roles of both COX-1 and COX-2 in skin tumorigenesis come from studies with resveratrol, a purported COX-1 inhibitor, and SC-58125, a COX-2-selective inhibitor, both of which reduced skin papilloma formation.[66,67]

The data obtained with the COX-knockout mice indicate that absence of either COX-1 or COX-2 decreases tumorigenesis in carcinogen-treated or genetically predisposed mice. The mechanisms by which COX-1 or COX-2 deficiency decrease tumorigenesis are unknown. PGs are known to have effects on a number of biological processes involved in carcinogenesis, including angiogenesis, cell proliferation, differentiation, and apoptosis.[7,36,68–70] Additionally, the COXs are known to metabolically activate certain classes of chemical carcinogens and/or to produce oxygen and peroxy radicals,[36] and both of these events would be reduced in COX-deficient mice. Alternatively, it is possible that the individual COX isoforms may lead to different profiles of PGs and/or channel the PGs to different signaling pathways.

CONCLUSIONS

The COX knockout mice have provided useful models for investigating the roles of the COX isoforms in normal physiology and various pathological states. However, the knockout of these genes leads to the decrease (heterozygous) or absence (homozygous null) of COX expression. As several diseases (cancer, inflammation) involve increased expression of COX activity, the development of mice that overexpress the COXs may lead to mice that are highly susceptible to these diseases. Furthermore, mice that overexpress COX-1 or COX-2, in combination with the COX-deficient mice, may facilitate identification of the mechanisms by which the COXs contribute to these diseases.

REFERENCES

1. DEWITT, D.L. & W.L. SMITH. 1988. Primary structure of prostaglandin G/H synthase from sheep vesicular gland determined from the complementary DNA sequence. Proc. Natl. Acad. Sci. USA **85:** 1412–1416.
2. MERLIE, J.P., D. FAGAN, J. MUDD & P. NEEDLEMAN. 1988. Isolation and characterization of the complementary DNA for sheep seminal vesicle prostaglandin endoperoxide synthase (cyclooxygenase). J. Biol. Chem. **263:** 3550–3553.
3. O'BANION, M.K., H.B. SADOWSKI, V. WINN & D.A. YOUNG. 1991. A serum- and glucocorticoid-regulated 4-kilobase mRNA encodes a cyclooxygenase-related protein. J. Biol. Chem. **266:** 23261–23267.
4. KUJUBU, D.A., B.S. FLETCHER, B.C. VARNUM, R.W. LIM & H.R. HERSCHMAN. 1991. TIS10, a phorbol ester tumor promoter-inducible mRNA from Swiss 3T3 cells, encodes a novel prostaglandin synthase/cyclooxygenase homologue. J. Biol. Chem. **266:** 12866–12872.
5. XIE, W.L., J.G. CHIPMAN, D.L. ROBERTSON, R.L. ERIKSON & D.L. SIMMONS. 1991. Expression of a mitogen-responsive gene encoding prostaglandin synthase is regulated by mRNA splicing. Proc. Natl. Acad. Sci. USA **88:** 2692–2696.
6. SIROIS, J., D.L. SIMMONS & J.S. RICHARDS. 1992. Hormonal regulation of messenger ribonucleic acid encoding a novel isoform of prostaglandin endoperoxide H synthase in rat preovulatory follicles. Induction *in vivo* and *in vitro*. J. Biol. Chem. **267:** 11586–11592.
7. SMITH, W.L. & D.L. DEWITT. 1996. Prostaglandin endoperoxide H synthases-1 and -2. Adv. Immunol. **62:** 167–215.
8. YAMAGATA, K., K.I. ANDREASSON, W.E. KAUFMANN, C.A. BARNES & P.F. WORLEY. 1993. Expression of a mitogen-inducible cyclooxygenase in brain neurons—Regulation by synaptic activity and glucocorticoids. Neuron **11:** 371–386.
9. WALENGA, R.W., M. KESTER, E. CORONEOS, S. BUTCHER, R. DWIVEDI & C. STATT. 1996. Constitutive expression of prostaglandin endoperoxide G/H synthetase (PGHS)-2 but not PGHS-1 in human tracheal epithelial cells *in vitro*. Prostaglandins **52:** 341–359.
10. HARRIS, R.C., J.A. MCKANNA, Y. AKAI, H.R. JACOBSON, R.N. DUBOIS & M.D. BREYER. 1994. Cyclooxygenase-2 is associated with the macula densa of rat kidney and increases with salt restriction. J. Clin. Invest. **94:** 2504–2510.
11. MORITA, I., M. SCHINDLER, M.K. REGIER, J.C. OTTO, T. HORI, D.L. DEWITT & W.L. SMITH. 1995. Different intracellular locations for prostaglandin endoperoxide H synthase-1 and -2. J. Biol. Chem. **270:** 10902–10908.
12. NEGISHI, M., Y. SUGIMOTO & A. ICHIKAWA. 1995. Molecular mechanisms of diverse actions of prostanoid receptors. Bba-Lipid. Lipid Metab. **1259:** 109–119.
13. BRUN, R.P., P. TONTONOZ, B.M. FORMAN, R. ELLIS, J. CHEN, R.M. EVANS & B.M. SPIEGELMAN. 1996. Differential activation of adipogenesis by multiple PPAR isoforms. Genes Dev. **10:** 974–984.
14. KLIEWER, S.A., S.S. SUNDSETH, S.A. JONES, P.J. BROWN, G.B. WISELY, C.S. KOBLE, P. DEVCHAND, W. WAHLI, T.M. WILLSON, J.M. LENHARD & J.M. LEHMANN. 1997. Fatty acids and eicosanoids regulate gene expression through direct interactions with peroxisome proliferator-activated receptors alpha and gamma. Proc. Natl. Acad. Sci. USA **94:** 4318–4323.

15. REDDY, S.T. & H.R. HERSCHMAN. 1997. Prostaglandin synthase-1 and prostaglandin synthase-2 are coupled to distinct phospholipases for the generation of prostaglandin D-2 in activated mast cells. J. Biol. Chem. **272:** 3231–3237.
16. VANE, J.R. 1971. Inhibition of prostaglandin synthesis as a mechanism of action for aspirin-like drugs. Nature New Biol. **231:** 232–235.
17. XIE, W., D.L. ROBERTSON & D.L. SIMMONS. 1992. Mitogen-inducible prostaglandin G/H synthase: A new target for nonsteroidal antiinflammatory drugs. Drug. Dev. Res. **25:** 249–265.
18. MEADE, E.A., W.L. SMITH & D.L. DEWITT. 1993. Differential inhibition of prostaglandin endoperoxide synthase (cyclooxygenase) isozymes by aspirin and other non-steroidal anti-inflammatory drugs. J. Biol. Chem. **268:** 6610–6614.
19. VANE, J. 1994. Pharmacology—Towards a better aspirin. Nature **367:** 215–216.
20. MITCHELL, J.A., M.G. BELVISI, P. AKARASEREENONT, R.A. ROBBINS, O.J. KWON, J. CROXTALL, P.J. BARNES & J.R. VANE. 1994. Induction of cyclo-oxygenase-2 by cytokines in human pulmonary epithelial cells: Regulation by dexamethasone. Br. J. Pharmacol. **113:** 1008–1014.
21. MASFERRER, J.L., P.C. ISAKSON & K. SEIBERT. 1996. Cyclooxygenase-2 inhibitors: A new class of anti-inflammatory agents that spare the gastrointestinal tract. Gastroenterol. Clin. North Am. **25:** 363–372.
22. KALGUTKAR, A.S., B.C. CREWS, S.W. ROWLINSON, C. GARNER, K. SEIBERT & L.J. MARNETT. 1998. Aspirin-like molecules that covalently inactivate cyclooxygenase-2. Science **280:** 1268–1270.
23. VANE, J.R. & R.M. BOTTING. 1998. Mechanism of action of nonsteroidal anti-inflammatory drugs. Am. J. Med. **104:** 2S–8S.
24. SMITH, C.J., Y. ZHANG, C.M. KOBOLDT, J. MUHAMMAD, B.S. ZWEIFEL, A. SHAFFER, J.J. TALLEY, J.L. MASFERRER, K. SEIBERT & P.C. ISAKSON. 1998. Pharmacological analysis of cyclooxygenase-1 in inflammation. Proc. Natl. Acad. Sci. USA **95:** 13313–13318.
25. ABRAMSON, S.B. & G. WEISSMANN. 1989. The mechanisms of action of nonsteroidal antiinflammatory drugs. Arthritis Rheum. **32:** 1–9.
26. ALBERTS, D.S., L. HIXSON, D. AHNEN, C. BOGERT, J. EINSPAHR, N. PARANKA, K. BRENDEL, P.H. GROSS, R. PAMUKCU & R.W. BURT. 1995. Do NSAIDs exert their colon cancer chemoprevention activities through the inhibition of mucosal prostaglandin synthetase? J. Cell. Biochem. Suppl. **22:** 18–23.
27. HANIF, R., A. PITTAS, Y. FENG, M.I. KOUTSOS, L. QIAO, L. STAIANO COICO, S.I. SHIFF & B. RIGAS. 1996. Effects of nonsteroidal anti-inflammatory drugs on proliferation and on induction of apoptosis in colon cancer cells by a prostaglandin-independent pathway. Biochem. Pharmacol. **52:** 237–245.
28. PIAZZA, G.A., D.S. ALBERTS, L.J. HIXSON, N.S. PARANKA, H. LI, T. FINN, C. BOGERT, J.M. GUILLEN, K. BRENDEL, P.H. GROSS, G. SPERL, J. RITCHIE, R.W. BURT, L. ELLSWORTH, D.J. AHNEN & R. PAMUKCU. 1997. Sulindac sulfone inhibits azoxymethane-induced colon carcinogenesis in rats without reducing prostaglandin levels. Cancer Res. **57:** 2909–2915.
29. PIAZZA, G.A., A.K. RAHM, T.S. FINN, B.H. FRYER, H. LI, A.L. STOUMEN, R. PAMUKCU & D.J. AHNEN. 1997. Apoptosis primarily accounts for the growth-inhibitory properties of sulindac metabolites and involves a mechanism that is independent of cyclooxygenase inhibition, cell cycle arrest, and p53 induction. Cancer Res. **57:** 2452–2459.
30. WECHTER, W.J., D. KANTOCI, E.D. MURRAY, JR., D.D. QUIGGLE, D.D. LEIPOLD, K.M. GIBSON & J.D. MCCRACKEN. 1997. R-flurbiprofen chemoprevention and treatment of intestinal adenomas in the APC(Min)/+ mouse model: Implications for prophylaxis and treatment of colon cancer. Cancer Res. **57:** 4316–4324.

31. LEHMANN, J.M., J.M. LENHARD, B.B. OLIVER, G.M. RINGOLD & S.A. KLIEWER. 1997. Peroxisome proliferator-activated receptors alpha and gamma are activated by indomethacin and other non-steroidal anti-inflammatory drugs. J. Biol. Chem. **272:** 3406–3410.

32. ELDER, D.J.E., D.E. HALTON, A. HAGUE & C. PARASKEVA. 1997. Induction of apoptotic cell death in human colorectal carcinoma cell lines by a cyclooxygenase-2 (COX-2)-selective nonsteroidal anti-inflammatory drug: Independence from COX-2 protein expression. Clin. Cancer Res. **3:** 1679–1683.

33. LANGENBACH, R., S.G. MORHAM, H.F. TIANO, C.D. LOFTIN, B.I. GHANAYEM, P.C. CHULADA, J.F. MAHLER, C.A. LEE, E.H. GOULDING, K.D. KLUCKMAN, H.S. KIM & O. SMITHIES. 1995. Prostaglandin synthase 1 gene disruption in mice reduces arachidonic acid-induced inflammation and indomethacin-induced gastric ulceration. Cell **83:** 483–492.

34. MORHAM, S.G., R. LANGENBACH, C.D. LOFTIN, H.F. TIANO, N. VOULOUMANOS, J.C. JENNETTE, J.F. MAHLER, K.D. KLUCKMAN, A. LEDFORD, C.A. LEE & O. SMITHIES. 1995. Prostaglandin synthase 2 gene disruption causes severe renal pathology in the mouse. Cell **83:** 473–482.

35. DINCHUK, J.E., B.D. CAR, R.J. FOCHT, J.J. JOHNSTON, B.D. JAFFEE, M.B. COVINGTON, N.R. CONTEL, V.M. ENG, R.J. COLLINS, P.M. CZERNIAK, S.A. GORRY & J.M. TRZASKOS. 1995. Renal abnormalities and an altered inflammatory response in mice lacking cyclooxygenase II. Nature **378:** 406–409.

36. MARNETT, L.J. 1992. Aspirin and the potential role of prostaglandins in colon cancer. Cancer Res. **52:** 5575–5589.

37. RAO, C.V., A. RIVENSON, B. SIMI, E. ZANG, G. KELLOFF, V. STEELE & B.S. REDDY. 1995. Chemoprevention of colon carcinogenesis by sulindac, a nonsteroidal anti-inflammatory agent. Cancer Res. **55:** 1464–1472.

38. THUN, M.J., M.M. NAMBOODIRI & C.W.J. HEATH. 1991. Aspirin use and reduced risk of fatal colon cancer. N. Engl. J. Med. **325:** 1593–1596.

39. THUN, M.J., M.M. NAMBOODIRI, E.E. CALLE, W.D. FLANDERS & C.W.J. HEATH. 1993. Aspirin use and risk of fatal cancer. Cancer Res. **53:** 1322–1327.

40. ROSENBERG, L., J.R. PALMER, A.G. ZAUBER, M.E. WARSHAUER, P.D. STOLLEY & S. SHAPIRO. 1991. A hypothesis: Nonsteroidal anti-inflammatory drugs reduce the incidence of large-bowel cancer. J. Natl. Cancer Inst. **83:** 355–358.

41. OSHIMA, M., J.E. DINCHUK, S.L. KARGMAN, H. OSHIMA, B. HANCOCK, E. KWONG, J.M. TRZASKOS, J.F. EVANS & M.M. TAKETO. 1996. Suppression of intestinal polyposis in Apc(Delta 716) knockout mice by inhibition of cyclooxygenase 2 (COX-2). Cell **87:** 803–809.

42. VERMA, A.K., C.L. ASHENDEL & R.K. BOUTWELL. 1980. Inhibition by prostaglandin synthesis inhibitors of the induction of epidermal ornithine decarboxylase activity, the accumulation of prostaglandins, and tumor promotion caused by 12-*O*-tetradecanoylphorbol-13-acetate. Cancer Res. **40:** 308–315.

43. FURSTENBERGER, G., M. GROSS & F. MARKS. 1989. Eicosanoids and multistage carcinogenesis in NMRI mouse skin: Role of prostaglandins E and F in conversion (first stage of tumor promotion) and promotion (second stage of tumor promotion). Carcinogenesis **10:** 91–96.

44. MULLER-DECKER, K., K. SCHOLZ, F. MARKS & G. FURSTENBERGER. 1995. Differential expression of prostaglandin H synthase isozymes during multistage carcinogenesis in mouse epidermis. Mol. Carcinog. **12:** 31–41.

45. SANO, H., Y. KAWAHITO, R.L. WILDER, A. HASHIRAMOTO, S. MUKAI, K. ASAI, S. KIMURA, H. KATO, M. KONDO & T. HLA. 1995. Expression of cyclooxygenase-1 and -2 in human colorectal cancer. Cancer Res. **55:** 3785–3789.

46. EBERHART, C.E., R.J. COFFEY, A. RADHIKA, F.M. GIARDIELLO, S. FERRENBACH & R.N. DUBOIS. 1994. Up-regulation of cyclooxygenase 2 gene expression in human colorectal adenomas and adenocarcinomas. Gastroenterology 107: 1183–1188.
47. DUBOIS, R.N., A. RADHIKA, B.S. REDDY & A.J. ENTINGH. 1996. Increased cyclooxygenase-2 levels in carcinogen-induced rat colonic tumors. Gastroenterology 110: 1259–1262.
48. BOOLBOL, S.K., A.J. DANNENBERG, A. CHADBURN, C. MARTUCCI, X.J. GUO, J.T. RAMONETTI, M. ABREUGORIS, H.L. NEWMARK, M.L. LIPKIN, J.J. DECOSSE & M.M. BERTAGNOLLI. 1996. Cyclooxygenase-2 overexpression and tumor formation are blocked by sulindac in a murine model of familial adenomatous polyposis. Cancer Res. 56: 2556–2560.
49. KARGMAN, S.L., G.P. O'NEILL, P.J. VICKERS, J.F. EVANS, J.A. MANCINI & S. JOTHY. 1995. Expression of prostaglandin G/H synthase-1 and -2 protein in human colon cancer. Cancer Res. 55: 2556–2559.
50. LIM, H., B.C. PARIA, S.K. DAS, J.E. DINCHUK, R. LANGENBACH, J.M. TRZASKOS & S.K. DEY. 1997. Multiple female reproductive failures in cyclooxygenase 2–deficient mice. Cell 91: 197–208.
51. GROSS, G.A., T. IMAMURA, C. LUEDKE, S.K. VOGT, L.M. OLSON, D.M. NELSON, Y. SADOVSKY & L.J. MUGLIA. 1998. Opposing actions of prostaglandins and oxytocin determine the onset of murine labor. Proc. Natl. Acad. Sci. USA 95: 11875–11879.
52. ROBERT, A. 1979. Cytoprotection by prostaglandins. Gastroenterology 77: 761–767.
53. BLACK, H.E. 1986. Renal toxicity of non-steroidal anti-inflammatory drugs. Toxicol. Pathol. 14: 83–90.
54. LICHTENSTEIN, D.R., S. SYNGAL & M.M. WOLFE. 1995. Nonsteroidal antiinflammatory drugs and the gastrointestinal tract. The double-edged sword. Arthritis Rheum. 38: 5–18.
55. MURRAY, M.D. & D.C. BRATER. 1993. Renal toxicity of the nonsteroidal anti-inflammatory drugs. Annu. Rev. Pharmacol. Toxicol. 33: 435–465.
56. DAVIS, B.J., D.E. LENNARD, C.A. LEE, H.F. TIANO, S.G. MORHAM, W.C. WETSEL, & R. LANGENBACH. 1999. Anovulation in cyclooxygenase-2-deficient mice is restored by prostaglandin E-2 and interleukin-1 beta. Endocrinology 140: 2685–2695.
57. WHELTON, A. 1995. Renal effects of over-the-counter analgesics. J. Clin. Pharmacol. 35: 454–463.
58. MITCHELL, J.A., S. LARKIN & T.J. WILLIAMS. 1995. Cyclooxygenase-2: Regulation and relevance in inflammation. Biochem. Pharmacol. 50: 1535–1542.
59. CIRINO, G. 1998. Multiple controls in inflammation. Extracellular and intracellular phospholipase A2, inducible and constitutive cyclooxygenase, and inducible nitric oxide synthase. Biochem. Pharmacol. 55: 105–111.
60. APPLETON, I., A. TOMLINSON, P.R. COLVILLE NASH & D.A. WILLOUGHBY. 1993. Temporal and spatial immunolocalization of cytokines in murine chronic granulomatous tissue. Implications for their role in tissue development and repair processes. Lab. Invest. 69: 405–414.
61. MOSER, A.R., H.C. PITOT & W.F. DOVE. 1990. A dominant mutation that predisposes to multiple intestinal neoplasia in the mouse. Science 247: 322–324.
62. SHOEMAKER, A.R., K.A. GOULD, C. LUONGO, A.R. MOSER & W.F. DOVE. 1997. Studies of neoplasia in the Min mouse. Biochim. Biophys. Acta 1332: F25–F48.
63. CHULADA, P.C., C. DOYLE, B. GAUL, H.F. TIANO, J.F. MAHLER, C.A. LEE, S.G. MORHAM & R. LANGENBACH. 1998. Cyclooxygenase-1 and -2 deficiency decrease spontaneous intestinal adenomas in the Min mouse. (Abstract). Proc. Am. Assoc. Cancer Res. 39: 195.

64. REDDY, B.S., C.V. RAO, A. RIVENSON & G. KELLOFF. 1993. Inhibitory effect of aspirin on azoxymethane-induced colon carcinogenesis in F344 rats. Carcinogenesis **14:** 1493–1497.

65. TIANO, H.F., P.C. CHULADA, J. SPALDING, C.A. LEE, C.D. LOFTIN, J.F. MAHLER, S.G. MORHAM & R. LANGENBACH. 1998. Effects of cyclooxygenase deficiency on inflammation and papilloma formation in mouse skin. (Abstract). Proc. Am. Assoc. Cancer Res. **38:** 257.

66. JANG, M., L. CAI, G.O. UDEANI, K.V. SLOWING, C.F. THOMAS, C.W. BEECHER, H.H. FONG, N.R. FARNSWORTH, A.D. KINGHORN, R.G. MEHTA, R.C. MOON & J.M. PEZZUTO. 1997. Cancer chemopreventive activity of resveratrol, a natural product derived from grapes. Science **275:** 218–220.

67. MULLERDECKER, K., A. KOPPSCHNEIDER, F. MARKS, K. SEIBERT & G. FURSTENBERGER. 1998. Localization of prostaglandin H synthase isoenzymes in murine epidermal tumors: Suppression of skin tumor promotion by inhibition of prostaglandin H synthase-2. Mol. Carcinog. **23:** 36–44.

68. TSUJII, M. & R.N. DUBOIS. 1995. Alterations in cellular adhesion and apoptosis in epithelial cells overexpressing prostaglandin endoperoxide synthase 2. Cell **83:** 493–501.

69. TSUJII, M., S. KAWANO, S. TSUJI, H. SAWAOKA, M. HORI & R.N. DUBOIS. 1998. Cyclooxygenase regulates angiogenesis induced by colon cancer cells. Cell **93:** 705–716.

70. NARKO, K., A. RISTIMAKI, A. MACPHEE, E. SMITH, C.C. HAUDENSCHILD & T. HLA. 1997. Tumorigenic transformation of immortalized ECV endothelial cells by cyclooxygenase-1 overexpression. J. Biol. Chem. **272:** 21455–21460.

Inhibition of Cyclooxygenase-2 Expression

An Approach to Preventing Head and Neck Cancer

JUAN R. MESTRE,[a,b] GEORGETTE CHAN,[c] FAN ZHANG,[a,d] EUN K. YANG,[c]
PETER G. SACKS,[b] JAY O. BOYLE,[b] JATIN P. SHAH,[b] DAVID EDELSTEIN,[e]
KOTHA SUBBARAMAIAH,[a,c] AND ANDREW J. DANNENBERG [a,c,f]

[a]Anne Fisher Nutrition Center at Strang Cancer Prevention Center

[b]Head and Neck Service, Department of Surgery,
Memorial Sloan-Kettering Cancer Center

Departments of [c]Medicine and [d]Thoracic Surgery, New York Presbyterian Hospital and
Weill Medical College of Cornell University

[e]Manhattan Eye, Ear and Throat Hospital, New York, New York 10021, USA

ABSTRACT: Cyclooxygenase (COX) catalyzes the formation of prostaglandins
(PG) from arachidonic acid. A large body of evidence has accumulated to suggest that COX-2, the inducible form of COX, is important in carcinogenesis. In
this study, we determined whether (1) COX-2 was overexpressed in squamous
cell carcinoma of the head and neck (HNSCC) and whether (2) retinoids, a
class of chemopreventive agents, blocked epidermal growth factor (EGF)-me-
diated activation of COX-2 expression. Levels of COX-2 mRNA were determined in 15 cases of HNSCC and 10 cases of normal oral mucosa. Nearly a 100-
fold increase in amounts of COX-2 mRNA was detected in HNSCC. By immunoblot analysis, COX-2 protein was detected in 6 of 6 cases of HNSCC but was
undetectable in normal mucosa. Because retinoids protect against oral cavity
cancer, we investigated whether retinoids could suppress EGF-mediated induction of COX-2 in cultured oral squamous carcinoma cells. Treatment with
EGF led to increased levels of COX-2 mRNA, COX-2 protein, and synthesis of
PG. These effects were suppressed by a variety of retinoids. Based on the results of this study, it will be important to establish whether newly developed selective COX-2 inhibitors are useful in preventing or treating HNSCC.
Moreover, the anticancer properties of retinoids may be due, in part, to inhibition of COX-2 expression. Combining a retinoid with a selective COX-2 inhibitor may be more effective than either agent alone in preventing cancer of
the upper aerodigestive tract.

INTRODUCTION

Head and neck cancer is a major, worldwide cause of morbidity and mortality.
Over 40,000 cases of squamous cell carcinoma of the head and neck (HNSCC) occur
each year in the United States alone.[1] Despite recent advances in radiotherapy and

[f]Address for communication: Andrew J. Dannenberg, M.D., New York Presbyterian Hospital-
Cornell, Division of Gastroenterology, Room F-206, 1300 York Avenue, New York, NY 10021.
Voice: 212-746-4403; fax: 212-746-4885.
    e-mail: ajdannen@mail.med.cornell.edu

chemotherapy, the survival of patients with HNSCC has not improved significantly. Moreover, patients who have been cured of one cancer of the head and neck develop second primary carcinomas of the head and neck, lung, or esophagus at a rate approaching 4% per year.[2] Hence, new molecular targets are needed for the prevention and treatment of HNSCC and related cancers.

Cyclooxygenases (COX)[1] catalyze the synthesis of prostaglandins (PG) from arachidonic acid. There are two isoforms of COX. One is constitutively expressed (COX-1), and the other is inducible (COX-2; ref. 3). The *COX-2* gene is an immediate, early response gene that is induced by growth factors, oncogenes, carcinogens, and tumor-promoting phorbol esters.[3–5] The constitutive isoform, COX-1, is essentially unaffected by these factors.

A large body of evidence from a variety of experimental systems suggests that COX-2 is important in carcinogenesis. COX-2 is upregulated in transformed cells[3,6] and in malignant tissue.[7-10] Oshima *et al.* showed that knocking out the *COX-2* gene caused a marked reduction in the number and size of intestinal polyps in a murine model of familial adenomatous polyposis, that is, $APC^{\Delta716}$ knockout mice.[11] COX-2 knockout mice also develop about 75% fewer chemically induced skin papillomas than control mice.[12] In addition to the genetic evidence implicating COX-2 in tumorigenesis, recently developed selective inhibitors of COX-2 inhibit intestinal tumor formation in experimental animals.[11,13]

In this study, we investigated whether COX-2 was overexpressed in HNSCC compared with normal oral mucosa from healthy volunteers. Additionally, we determined whether retinoids, a class of chemopreventive agents, suppressed the induction of COX-2 in oral epithelial cells.[14,15]

MATERIAL AND METHODS

Material

COX-2 primers, Dulbecco's modified Eagle medium, nutrient mixture F-12 (DMEM/F-12), and fetal bovine serum (FBS) were from Life Technologies, Inc. (Grand Island, NY). RNeasy Mini kits were from Qiagen Inc. (Santa Clarita, CA). GeneAmp RNA PCR kits were from Perkin Elmer (Norwalk, CT). GenElute™ Agarose Spin Columns were from Supelco (Bellefonte, PA). Lowry protein assay kits, retinoids, epidermal growth factor (EGF), sodium arachidonate and secondary antibody to IgG conjugated to horseradish peroxidase were from Sigma Chemical Co. (St. Louis, MO). The COX-2 standard for immunoblotting was from Cayman Chemical Co. (Ann Arbor, MI). The COX-2 polyclonal antibody, PG-27, was from Oxford Biomedical Research, Inc. (Oxford, MI). Western blotting detection reagents (ECL) were from Amersham Pharmacia Biotech. Enzyme immunoassay reagents for PGE_2 analysis were from Cayman Co. (Ann Arbor, MI).

Patient Samples

HNSCC was obtained from 15 patients who underwent resection of their tumors at Memorial Sloan-Kettering Cancer Center; 2 mm × 2 mm pieces of HNSCC were sharply excised, placed in sterile tubes, and frozen immediately in liquid nitrogen. Normal oral mucosa was obtained from 10 subjects; these individuals were nonsmoking, nondrinking healthy volunteers and patients undergoing ear, nose, and throat procedures for benign disease. All tissue samples for RT-PCR and Western blotting were stored at −80°C until analysis. Informed consent was obtained from each patient. The study was approved by the Committees on Human Rights in Research at the participating institutions.

Cell Line

1483 squamous carcinoma cells have been described previously.[16] Treatment with vehicle (0.01% DMSO), retinoids, or EGF was carried out under serum-free conditions.[15]

PGE_2 Production

To determine production of PGE_2, 10 µg of cellular lysate protein was incubated in 2 mL HEPES-buffered saline solution containing 100 µM sodium arachidonate at 37°C for 4 minutes; 50 µL was then removed for determination of PGE_2 by EIA.[14,15]

Western Blotting

Frozen tissue was thawed in ice-cold lysis buffer containing 150 mM NaCl, 100 mM Tris-buffered saline (pH 8), 1% Tween-20, 50 mM diethyldithiocarbamate, 1 mM EDTA and 1 mM phenylmethylsulfonyl fluoride. Tissues were sonicated for 20 sec on ice and centrifuged at $10,000 \times g$ for 10 min at 4°C to remove the particulate material. The protein concentration of the supernatant was measured using the Lowry protein assay kit. Lysates of 1483 cells were prepared as in previous studies.[14,15] Immunoblot analysis for COX-2 was performed as in previous studies.[14,15]

Northern Blotting

Analysis was done with a radiolabeled human COX-2 cDNA as described in reference 15.

Construction of a COX-2 Competitor Template Containing a Nucleotide Deletion

A competitive RT-PCR deletion construct (mimic) for COX-2 was synthesized using a mutant sense primer (nts 932-955 attached to nts 1111-1130; 5′-GGTCTG-GTGCCTGGTCTGATGATGGAGTGGCTATCACTTCAAAC-3′) and an antisense primer (nts 1634-1655; 5′-GTCCTTTCAAGGAGAATGGTGC-3′), producing a 569-bp PCR product. The mutant sense primer contains the primer-binding sequence of endogenous target (from nt 932 to 955) attached to the end of an intervening DNA sequence (a 156-bp deletion from nt 956 to nt 1110). Thus, the mimic DNA has primer-binding sequences identical to the target cDNA. The 569-bp mimic was further amplified using the sense primer (5′-GGTCTGGTGCCTGGTCTGATGATG-3′) and the antisense primer (5′-GTCCTTTCAAGGAGAATGGTGC-3′) in a reaction mixture containing 10 mM Tris-HCl (pH 8.3), 50 mM KCl, 2 mM $MgCl_2$, 0.2 mM deoxynucleotide triphosphate, 2.5 units AmpiTaq DNA polymerase, and 400 nM primers for 35 cycles consisting of denaturation at 94°C for 20 sec, annealing at 60°C for 20 sec, and extension at 72°C for 30 sec in a Perkin Elmer 2400 thermal cycler. The PCR products were electrophoresed on 1% agarose gels and gel-purified using GenElute[TM] Agarose Spin Columns according to the manufacturer's protocol.

RNA Isolation and Reverse Transcription

Total RNA was isolated from head and neck tissue (approximately 50 mg) using RNeasy Mini Kits from Qiagen; 0.6 µg of total RNA was reverse transcribed using the GeneAmp RNA PCR kit according to the manufacturer's protocol.

Quantitative Polymerase Chain Reaction for COX-2 in Human Head and Neck Tissue

Each PCR was carried out in 25 µL of a reaction mix, containing 10 mM Tris-HCl (pH 8.3), 50 mM KCl, 2 mM $MgCl_2$, 0.2 mM deoxynucleotide triphosphate, 2.5 units Amplitaq DNA polymerase, and 400 nM primers (the sense primer: 5'-GGTCTGGTGCCTGGTCTGATGATG-3' and the antisense primer: 5'-GTC-CTTTCAAGGAGAATGGTGC-3'). Five µL aliquots of the reverse-transcribed cDNA samples and various known amounts of COX-2 mimic (between 0.001 pg and 0.05 pg), adjusted to the abundance of the target cDNA, were added to the reaction mix and coamplified for 35 cycles: denaturation at 94°C for 20 sec, annealing at 65°C for 20 sec, extension at 72°C for 90 sec, and final extension at 72°C for 10 minutes. Ten µL of PCR products, 724-bp fragments from endogenous target cDNA and 569-bp fragments from mimic COX-2, were then separated by electrophoresis on 1% agarose gels and visualized by ethidium bromide staining. A computer densitometer (Eagle Eye II; Stratagene, La Jolla, CA) was used to determine the density of the bands. A comparison of the band densities yields the quantity of COX-2 mRNA in the reaction.

Statistics

Comparisons between groups were made by the Student's *t*-test. A difference between groups of $p < 0.05$ was considered significant.

RESULTS

Cyclooxygenase-2 Is Overexpressed in HNSCC

To analyze the expression of COX-2 in tissue, we developed a sensitive competitive RT-PCR assay in which the amount of COX-2 mRNA could be measured from small quantities of RNA. This method relies on the coamplification in the same tube of known amounts of competitor DNA with COX-2 cDNA obtained after reverse transcription from total tissue RNA. The competitor and target use the same PCR primers but yield amplicons with a different size, allowing their separation on a gel at the end of the reaction. There was nearly a 100-fold increase in amounts of COX-2 mRNA in HNSCC (mean 353 fg/µg total RNA) versus normal mucosa (mean 3.7 fg/µg total RNA) (FIG. 1). Increased expression of COX-2 was detected in HNSCC from all sites in the head and neck, including the tongue, hypopharynx, larynx, and oral cavity.

To determine whether amounts of COX-2 protein were also increased in HNSCC, Western blot analysis was performed. An immunoblot comparing 6 samples of HNSCC versus 6 samples of normal oral mucosa from healthy volunteers is shown

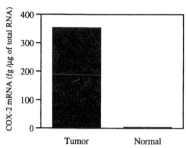

FIGURE 1. Increased levels of COX-2 mRNA in HNSCC. Quantitative RT-PCR was used to determine amounts of COX-2 mRNA in 15 cases of HNSCC and 10 cases of normal oral mucosa. A nearly 100-fold increase in amounts of COX-2 mRNA was detected in HNSCC versus normal oral mucosa ($p < 0.001$).

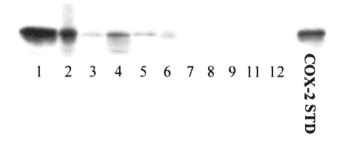

FIGURE 2. Levels of COX-2 protein are increased in HNSCC. Immunoblotting was performed on HNSCC from 6 patients (lanes 1–6) and normal oral mucosa from 6 healthy volunteers (lanes 7–12). Equal amounts of protein (100 μg/lane) were loaded onto a 10% SDS-polyacrylamide gel, electrophoresed, and subsequently transferred onto nitrocellulose. The immunoblot was probed with antibody specific for COX-2. Purified ovine COX-2 was used as a standard.

in FIGURE 2. COX-2 protein was detected in 6 of 6 cases of HNSCC but was undetectable in normal mucosa.

Retinoids Suppress Epidermal Growth Factor–mediated Induction of COX-2 in Human Oral Squamous Carcinoma Cells

Deregulated signaling through the epidermal growth factor receptor (EGFR) pathway is an early event in the development of head and neck cancers[17] and may contribute to the overexpression of COX-2 in HNSCC (FIGS. 1 and 2). Retinoids, a group of naturally occurring and synthetic analogues of vitamin A, suppress carcinogenesis in the oral cavity.[18,19] Hence, we wondered whether retinoids would suppress EGF-mediated induction of COX-2 in cultured oral squamous carcinoma cells.

Treatment with EGF led to approximately a 100% increase in production of PGE_2. This effect of EGF was suppressed by treatment with all-*trans*-retinoic acid (RA), 13-*cis*-RA, retinyl acetate, and 9-*cis*-RA (FIG. 3). To determine whether these differences in production of PGE_2 could be related to differences in amounts of COX, Western blotting was done. FIGURE 4 shows that EGF upregulated COX-2 by

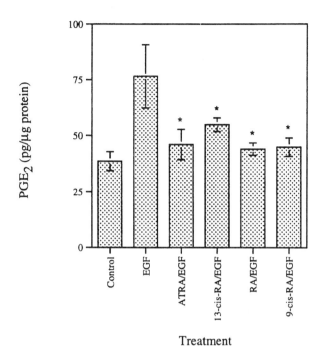

Treatment

FIGURE 3. Retinoids suppress EGF-mediated increases in production of PGE_2. 1483 cells were treated with 1 μM all-*trans*-RA (ATRA), 13-*cis*-RA, retinyl acetate, 9-*cis*-RA, or vehicle (0.01% DMSO). Twenty-four hours later, the medium was replaced with DMEM/F-12 with or without EGF (1 ng/mL) for 5 hours. Production of PGE_2 was determined by enzyme immunoassay. Columns, means; bars, SD; n = 3. *, $p < 0.01$ versus EGF treatment. (Mestre *et al.*[15] With permission from *Cancer Research*.)

about 200 percent. This effect was suppressed by pretreatment with each of the retinoids. In separate experiments, we showed that retinoids inhibited EGF-mediated induction of COX-2, even when the two agents were administered simultaneously.

Changes in amounts of COX-2 enzyme could reflect altered protein synthesis or degradation. Northern blotting was done to investigate whether retinoids suppressed EGF-mediated induction of COX-2 via a pretranslational mechanism. Treatment with EGF increased levels of COX-2 mRNA. This effect was inhibited by 1 μM retinoids (FIG. 5). Retinoids suppressed EGF-mediated induction of COX-2 mRNA even when the retinoids and EGF were administered simultaneously (data not shown). As shown in FIGURE 6, concentrations of all-*trans*-RA ranging from 0.01–10 μM blocked EGF-mediated induction of COX-2 mRNA.

DISCUSSION

This study demonstrates that COX-2 is overexpressed in HNSCC, which is likely to cause the increased levels of PG observed in HNSCC.[20,21] Several different mech-

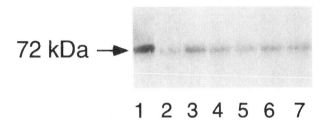

FIGURE 4. Retinoids inhibit EGF-mediated induction of COX-2. 1483 cells were treated with vehicle (0.01% DMSO; lanes 2 and 3) or 1 µM all-*trans*-RA, 13-*cis*-RA, retinyl acetate, or 9-*cis*-RA (lanes 4–7) for 24 hours. The medium was replaced with DMEM/F-12 (lane 2) or DMEM/F-12 and EGF (1 ng/mL; lanes 3–7) for 5 hours. Lane 1, ovine COX-2 standard. Lysate protein (25 µg/lane) was loaded onto a 10% SDS-polyacrylamide gel, electrophoresed, and subsequently transferred onto nitrocellulose. Immunoblots were probed with antibody specific for COX-2. Results of densitometry in arbitrary units were as follows: Lane 2, 24 ± 11; lane 3, 73 ± 9; lane 4, 45 ± 3;[a] lane 5, 48 ± 6;[b] lane 6, 42 ± 2;[a] lane 7, 34 ± 2.[a] Values are means ± SD; n = 3. [a] $p < 0.01$ compared with EGF treatment; [b] $p = 0.01$ compared with EGF treatment. (Mestre *et al.*[15] With permission from *Cancer Research*.)

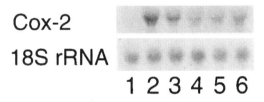

FIGURE 5. Retinoids inhibit EGF-mediated induction of COX-2 mRNA. 1483 cells were treated with vehicle (0.01% DMSO; lanes 1 and 2) or 1 µM all-*trans*-RA, 13-*cis*-RA, retinyl acetate, or 9-*cis*-RA (lanes 3–6) for 24 hours. The medium was replaced with DMEM/F-12 (lane 1) or DMEM/F-12 and EGF (1 ng/mL; lanes 2–6) for 3 hours. Total cellular RNA was isolated. Each lane contained 6 µg of RNA. The Northern blot was probed sequentially with probes that recognized COX-2 mRNA and 18S rRNA. Results of densitometry expressed in arbitrary units were as follows: Lane 1, 20; lane 2, 796; lane 3, 281; lane 4, 133; lane 5, 178; and lane 6, 179. (Mestre *et al.*[15] With permission from *Cancer Research*.)

anisms could provide an important link between COX-2 and HNSCC. Enhanced synthesis of PG, a consequence of upregulation of COX-2, can increase cell proliferation,[22] promote angiogenesis,[23] and inhibit immune surveillance.[24] All of these effects favor the growth of malignant cells. Additionally, overexpression of COX-2 inhibits apoptosis[25] and enhances invasiveness.[26] In extrahepatic tissues, like the head and neck, which have low mixed function oxidase activity,[27] COX-2 may also be important for activating xenobiotics to reactive electrophiles that are carcinogenic. For example, COX catalyzes the oxidation of the tobacco procarcinogen B[a]P-7,8-dihydrodiol, to B[a]P-diolepoxide, which is a highly reactive and strongly mutagenic carcinogen.[28] Additional studies are needed to determine which of these mechanisms are important in HNSCC.

Cox-2

18S rRNA

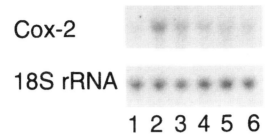

1 2 3 4 5 6

FIGURE 6. All-*trans*-RA inhibits EGF-mediated induction of COX-2. 1483 cells were treated with vehicle (0.01% DMSO; lanes 1 and 2) or a range of concentrations of all-*trans*-RA (0.01, 0.1, 1, or 10 µM; lanes 3–6) for 24 hours. The medium was replaced with DMEM/F-12 (lane 1) or DMEM/F-12 and EGF (1 ng/mL; lanes 2–6) for 3 hours. Total cellular RNA was isolated. Each lane contained 6 µg of RNA. The Northern blot was probed sequentially with probes that recognized COX-2 mRNA and 18S rRNA. Results of densitometry expressed in arbitrary units were as follows: Lane 1, 33; lane 2, 1285; lane 3, 531; lane 4, 400; lane 5, 100; and lane 6, 105. (Mestre *et al.*[15] With permission from *Cancer Research.*)

Nonselective inhibitors of COX-1 and COX-2, such as piroxicam and indomethacin prevent HNSCC in experimental animals.[29] Recently, selective inhibitors of COX-2 have been developed. These compounds possess anticancer properties[11,13] and appear to be safer than traditional nonsteroidal antiinflammatory drugs. Based on the results of this study, it will be important to establish whether selective inhibitors of COX-2 are useful in preventing or treating HNSCC.

Retinoids are effective in treating oral leukoplakia[18] and preventing second primary malignancies in patients with a history of head and neck cancer.[19] The basis for these effects is not completely understood, although RA downregulates EGFR and transforming growth factor alpha,[30] inhibits cellular proliferation,[31] and induces apoptosis.[32] Our observation that retinoids inhibit EGF-mediated induction of COX-2 may also be important for understanding the chemopreventive properties of retinoids. Ultimately, combining a retinoid with a selective inhibitor of COX-2 may be more effective than either agent alone in preventing cancer of the upper aerodigestive tract.

ACKNOWLEDGMENTS

This work was supported by a Grant from the Singapore Cancer Society. J.R. Mestre was a fellow of the Cancer Research Foundation of America. Some of the data in this paper were previously reported in *Cancer Research.*[15]

REFERENCES

1. LANDIS, S.H., T. MURRAY, S. BOLEN & P.A. WINGO. 1998. Cancer statistics, 1998. CA Cancer J. Clin. **48:** 6–29.
2. DAY, G.L. & W.J. BLOT. 1992. Second primary tumors in patients with oral cancer. Cancer **70:** 14–19.

3. HERSCHMAN, H.R. 1996. Prostaglandin synthase 2. Biochim. Biophys. Acta **1299:** 125–140.
4. SUBBARAMAIAH, K., N. TELANG, J.T. RAMONETTI, R. ARAKI, B. DEVITO, B.B. WEKSLER & A.J. DANNENBERG. 1996. Transcription of cyclooxygenase-2 is enhanced in transformed mammary epithelial cells. Cancer Res. **56:** 4424–4429.
5. KELLEY, D.J., J.R. MESTRE, K. SUBBARAMAIAH, P.G. SACKS, S.P. SCHANTZ, T. TANABE, H. INOUE, J.T. RAMONETTI & A.J. DANNENBERG. 1997. Benzo[a]pyrene upregulates cyclooxygenase-2 gene expression in oral epithelial cells. Carcinogenesis **18:** 795–799.
6. KUTCHERA, W., D.A. JONES, N. MATSUNAMI, J. GRODEN, T.M. MCINTYRE, G.A. ZIMMERMAN, R.L. WHITE & S.M. PRESCOTT. 1996. Prostaglandin H synthase-2 is expressed abnormally in human colon cancer: Evidence for a transcriptional effect. Proc. Natl. Acad. Sci. USA **93:** 4816–4820.
7. EBERHART, C.E., R.J. COFFEY, A. RADHIKA, F.M. GIARDIELLO, S. FERRENBACH & R.N. DUBOIS. 1994. Up-regulation of cyclooxygenase 2 gene expression in human colorectal adenomas and adenocarcinomas. Gastroenterology **107:** 1183–1188.
8. RISTIMAKI, A., N. HONKANEN, H. JANKALA, P. SIPPONEN & M. HARKONEN. 1997. Expression of cyclooxygenase-2 in human gastric carcinoma. Cancer Res. **57:** 1276–1280.
9. WILSON, K.T., S. FU, K.S. RAMANUJAM & S.J. MELTZER. 1998. Increased expression of inducible nitric oxide and cyclooxygenase-2 in Barrett's esophagus and associated adenocarcinomas. Cancer Res. **58:** 2929–2934.
10. HIDA, T., Y. YATABE, H. ACHIWA, H. MURAMATSU, K. KOZAKI, S. NAKAMURA, M. OGAWA, T. MITSUDOMI, T. SUGIURA & T. TAKAHASHI. 1998. Increased expressed of cyclooxygenase 2 occurs frequently in human lung cancers, specifically in adenocarcinomas. Cancer Res. **58:** 3761–3764.
11. OSHIMA, M., J.E. DINCHUK, S.L. KARGMAN, H. OSHIMA, B. HANCOCK, E. KWONG, J.M. TRZASKOS, J.F. EVANS & M.M. TAKETO. 1996. Suppression of intestinal polyposis in Apc$^{\Delta 716}$ knockout mice by inhibition of cyclooxygenase 2 (COX-2). Cell **87:** 803–809.
12. TIANO, H., P. CHULADA, J. SPALDING, C. LEE, C. LOFTIN, J. MAHLER, S. MORHAM & R. LANGENBACH. 1997. Effects of cyclooxygenase deficiency on inflammation and papilloma development in mouse skin. Proc. Am. Assoc. Cancer Res. **38:** 1727.
13. KAWAMORI, T., C.V. RAO, K. SEIBERT & B.S. REDDY. 1998. Chemopreventive activity of celecoxib, a specific cyclooxygenase-2 inhibitor, against colon carcinogenesis. Cancer Res. **58:** 409–412.
14. MESTRE, J.R., K. SUBBARAMAIAH, P.G. SACKS, S.P. SCHANTZ, T. TANABE, H. INOUE & A.J. DANNENBERG. 1997. Retinoids suppress phorbol ester-mediated induction of cyclooxygenase-2. Cancer Res. **57:** 1081–1085.
15. MESTRE, J.R., K. SUBBARAMAIAH, P.G. SACKS, S.P. SCHANTZ, T. TANABE, H. INOUE & A.J. DANNENBERG. 1997. Retinoids suppress epidermal growth factor-induced transcription of cyclooxygenase-2 in human oral squamous carcinoma cells. Cancer Res. **57:** 2890–2895.
16. SACKS, P.G., S.M. PARNES, G.E. GALLICK, Z. MANSOURI, R. LICHTNER, K.L. SATYAPRAKASH, S. PATHAK & D.F. PARSONS. 1988. Establishment and characterization of two new squamous cell carcinoma cell lines derived from tumors of the head and neck. Cancer Res. **48:** 2858–2866.
17. SHIN, D.M., J.Y. RO, W.K. HONG & W.N. HITTELMAN. 1994. Dysregulation of epidermal growth factor receptor expression in premalignant lesions during head and neck tumorigenesis. Cancer Res. **54:** 3153–3159.
18. HONG, W.K., J. ENDICOTT, L.M. ITRI, W. DOOS, J.G. BATSAKIS, R. BELL, S. FOFONOFF, R. BYERS, E.N. ATKINSON, C. VAUGHAN, B.B. TOTH, A. KRAMER, I.W. DIMERY, P. SKIPPER & S. STRONG. 1986. 13-*cis*-retinoic acid in the treatment of oral leukoplakia. N. Engl. J. Med. **315:** 1501–1505.

19. HONG, W.K., S.M. LIPPMAN, L.M. ITRI, D.D. KARP, J.S. LEE, R. BYERS, S.P. SCHANTZ, A.M. KRAMER, R. LOTAN, L.J. PETERS, I.W. DIMERY, B.W. BROWN & H. GOEPFERT. 1990. Prevention of second primary tumors with isotretinoin in squamous-cell carcinoma of the head and neck. N. Engl. J. Med. **323:** 795–801.

20. KARMALI, R.A., T. WUSTROW, H.T. THALER & E.W. STRONG. 1984. Prostaglandins in carcinomas of the head and neck. Cancer Lett. **22:** 333–336.

21. JUNG, T.T.K., N.T. BERLINGER & S.K. JUHN. 1985. Prostaglandins in squamous cell carcinoma of the head and neck: A preliminary study. Laryngoscope **95:** 307–312.

22. SHENG, H., J. SHAO, J.D. MORROW, R.D. BEAUCHAMP & R.N. DuBOIS. 1998. Modulation of apoptosis and Bcl-2 expression by prostaglandin E_2 in human colon cancer cells. Cancer Res. **58:** 362–366.

23. TSUJII, M., S. KAWANO, S. TSUJI, H. SAWAOKA, M. HORI & R.N. DuBOIS. 1998. Cyclooxygenase regulates angiogenesis induced by colon cancer cells. Cell **93:** 705–716.

24. HUANG, M., M. STOLINA, S. SHARMA, J.T. MAO, L. ZHU, P.W. MILLER, J. WOLLMAN, H. HERSCHMAN & S.M. DUBINETT. 1998. Non-small cell lung cancer cyclooxygenase-2-dependent regulation of cytokine balance in lymphocytes and macrophages: Up-regulation of interleukin 10 and down-regulation of interleukin 12 production. Cancer Res. **58:** 1208–1216.

25. TSUJII, M. & R.N. DuBOIS. 1995. Alterations in cellular adhesion and apoptosis in epithelial cells overexpressing prostaglandin endoperoxide synthase 2. Cell **83:** 493–501.

26. TSUJII, M., S. KAWANO & R.N. DuBOIS. 1997. Cyclooxygenase-2 expression in human colon cancer cells increases metastatic potential. Proc. Natl. Acad. Sci. USA **94:** 3336–3340.

27. JANOT, F., L. MASSAAD, V. RIBRAG, I. DE WAZIERS, P.H. BEAUNE, B. LUBOINSKI, O. PARISE, A. GOUYETTE & G.G. CHABOT. 1993. Principal xenobiotic-metabolizing enzyme systems in human head and neck squamous cell carcinoma. Carcinogenesis **14:** 1279–1283.

28. ELING, T.E., D.C. THOMPSON, G.L. FOUREMAN, J.F. CURTIS & M.F. HUGHES. 1990. Prostaglandin H synthase and xenobiotic oxidation. Annu. Rev. Pharmacol. Toxicol. **30:** 1–45.

29. TANAKA, T., A. NISHIKAWA, Y. MORI, Y. MORISHITA & H. MORI. 1989. Inhibitory effects of non-steroidal anti-inflammatory drugs, piroxicam and indomethacin on 4-nitroquinoline 1-oxide-induced tongue carcinogenesis in male ACI/N rats. Cancer Lett. **48:** 177–182.

30. RUBIN GRANDIS, J., Q. ZENG & D.J. TWEARDY. 1996. Retinoic acid normalizes the increased gene transcription rate of TGF-α and EGFR in head and neck cancer cell lines. Nature Med. **2:** 237–240.

31. SACKS, P.G., V. OKE, B. AMOS, T. VASEY & R. LOTAN. 1989. Modulation of growth, differentiation and glycoprotein synthesis by β-all-*trans*-retinoic acid in a multicellular tumor spheroid model for squamous carcinoma of the head and neck. Int. J. Cancer **44:** 926–933.

32. ORIDATE, N., D. LOTAN, X-C. XU, W.K. HONG & R. LOTAN. 1996. Differential induction of apoptosis by all-*trans*-retinoic acid and *N*-(4-hydroxyphenyl)retinamide in human head and neck squamous cell carcinoma cell lines. Clin. Cancer Res. **2:** 855–863.

The Role of COX-2 in Intestinal Cancer

CHRISTOPHER WILLIAMS,[a] REBECCA L. SHATTUCK-BRANDT,[a] AND RAYMOND N. DuBOIS[a,b,c]

Departments of [a]Cell Biology and [b]Medicine, Division of Gastroenterology, Vanderbilt School of Medicine, Veterans Administration Medical Center, Nashville, Tennessee 37232, USA

ABSTRACT: Cyclooxygenase (COX), the key regulatory enzyme for prostaglandin synthesis is transcribed from two distinct genes. COX-1 is expressed constitutively in most tissues, and COX-2 is induced by a wide variety of stimuli and was initially identified as an immediate-early growth response gene. In addition, COX-2 expression is markedly increased in 85–90% of human colorectal adenocarcinomas, whereas COX-1 levels remain unchanged. Several epidemiological studies have reported a 40–50% reduction in the risk of developing colorectal cancer in persons who chronically take such nonsteroidal anti-inflammatory drugs (NSAIDs) as aspirin, which are classic inhibitors of cyclooxygenase. Genetic evidence also supports a role for COX-2, since mice null for COX-2 have an 86% reduction in tumor multiplicity in a background containing a mutated APC allele. These results strongly suggest that COX-2 contributes to the development of intestinal tumors and that inhibition of COX is chemopreventative.

INTRODUCTION

Colorectal cancer is the second leading cause of cancer-related deaths in Western civilizations, claiming about 55,000 lives in the United States in 1998. Americans have a 5% risk of developing this disease, and approximately one in ten have a family member who develops colorectal cancer.[1] Recent studies have implicated increased expression of prostaglandin G/H synthase-2 (PGHS-2, cyclooxygenase-2) and associated abnormalities in eicosanoid metabolism with gastrointestinal tumor progression. In this review, we will discuss the potential role of cyclooxygenase-2 (COX-2) and nonsteroidal anti-inflammatory drugs in colorectal carcinogenesis.

EICOSANOID BIOSYNTHESIS

Arachidonic acid metabolism by cyclooxygenase results in the generation of such eicosanoid products as prostaglandins and thromboxanes. The functions of these bioactive lipid molecules include processes such as inflammation, ovulation, mitogenesis, and differentiation. These effects result from modulation of a number of signaling pathways that control distinct physiologic activities.

[c]Address for communication: Department of Cell Biology, Vanderbilt University, MCN C-2104, 1161 21st Avenue South, Nashville, TN 37232. Voice: 615-343-2865; fax: 615-343-6629.
e-mail: raymond.dubois@mcmail.vanderbilt.edu

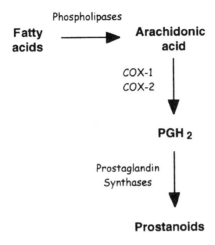

FIGURE 1. Eicosanoid.

There are multiple steps in the eicosanoid biosynthetic pathway. The first step in this pathway is the liberation of arachidonic acid from membrane phospholipids as a result of phospholipase activity. The key step in prostaglandin synthesis is believed to occur at the conversion of arachidonic acid to prostaglandin H_2 (PGH_2) (FIG. 1). PGH_2 is the immediate substrate for a number of cell-specific prostaglandin synthesis that ultimately generate such prostanoids as PGE_2, PGD_2, $PGF_{1\alpha}$, prostacyclin (PGI_2), as well as thromboxane A_2 (TXA_2).

COX-1, purified to homogeneity from bovine vesicular glands in 1976,[2] is often referred to as the constitutive cyclooxygenase, inasmuch as COX-1 mRNA and protein are present at relatively stable levels in most tissues. It is widely believed that COX-1 contributes to the production of prostaglandins that are important in normal homeostatic functions. For example, it is believed that cytoprotective prostaglandins in the gastric mucosa, such as prostacyclin, are produced predominately via COX-1.[3]

In 1989 an inducible form of cyclooxygenase (COX-2) was identified.[4] This 70 kDa cyclooxygenase isoform was independently identified by differential screening of a phorbol ester–stimulated Swiss 3T3 fibroblast cDNA library.[5] COX-2 is often referred to as the inducible cyclooxygenase, because COX-2 expression is influenced by a wide range of extracellular and intracellular stimuli, including LPS,[6–8] forskolin,[9] IL-1, tumor necrosis factor,[10–12] serum,[13,14] EGF,[15] TGFα,[16] IFN-γ,[17] retinoic acid,[18] and endothelin.[19] In many cell lines mitogenic stimulation induces the formation of prostaglandins, and increased prostaglandin levels closely coincide with a significant increase in COX-2 protein. Rat intestinal epithelial cells (RIE-1) exhibit a large increase in prostaglandin production following stimulation with such mitogens as TGFα or EGF.[16] Under resting conditions, these cells have no detectable COX-1 or COX-2, hence prostaglandins are not produced. The COX-2 levels are rate limiting with regard to prostanoid production in the RIE-1 cells.

NONSTEROIDAL ANTI-INFLAMMATORY DRUGS
AND CYCLOOXYGENASES

In 1971 John Vane reported the seminal observation that two different nonsteroidal anti-inflammatory drugs (NSAIDs), sodium salicylate and indomethacin, inhibited prostaglandin production and that prostaglandin blockade likely accounted for their therapeutic effects.[20] Increased prostaglandin production is common in many pathophysiological states. For example, such prostaglandins as PGE_2, PGF_2, PGD_2, PGI_2, and TXA_2 are elevated at sites of inflammation, and NSAIDs prevent this pathologic increase in prostaglandins. However, as noted above, a variety of prostaglandin products contribute to normal physiologic functions, such as cytoprotection of the gastric mucosa, modulation of water, electrolyte transport in the kidney, and maintenance of vascular tone. It is the chronic blockade of protective prostacyclin and/or PGE_2 in the stomach by NSAIDs that is believed to contribute to ulceration and erosion of the gastric mucosa.[3] As of January 1997 there were many different nonsteroidal anti-inflammatory drugs under development or in clinical trials[21] as a result of the recent emphasis on the development of COX-2-selective inhibitors.[22] The more commonly used COX-2 inhibitors can be divided into two distinct structural classes: NS-398 and L-745,337 are members of the acidic sulfonamides, which are also referred to as the methanesulfonanilide class of inhibitors; and SC58125, SC-57666, and celecoxib, which are examples of heterocycles or tricyclic inhibitors.

A number of assay systems have been developed to evaluate the ability of NSAIDs to inhibit COX. These include purified enzyme assays, microsomal membrane preparations from cells expressing COXs, disrupted cells, whole cells, and whole blood, to name a few. The selectivity for each isoform can be expressed as the COX-2/COX-1 IC_{50} ratio. Inasmuch as the absolute IC_{50}'s and selectivity ratios will vary from assay to assay, it is impossible to directly compare IC_{50}'s. However, rank order of selective inhibitors can be compared in different models.

CYCLOOXYGENASE AND COLORECTAL CANCER

The first indication that COX might be involved in colorectal cancer came from the results of NSAID treatment studies of animal models.[23–25] This was followed by the observation that a patient with Gardner's syndrome, a familial form of colorectal cancer, showed profound reduction in the number of rectal polyps following prolonged treatment with a NSAID.[26] This observation was followed by reports that NSAID use led to a 40–50% reduction in risk for colorectal cancer.

The protective effect of NSAIDs suggested that an abnormality in eicosanoid metabolism may contribute to tumor growth. Furthermore, it has been reported that PGE_2 and 6-keto $PGF_{1\alpha}$ were elevated in colorectal cancers.[27,28] Prostaglandin production could be influenced by variations in the levels of COX-2, and increases in COX-2 protein might then account for the increased prostaglandins observed in solid tumors. Indeed, our laboratory, and others, have observed an increase in COX-2 mRNA and protein in surgically resected adenocarcinomas. Eighty-five percent of the adenocarcinomas analyzed exhibited elevated COX-2.[29–32] COX-1 generally was not found expressed in either normal intestinal mucosa or in premalignant or malignant lesions. Fifty percent of benign polyps showed increased expression of

TABLE 1. Tumor burden is inversely related to COX-2 genotype[37]

Genotype	Number of Polyps
APC $^{-/+}$; COX-2 $^{+/+}$	682
APC $^{-/+}$; COX-2 $^{+/-}$	224
APC $^{-/+}$; COX-2 $^{-/+}$	83

COX-2,[29] indicating that dysregulation of COX-2 is an early event in the progression from normal epithelium to a malignant lesion.

COX-2 is also increased in the tumors from two animal models for colorectal cancer. One such animal model is the Min (multiple intestinal neoplasia) mouse, which is a mouse model for the genetic disease familial adenomatous polyposis (FAP). Both the human and mouse forms of FAP have germline mutations in the adenomatous polyposis coli (APC) gene and somatic inactivation of the remaining wildtype allele, which leads to the development of multiple intestinal tumors.[33] A second animal model for colorectal tumorigenesis involves carcinogen treatment of rodents. Treatment of rats or mice with the potent carcinogen azoxymethane (AOM) results in colorectal cancers within 52 weeks. The tumors found in both the Min mouse and the AOM-treated rat contain elevated levels of COX-2.[34–36]

Perhaps the most compelling evidence that COX-2-mediated activity contributes positively to tumor biology was reported in 1996 by Oshima *et al.*[37] This study addressed the question of whether the effect of NSAIDs on tumor size and multiplicity was achieved through a cyclooxygenase-dependent or -independent mechanism. This study used mice carrying a germline mutation within the APC gene. APC$^{\Delta716}$ heterozygote mice exhibited a tumor pattern similar to the distribution of polyps observed in the Min mouse model, but the overall tumor burden was significantly increased. When the APC$^{\Delta716}$ mutant mice were bred with mice nullizygous for COX-2, the number of polyps was significantly reduced in a COX-2 gene dose-dependent manner (TABLE 1). Interestingly, when COX-2 was completely eliminated from the genetic constitution of the APC mutant mice, complete elimination of tumor formation did not occur. This suggests that COX-2 activity may not be an absolute requirement for polyp formation in this model but rather may be acting as a tumor promoter. Nevertheless, these data strongly suggest that COX-2 can contribute to the multiplicity of tumors in this animal model of colorectal cancer.

The precise mechanism(s) whereby COX-2 levels are increased and maintained in the developing adenoma have yet to be determined. Secretion of growth factors is a common feature of many tumors. Therefore, increased local production of growth factors from the tumor could result in upregulation of COX-2 via an auto- or paracrine mechanism. Such growth factors as TGF-α or TGF-β can induce COX-2 in a number of cell lines.

NSAIDs AND GASTROINTESTINAL TUMORIGENESIS

The effects of NSAIDs on tumor growth have been evaluated in both the Min and AOM-treated mouse models (TABLE 2). Experiments evaluating the effectiveness of such nonselective NSAIDs as piroxicam, sulindac, and aspirin at reducing tumor

TABLE 2. NSAID treatment of animal models of colorectal cancer

Animal Model	NSAID Used	Outcome	Reference
Min mouse	Piroxicam	↓ Tumor multiplicity no Δ in ACF #	Jacoby et al. 1996 [38]
	Sulindac	↓ Tumor multiplicity	Beazer-Barclay, 1996[41] Boolbol, 1996[39] Chiu, 1997[40]
	Sulindac sulfide	↓ Tumor multiplicity	Mahmoud, 1998[43]
	Sulindac sulfone	No effect	Mahmoud, 1998[43]
	Aspirin	↓ Multiplicity	Barnes, 1998[42]
AOM rat	Sulindac	↓ Incidence	Samaha, 1997[46] Piazza, 1997[45]
		↓ Multiplicity	
	Sulindac sulfone	↓ Multiplicity	Piazza, 1997[45]
		↓ Incidence	
	Piroxicam	↓ Multiplicity	Pereira, 1996[76]
		↓ ACF	Piazza, 1997[45]
		↓ Incidence	
	Celecoxib	↓ ACF	Reddy, 1996[47]
		↓ Multiplicity	
	NS-398	↓ ACF	Yoshimi, 1997[49]
Xenograft models	SC-58125	↓ Tumor growth	Sheng, 1997[60]
	Indomethacin	↓ Tumor growth[a]	Tsujii, 1998[67]
	NS-398	No effect[a]	Tsujii, 1998[67]
APC mutant mouse	MF tricyclic or sulindac	↓ Multiplicity	Oshima, 1996[37]

[a]Using HCT-116 cells, which do not express COX-1 or COX-2.

burden in the Min, APC$^{\Delta 716}$, or AOM-treated mouse have been performed.[37–46] These studies all concluded that NSAID usage resulted in a significant reduction in the overall tumor multiplicity. In addition, selective inhibition of COX-2 was effective at reducing the number and size of aberrant crypt foci as well as tumor burden in the AOM rat model.[47–49] These data, combined with the FAP patient trials with sulindac, demonstrate that gastrointestinal tumorigenicity can be controlled by treatment with nonsteroidal anti-inflammatory drugs.

MECHANISMS FOR THE PROTECTIVE EFFECT OF NSAIDs

The effect of NSAIDs on tumor growth are most likely multifactorial consisting of both tumor-specific effects and/or host effects. One of the first reported mechanisms for their effect was that of NSAID-induced apoptosis. Studies performed in the Min and AOM-treated rodent models and in human FAP clinical trials indicate that the non-selective COX inhibitor, sulindac, decreased tumor multiplicity and increased the apoptotic index.[39,43,46,50] Moreover, these effects were accompanied by changes in tissue PGE_2[39,43] but not by changes in cellular proliferation.[50]

The mechanism(s) contributing to this increase in apoptosis are still under debate. A number of studies using the HT-29 colorectal cancer cell line and sulindac sulfide have suggested that NSAID treatment increases apoptosis and G_0/G_1 arrest in a COX-independent manner.[51–58] However, it is important to note that in all these studies, the HT-29 cells were treated with high doses of sulindac sulfide (>100 μM) and, with the exception of the report by Hanif *et al.*, COX-2 mRNA, protein, or prostaglandin levels were not measured. Furthermore, Hanif *et al.* only measured prostaglandin levels without determining which COX isoforms were present in the cells. In contrast to the results obtained with sulindac sulfide, studies using two structurally distinct COX-2 selective inhibitors, NS-398 and SC-58125, suggest that changes in cellular proliferation or apoptosis are COX-2-dependent. In 1995, Tsuji *et al.* reported that NS-398 suppressed the proliferation of two cell lines that expressed high COX-1 and COX-2 levels (MKN45 and CACO-2), and minimal effects were seen in cell lines that expressed only high levels of COX-1 (DLDI, LoVo, MKN28, and KATO III).[59] Furthermore, Sheng *et al.* reported that in HCA-7 cells, which express high levels of COX-2 mRNA and protein, the COX-2-selective inhibitor, SC-58125, inhibited cell growth and increased apoptosis and that these effects could be reversed by the addition of PGE_2.[60]

The regulation of apoptosis by arachidonic acid metabolites is still under investigation. Inhibition of COX-2 by NSAIDs could lead to an increase in the free pool of arachidonate in the cell, which would increase the available substrate for other arachidonic acid metabolic pathways. It has been reported that this increase in arachidonate activates sphingomyelinase, leading to production of ceramide, which is a potent apoptosis-inducing agent.[61] In addition, Tang *et al.* reported that the lipoxygenase pathway functions as a regulator of apoptosis.[62]

A recent report also implicates NSAIDs in restoring genomic stability in colorectal cancer cell lines exhibiting mismatch repair (MMR) phenotypes.[63] Microsatellite instability (MSI) and apoptosis were assessed in colorectal cancer cells with defined mutations in mismatch repair genes, which were treated for extended periods with either aspirin or sulindac. A significant reduction in MSI was observed that inversely correlated with an increase in the apoptotic index. When the cells were separated into two pools, it became evident that MSI remained constant in the apoptotic cells, whereas MSI decreased in the nonapoptotic cells, which suggests that treatment by aspirin or sulindac induces a genetic selection for cells that retain stable microsatellites. Whether sensitization of MMR action is a common feature of different classes of NSAIDs has yet to be tested, and whether NSAIDs protect MMR-deficient cells at sporadic loci remains to be evaluated. However, if NSAIDs selectively targets cells with microsatellite instability for apoptosis, chemopreventative use of NSAIDs in HNPCC patients may be efficacious.

Attenuation of tumor growth by NSAID treatment results, in part, via such modulation of host processes as angiogenesis or immune surveillance. PGE_2 can downregulate the nonspecific tumoricidal activity of activated macrophages. Indomethacin treatment of activated macrophages increases their cytotoxic activity in tumor cell–killing assays. The enhanced cytotoxic activity observed with indomethacin treatment is reversed by addition of PGE_2.[64,65] Lewis Lung Carcinoma cells xenografted into mice showed a progressive decrease in natural killer cell activity that correlated with increasing plasma concentrations of PGE_2. Treatment with indomethacin decreased plasma PGE_2 levels and relieved natural killer suppression.[66] Therefore, the inhibitory effect of NSAIDs on tumor growth may partly be explained by enhanced humoral and cell-mediated tumoricidal activity achieved via inhibiting production of immunosuppressive prostaglandins.

Expression of angiogenic factors like VEGF and bFGF are upregulated in colorectal cancer cells engineered to overexpress COX-2.[67] These increases were reversible when the cells were treated with NS-398. Overexpression of COX-2 in the tumor cells resulted in an increase in COX-1 expression in endothelial cells, which was reversible by treatment with neutralizing antibodies to angiogenic factors. Furthermore, NSAID-repressible endothelial cell migration and tube formation was enhanced when human umbilical vein endothelial cells were cocultured with COX-2-expressing colorectal cancer cells. Therefore, NSAIDs may affect the expression of pro-proliferative prostaglandins from the endothelial cells and thus effect the migration and growth of vascular structures in the tumor. Further studies determining whether tumor-derived prostaglandins contribute to *in vivo* vascularization of the tumor and whether or not NSAID treatment blocks this process need to be conducted.

DISCUSSION

Genetic and epidemiological studies strongly implicate COX-2 in the pathogenesis of intestinal cancer.[37,68–71] This is further supported by the observation that NSAIDs effectively reduce the tumor burden in FAP patients[50,72–75] as well as in the Min and AOM-treated mice.[37–46] However, many of these studies have used only the nonselective COX inhibitors. Few of the trials involving the COX-2-selective inhibitors are designed to include patients with colorectal cancer. We hope that over the next few years more studies will use COX-2-selective inhibitors in the clinical setting, now that there is an increased availability of COX-2-selective inhibitors and increased awareness of the importance of COX-2 in the pathogenesis of colorectal cancer.

The precise role that COX-2 and NSAIDs have in the pathogenesis of colorectal cancer is still under investigation. Elucidation of the effects of NSAIDs on intestinal tumorigenesis has been complicated by the suggestion that NSAIDs may be working through a COX-independent mechanism.[51–58] However, it is important to remember that many of these conclusions have been based on cell-culture models that only use the sulindac metabolite (sulindac sulfone) and that conclusions have been drawn from experiments in which prostaglandin levels have not been monitored. By contrast, experiments using two structurally distinct COX-2-selective inhibitors and COX-2-nullizygous mice suggest that reduction of prostaglandin levels through the inhibition of COX-2 effectively decreases the tumor burden in animals.[59,60] Studies using NS-398 and SC-58125 suggest that the decrease in tumor burden is due, in part, to an increase in apoptosis within the tumor.

Although these studies do suggest that COX-2 is playing an important role in intestinal tumorigenesis, they do not rule out the additional possibility that COX-1 plays a role in intestinal tumorigenesis. The results published by Tsujii *et al.* suggest that COX-1 may play some role in regulating angiogenesis.[67] In addition, this is one of the few reports that attempts to determine if the effects of NSAIDs are tumor specific or if they are affecting tumor–host interactions. However, these results were obtained through an *in vitro* assay, and it will be very important to determine the role of COX-1 and host interactions *in vivo*. Finally, the effects of prostaglandins on intestinal epithelial cell transformation has remained virtually uninvestigated. One of the first steps in determining the effects of prostaglandins on epithelial cells will be determining which prostaglandin receptors and signaling pathways are involved. It is only once we gain an understanding of the signaling pathways involved in epithelial transformation that more rational treatments can be devised.

REFERENCES

1. LANDIS, S.H., T. MURRAY, S. BOLDEN & P.A. WINGO. 1999. Cancer statistics. CA Cancer J. Clin. **49:** 8–31.
2. MIYAMOTO, T., N. OGINO, S. YAMAMOTO & O. HAYAISHI. 1976. Purification of prostaglandin endoperoxide synthetase from bovine vesicular gland microsomes. J. Biol. Chem. **251:** 2629–2636.
3. MILLER, T.A. 1983. Protective effects of prostaglandins against gastric mucosal damage: Current knowledge and proposed mechanisms. Am. J. Physiol. **245:** G601–623.
4. SIMMONS, D.L., D.B. LEVY, Y. YANNONI & R.L. ERIKSON. 1989. Identification of a phorbol ester-repressible v-*src*-inducible gene. Proc. Natl. Acad. Sci. USA **86:** 1178–1182.
5. KUJUBU, D.A., B.S. FLETCHER, B.C. VARNUM, R.W. LIM & H.R. HERSCHMAN. 1991. TISIO, a phorbol ester tumor promoter-inducible MRNA from Swiss 3T3 cells, encodes a novel prostaglandin synthase/cyclooxygenase homologue. J. Biol. Chem. **266:** 12866–12872.
6. FU, J.Y., J.L. MASFERRER, K. SEIBERT, A. RAZ & P. NEEDLEMAN. 1990. The induction and suppression of prostaglandin H2 synthase (cyclooxygenase) in human monocytes. J. Biol. Chem. **265:** 16737–16740.
7. O'SULLIVAN, M.G., F.H. CHILTON, E.M. HUGGINS & C.E. McCALL. 1992. Lipopolysaccharide priming of alveolar macrophages for enhanced synthesis of prostanoids involves induction of a novel prostaglandin H synthase. J. Biol. Chem. **267:** 14547–14550.
8. LEE, S.H., E. SOYOOLA, P. CHANMUGAM, S. HART, W. SUN, H. ZHONG, S. LIOU, D. SIMMONS & D. HWANG. 1992. Selective expression of mitogen-inducible cyclooxygenase in macrophages stimulated with lipopolysaccharide. J. Biol. Chem. **267:** 25934–25938.
9. KUJUBU, D.A. & H.R. HERSCHMAN. 1992. Dexamethasone inhibits mitogen induction of the TISIO prostaglandin synthase/cyclooxygenase gene. J. Biol. Chem. **267:** 7991–7994.
10. COYNE, D.W., M. NICKOLS, W. BERTRAND, AND A.R. MORRISON. 1992. Regulation of mesangial cell cyclooxygenase synthesis by cytokines and glucocorticoids. Am. J. Physiol. **263:** F97–102.
11. JONES, D.A., D.P. CARLTON, T.M. McINTYRE, G.A. ZIMMERMAN & S.M. PRESCOTT. 1993. Molecular cloning of human prostaglandin endoperoxide synthase type 11 and demonstration of expression in response to cytokines. J. Biol. Chem. **268:** 9049–9054.
12. GENG, Y., F. BLANCO, M. CORNELISSON & M. LOTZ. 1995. Regulation of cyclooxygenase-2 expression in normal human articular chondrocytes. J. Immunol. **155:** 796–801.
13. RYSECK, R.P., C. RAYNOSCHEK, H. MACDONALD-BRAVO, K. DORFMAN, M.G. MATTEI & R. BRAVO. 1992. Identification of an immediate early gene, pghs-B, whose protein product has prostaglandin synthase/cyclooxygenase activity. Cell Growth & Differen. **3:** 443–450.
14. DEWITT, D.L. & E.A. MEADE. 1993. Serum and glucocorticoid. regulation of gene transcription and expression of prostaglandin H synthase-1 and prostaglandin H synthase-2 isozymes. Arch. Biochem. Biophys. **306:** 94–102.

15. HAMASAKI, Y., J. KITZLER, R. HARDMAN, P. NETTESHEIM & T.E. ELING. 1993. Phorbol ester and epidermal growth factor enhance the expression of two inducible prostaglandin H synthase genes in rat tracheal epithelial cells. Arch. Biochem. Biophys. **304:** 226–234.

16. DUBOIS, R.N., J. AWAD, J. MORROW, L.J. ROBERTS & P.R. BISHOP. 1994. Regulation of eicosanoid production and mitogenesis in rat intestinal epithelial cells by transforming growth factor-α and phorbol ester. J. Clin. Invest. **93:** 493–498.

17. RIESE, J., T. HOFF, A. NORDHOFF, D.L. DEWITT, K. RESCH & V. KAEVER. 1994. Transient expression of prostaglandin endoperoxide synthase-2 during mouse macrophage activation. J. Leukocyte Biol. **55:** 476–482.

18. BAZAN, N.G., B.S. FLETCHER, H.R. HERSCHMAN & P.K. MUKHERJEE. 1994. Platelet-activating factor and retinoic acid synergistically activate the inducible prostaglandin synthase gene. Proc. Natl. Acad. Sci. USA **91:** 5252–5256.

19. KESTER, M., E. CORONEOS, P.J. THOMAS & M.J. DUNN. 1994. Endothelin stimulates prostaglandin endoperoxide synthase-2 MRNA expression and protein synthesis through a tyrosine kinase-signaling pathway in rat mesangial cells. J. Biol. Chem. **269:** 22574–22580.

20. VANE, J.R. 1971. Inhibition of prostaglandin synthesis as a mechanism of action for aspirin-like drugs. Nature New Biol. **231:** 232–235.

21. Non-Steroidal Anti-Inflammatory Drugs: Cyclooxygenase Inhibitors. 1997. Drug Market Development **8:** 8–15.

22. PENNISI, E. 1998. Building a better aspirin. Science **280:** 1191–1192.

23. HIAL, V., Z. HORAKOVA, F.E. SHAFF & M.A. BEAVEN. 1976. Alteration of tumor growth by aspirin and indomethacin: Studies with two transplantable tumors in mouse. Eur. J. Pharmacol. **37:** 367–376.

24. POLLARD, M. & P.H. LUCKERT. 1980. Indomethacin treatment of rats with dimethyl-hydrazine-induced intestinal tumors. Cancer Treat. Rep. **64:** 1323–1327.

25. POLLARD, M. & P.H. LUCKERT. 1981. Effect of indomethacin on intestinal tumors induced in rats by the acetate derivative of dimethylnitrosamine. Science **214:** 558–559.

26. WADDELL, W.R. & R.W. LOUGHRY. 1983. Sulindac for polyposis of the colon. J. Surg. Oncol. **24:** 83–87.

27. RIGAS, B., I.S. GOLDMAN & L. LEVINE. 1993. Altered eicosanoid levels in human colon cancer. J. Lab. Clin. Med. **122:** 518–523.

28. BENNETT, A., A. CIVIER, C.N. HENSBY, P.B. MELHUISH & I.F. STAMFORD. 1987. Measurement of arachidonate and its metabolites extracted from human normal and malignant gastrointestinal tissues. Gut **28:** 315–318.

29. EBERHART, C.E., R.J. COFFEY, A. RADHIKA, F.M. GIARDIELLO, S. FERRENBACH & R.N. DUBOIS. 1994. Up-regulation of cyclooxygenase 2 gene expression in human colorectal adenomas and adenocarcinomas. Gastroenterology **107:** 1183–1188.

30. SANO, H., Y. KAWAHITO, R.L. WILDER, A. HASHIRAMOTO, S. MUKAI, K. ASAI, S. KIMURA, H. KATO, M. KONDO & T. HLA. 1995. Expression of cyclooxygenase-1 and -2 in human colorectal cancer. Cancer Res. **55:** 3785–3789.

31. KUTCHERA, W., D.A. JONES, N. MATSUNAMI, J. GRODEN, T.M. MCINTYRE, G.A. ZIMMERMAN, R.L. WHITE & S.M. PRESCOTT. 1996. Prostaglandin H synthase-2 is expressed abnormally in human colon cancer: Evidence for a transcriptional effect. Proc. Natl. Acad. Sci. USA **93:** 4816–4820.

32. KARGMAN, S., G. O'NEILL, P. VICKERS, J. EVANS, J. MANCINI & S. JOTHY. 1995. Expression of prostaglandin G/H synthase-1 and -2 protein in human colon cancer. Cancer Res. **55:** 2556–2559.

33. SU, L.K., K.W. KINZLER, B. VOGELSTEIN, A.C. PREISINGER, A.R. MOSER, C. LUONGO, K.A. GOULD & W.F. DOVE. 1992. Multiple intestinal neoplasia caused by a mutation in the murine homolog of the APC gene. Science **256:** 668–670.

34. SINGH, J., R. HAMID & B.S. REDDY. 1997. Dietary fat and colon cancer: Modulation of cyclooxygenase-2 by types and amount of dietary fat during the postinitiation stage of colon carcinogenesis. Cancer Res. **57:** 3465–3470.

35. WILLIAMS, C.W., C. LUONGO, A. RADHIKA, T. ZHANG, L.W. LAMPS, L.B. NANNEY, R.D. BEAUCHAMP & R.N. DUBOIS. 1996. Elevated cyclooxygenase-2 levels in Min mouse adenomas. Gastroenterology **111:** 1134–1140.

36. DUBOIS, R.N., A. RADHIKA, B.S. REDDY & A.J. ENTINGH. 1996. Increased cyclooxygenase-2 levels in carcinogen-induced rat colonic tumors. Gastroenterology **110:** 1259–1262.

37. OSHIMA, M., J.E. DINCHUK, S.L. KARGMAN, H. OSHIMA, B. HANCOCK, E. KWONG, J.M. TRZASKOS, J.F. EVANS & M.M. TAKETO. 1996. Suppression of intestinal polyposis in APC$^{\Delta 716}$ knockout mice by inhibition of prostaglandin endoperoxide synthase-2 (COX-2). Cell **87:** 803–809.

38. JACOBY, R.F., D.J. MARSHALL, M.A. NEWTON, K. NOVAKOVIC, K. TUTSCH, C.E. COLE, R.A. LUBET, G.J. KELLOF, A. VERMA, A.R. MOSER & W.F. DOVE. 1996. Chemoprevention of spontaneous intestinal adenomas in the Apc^{Min} mouse model by the nonsteroidal anti-inflammatory drug piroxicam. Cancer Res. **56:** 710–714.

39. BOOLBOL, S.K., A.J. DANNENBERG, A. CHADBURN, C. MARTUCCI, X.J. GUO, J.T. RAMONETTI, M. ABREU-GORIS, H.L. NEWMARK, M.L. LIPKIN, J.J. DECOSSE & M.M. BERTAGNOLL. 1996. Cyclooxygenase-2 overexpression and tumor formation are blocked by sulindac in a murine model of familial adenomatous polyposis. Cancer Res. **56:** 2556–2560.

40. CHIU, C.H., M.F. MCENTEE & J. WHELAN. 1997. Sulindac causes rapid regression of preexisting tumors in Min/+ mice independent of prostaglandin biosynthesis. Cancer Res. **57:** 4267–4273.

41. BEAZER-BARCLAY, Y., D.B. LEVY, A.R. MOSER, W.F. DOVE, S.R. HAMILTON, B. VOGELSTEIN & K.W. KINZLER. 1996. Sulindac suppresses tumorigenesis in the min mouse. Carcinogenesis **17:** 1757–1760.

42. BARNES, C.J. & M. LEE. 1998. Chemoprevention of spontaneous intestinal adenomas in the adenomatous polyposis coli Min mouse model with aspirin. Gastroenterology **114:** 873–877.

43. MAHMOUD, N.N., S.K. BOOLBOL, A.J. DANNENBERG, J.R. MESTRE, R.T. BILINSKI, C. MARTUCCI, H.L. NEWMARK, A. CHADBURN & M.M. BERTAGNOLLI. 1998. The sulfide metabolite of sulindac prevents tumors and restores enterocyte apoptosis in a murine model of familial adenomatous polyposis. Carcinogenesis **19:** 87–91.

44. RAO, C.V., A. RIVENSON, B. SIMI, E. ZANG, G. KELLOFF, V. STEELE & B.S. REDDY. 1995. Chemoprevention of colon carcinogenesis by sulindac, a nonsteroidal antiinflammatory agent. Cancer Res. **55:** 1464–1472.

45. PIAZZA, G.A., D.S. ALBERTS, L.J. HIXSON, N.S. PARANKA, H. LI, T. FINN, C. BOGERT, J.M. GUILLEN, K. BRENDEL, P.H. GROSS, G. SPERL, J. RITCHIE, R.W. BURT, L. ELLSWORTH, D.J. AHNEN & R. PAMUKCU. 1997. Sulindac sulfone inhibits azoxymethane-induced colon carcinogenesis in rats without reducing prostaglandin levels. Cancer Res. **57:** 2909–2915.

46. SAMAHA, H.S., G.J. KELLOFF, V. STEELE, C.V. RAO & B.S. REDDY. 1997. Modulation of apoptosis by sulindac, curcumin, phenylethyl-3-methylcaffeate, and 6-phenylhexyl isothiocyanate: Apoptotic index as a biomarker in colon cancer chemoprevention and promotion. Cancer Res. **57:** 1301–1305.

47. REDDY, B.S., C.V. RAO & K. SEIBERT. 1996. Evaluation of cyclooxygenase-2 inhibitor for potential chemopreventive properties in colon carcinogenesis. Cancer Res. **56:** 4566–4569.

48. KAWAMORI, T., C.V. RAO, K. SEIBERT & B.S. REDDY. 1998. Chemopreventive activity of celecoxib, a specific cyclooxygenase-2 inhibitor, against colon carcinogenesis. Cancer Res. **58:** 409–412.
49. YOSHIMI, N., K. KAWABATA, A. HARA, K. MATSUNAGA, Y. YAMADA & H. MORE. 1997. Inhibitory effect of NS-398, a selective cyclooxygenase-2 inhibitor, on azoxymethane-induced aberrant crypt foci in colon carcinogenesis of F344 rats. Jpn. J. Cancer Res. **88:** 1044–1051.
50. PASRICHA, P.J., A. BEDI, K. O'CONNOR, A. RASHID, A.J. AKHTAR, M.L. ZAHURAK, S. PIANTADOSI, S.R. HAMILTON & F.M. GIARDIELLO. 1995. The effects of sulindac on colorectal proliferation and apoptosis in familial adenomatous polyposis [see comments]. Gastroenterology **109:** 994–998.
51. SHIFF, S.J., L. QIAO, L.L. TSAI & B. RIGAS. 1995. Sulindac sulfide, an aspirin-like compound, inhibits proliferation, causes cell cycle quiescence, and induces apoptosis in HT-29 colon adenocarcinoma cells. J. Clin. Invest. **96:** 491–503.
52. QIAO, L., R. HANIF, E. SPHICAS, S.J. SHIFF & B. RIGAS. 1998. Effect of aspirin on induction of apoptosis in HT-29 human colon adenocarcinoma cells. Biochem. Pharmacol. **55:** 53–64.
53. PIAZZA, G.A., A.K. RAHM, T.S. FINN, B.H. FRYER, H. LI, A.L. STOUMEN, R. PAMUKCU & D.J. AHNEN. 1997. Apoptosis primarily accounts for the growth-inhibitory properties of sulindac metabolites and involves a mechanism that is independent of cyclooxygenase inhibition, cell cycle arrest, and p53 induction. Cancer Res. **57:** 2452–2459.
54. PIAZZA, G.A., A.L. RAHM, M. KRUTZSCH, G. SPERL, N.S. PARANKA, P.H. GROSS, K. BRENDEL, R.W. BURT, D.S. ALBERTS, R. PAMUKCU et al. 1995. Antineoplastic drugs sulindac sulfide and sulfone inhibit cell growth by inducing apoptosis. Cancer Res. **55:** 3110–3116.
55. GOLDBERG, Y., I.I. NASSIF, A. PITTAS, L.L. TSAI, B.D. DYNLACHT, B. RIGAS & S.J. SHIFF. 1996. The anti-proliferative effect of sulindac and sulindac sulfide on HT-29 colon cancer cells: Alterations in tumor suppressor and cell cycle-regulatory proteins. Oncogene **12:** 893–901.
56. HIXSON, L.J., D.S. ALBERTS, M. KRUTZSCH, J. EINSPHAR, K. BRENDEL, P.H. GROSS, N.S. PARANKA, M. BAIER, S. EMERSON, R. PAMUKCU et al. 1994. Antiproliferative effect of nonsteroidal antiinflammatory drugs against human colon cancer cells. Cancer Epidemiol. Biomarkers Prev. **3:** 433–438.
57. HANIF, R., A. PITTAS, Y. FENG, M.I. KOUTSOS, L. QIAO, L. STAIANO-COICO, S.I. SHIFF & AND B. RIGAS. 1996. Effects of nonsteroidal anti-inflammatory drugs on proliferation and on induction of apoptosis in colon cancer cells by a prostaglandin-independent pathway. Biochem. Pharmacol. **52:** 237–245.
58. QIAO, L., S.J. SHIFF & B. RIGAS. 1997. Sulindac sulfide inhibits the proliferation of colon cancer cells: Diminished expression of the proliferation markers PCNA and Ki-67. Cancer Lett. **115:** 229–234.
59. TSUJI, S., S. KAWANO, H. SAWAOKA, Y. TAKEI, I. KOBAYASHI, K. NAGANO, H. FUSAMOTO & T. KAMADA. 1996. Evidences for involvement of cyclooxygenase-2 in proliferation of two gastrointestinal cancer cell lines. Prostaglandins Leukotrienes Essent. Fatty Acids **55:** 179–183.
60. SHENG, H., J. SHAO, S.C. KIRKLAND, P. ISAKSON, R. COFFEY, J. MORROW, R.D. BEAUCHAMP & R.N. DUBOIS. 1997. Inhibition of human colon cancer cell growth by selective inhibition of cyclooxygenase-2. J. Clin. Invest. **99:** 2254–2259.
61. CHAN, T.A., P.J. MORIN, B. VOGELSTEIN & K.W. KINZLER. 1998. Mechanisms underlying nonsteroidal antiinflammatory drug-mediated apoptosis. Proc. Natl. Acad. Sci. USA **95:** 681–686.

62. TANG, D.G., Y.Q. CHEN & K.V. HONN. 1996. Arachidonate lipoxygenases as essential regulators of cell survival and apoptosis. Proc. Natl. Acad. Sci. USA **93:** 5241–5246.

63. RÜSCHOFF, J., S. WALLINGER, W. DIETMAIER, T. BOCKER, G. BROCKHOFF, F. HOFSTDDTER & R. FISHEL. 1998. Aspirin suppresses the mutator phenotype associated with hereditary nonpolyposis colorectal cancer by genetic selection. Proc. Natl. Acad. Sci. USA **95:** 11301–11306.

64. TAFFET, S., J. PACE & S. RUSSELL. 1981. Lymphokine maintains macrophage activation for tumor cell killing by interfering with the negative regulatory effect of prostaglandin E2. J. Immunol. **127:** 121–124.

65. TAFFET, S. & S. RUSSELL. 1981. Macrophage-mediated tumor cell killing: Regulation of expression of cytolytic activity by prostaglandin E. J. Immunol. **126:** 424–427.

66. YOUNG, M., E. WHEELER & M. NEWBY. 1986. Macrophage-mediated suppression of natural killer cell activity in mice bearing Lewis lung carcinoma. J. Natl. Cancer Inst. **76:** 745–750.

67. TSUJII, M., S. KAWANO, S. TSUJI, H. SAWAOKA, M. HORI & R.N. DUBOIS. 1998. Cyclooxygenase regulates angiogenesis induced by colon cancer cells. Cell **93:** 705–716.

68. PELEG, I.I., M.F. LUBIN, G.A. COTSONIS, W.S. CLARK & C.M. WILCOX. 1996. Long-term use of nonsteroidal antiinflammatory drugs and other chemopreventors and risk of subsequent colorectal neoplasia. Dig. Dis. Sci. **41:** 1319–1326.

69. GIOVANNUCCI, E., E.B. RIMM, M.J. STAMPFER, G.A. COLDITZ, A. ASCHERIO & W.C. WILLETT. 1994. Aspirin use and the risk for colorectal cancer and adenoma in male health professionals. Ann. Intern. Med. **121:** 241–246.

70. GIOVANNUCCI, E., K.M. EGAN, D.J. HUNTER, M.J. STAMPFER, G.A. COLDITZ, W.C. WILLETT & F.E. SPEIZER. 1995. Aspirin and the risk of colorectal cancer in women. N. Engl. J. Med. **333:** 609–614.

71. GANN, P.H., J.E. MANSON, R.J. GLYNN, J.E. BURING & C.H. HENNEKENS. 1993. Low-dose aspirin and incidence of colorectal tumors in a randomized trial. J. Natl. Cancer Inst. **85:** 1220–1224.

72. LABAYLE, D., D. FISCHER, P. VIELH, F. DROUHIN, A. PARIENTE, C. BORIES, 0. DUHAMEL, M. TROUSSET & P. ATTALI. 1991. Sulindac causes regression of rectal polyps in familial adenomatous polyposis. Gastroenterology **101:** 635–639.

73. GIARDIELLO, F.M., S.R. HAMILTON, A.J. KRUSH, S. PIANTADOSI, L.M. HYLIND, P. CELANO, S.V. BOOKER, C.R. ROBINSON & G.J. OFFERHAUS. 1993. Treatment of colonic and rectal adenomas with sulindac in familial adenomatous polyposis. N. Engl. J. Med. **328:** 1313–1316.

74. NUGENT, K.P., K.C. FARMER, A.D. SPIGELMAN, C.B. WILLIAMS & R.K. PHILLIPS. 1993. Randomized controlled trial of the effect of sulindac on duodenal and rectal polyposis and cell proliferation in patients with familial adenomatous polyposis. Br. J. Surg. **80:** 1618–1619.

75. GIARDIELLO, F.M., E.W. SPANNHAKE, R.N. DUBOIS, L.M. HYLIND, C.R. ROBINSON, W.C. HUBBARD, S.R. HAMILTON & V.W. YANG. 1998. Prostaglandin levels in human colorectal mucosa: Effects of sulindac in patients with familial adenomatous polyposis. Dig. Dis. Sci. **43:** 311–316.

76. PEREIRA, M.A., L.H. BARNES, V.E. STEELE, G.V. KELLOFF & R.A. LUBET. 1996. Piroxicam-induced regression of azoxymethane-induced aberrant crypt foci and prevention of colon cancer in rats. Carcinogenesis **17:** 373–376.

COX-2 Inhibitors

A New Class of Antiangiogenic Agents

JAIME L. MASFERRER,[a] ALANE KOKI, AND KAREN SEIBERT

Discovery Pharmacology and Analytical Sciences Center,
G.D. Searle / Monsanto Company, St. Louis, Missouri 63167, USA

ABSTRACT: The formation of new blood vessels by angiogenesis to provide adequate blood supply is a key requirement for the growth of many tumors. While normal blood vessels expressed the COX-1 enzyme, new angiogenic endothelial cells expressed the inducible COX-2. We evaluated the role of COX inhibitors in the mouse corneal micropocket assay in which angiogenesis is driven by the addition of a Hydron pellet containing basic fibroblast growth factor (bFGF). Neovascular areas were measured with a slit lamp five days after pellet implantation into the corneal stroma. All animals containing implants with bFGF (90 ng) developed intensive areas of neovascularization, whereas the controls implanted with the Hydron pellet alone did not. Indomethacin (a nonselective COX-1/COX-2 inhibitor) and SC-236 (a COX-2-selective inhibitor) inhibited angiogenesis in a dose-dependent manner. Importantly, the indomethacin-treated mice developed severe gastrointestinal toxicity at the efficacious dose of 3 mg/kg/day. By contrast, gastrointestinal lesions were not observed, and platelet COX-1 activity was unaffected, at antiangiogenic doses of SC-236 (1–6 mg/kg/day). Furthermore, a COX-1-selective inhibitor, SC-560, was ineffective at doses up to 10 mg/kg, a dose that completely blocked platelet COX-1 activity in these mice. SC-236 was also effective in reducing angiogenesis driven by bFGF, vascular endothelium growth factor (VEGF), or carrageenan in the matrigel rat model. Finally, in several tumor models, SC-236 consistently and effectively inhibited tumor growth and angiogenesis. This novel antiangiogenic activity of COX-2 inhibitors indicates their potential therapeutic utility in several types of cancer.

The formation of new blood vessels by angiogenesis is thought to be a key requirement for the growth of many tumors. Based on this hypothesis, a new field of research was generated and pioneered by the work of Dr. Judah Folkman.[1] This research has led to the identification of several new drugs that target different mediators and receptors linked to the angiogenesis process. These new agents are expected to limit the blood supply to the cancerous cells and therefore indirectly limit tumor growth by affecting cell proliferation and/or inducing apoptosis. Thus, antiangiogenic and cytotoxic agents may exhibit potent synergistic antitumor activity in dual therapy by impacting on two independent mechanisms essential to tumor maintenance

[a]Address for correspondence: Group Leader/Project Leader, Discovery Pharmacology, 800 N. Lindbergh Boulevard, Mail Zone T3G, St. Louis, MO 63167. Voice: 314-694-8950; fax: 314-694-3415.
e-mail: jlmasf@monsanto.com

and growth (i.e., neovascularization and neoplastic cell maintenance/proliferation). As a monotherapeutic agent, antiangiogenics are expected to be much safer and better tolerated than traditional chemotherapeutic drugs and may hence be ideal candidates for use in the prevention of cancer. In this modality, antiangiogenic agents could also be effectively used in secondary prevention modalities in patients who are in remission following surgical resection, radiation, or chemotherapy.

Prostaglandins are formed via the cyclooxygenase (COX) pathway and are known to be potent proangiogenic molecules.[2,3] It has been postulated that the elevated levels of PGE_2 found in the joints of rheumatoid arthritis patients play a critical role in promoting neovascularization essential to pannus formation.[4] PGE_2 has also been shown to potently induce the growth of new blood vessels in the corneal micropocket model.[5] Because large amounts of PGE_2 are also generated by different tumors, one could hypothesize a similar role for PGE_2 in tumor angiogenesis.

While mature blood vessels express COX-1, new angiogenic endothelial cells express the inducible COX-2.[6] Based on these observations, we hypothesized that tumor-derived growth factors promote angiogenesis by inducing the production of COX-2-derived PGE_2. To evaluate this hypothesis, we studied the effect of COX inhibitors on basic fibroblast growth factor (bFGF)-induced angiogenesis in the mouse and rat corneal micropocket assay. Hydron pellets impregnated with bFGF induced intensive areas of neovascularization in the corneal stroma, which were measured with a slit lamp five days following implantation. Indomethacin, a nonsteroidal antiinflammatory (NSAID) drug that nonselectivily inhibits both COX-1 and COX-2, dose-dependently blocked angiogenesis, indicating that prostaglandins play a important role in the angiogenic process. To further determine the role of COX-1 and COX-2 in the regulation of the angiogenic process, specific inhibitors of each isoform were evaluated in the corneal micropocket assay. The COX-1 selective inhibitor, SC-560, was completely ineffective in blocking angiogenesis at doses up to 10 mg/kg, a dose that completely blocked platelet and gastric COX-1 activity in these mice. By contrast, the specific COX-2 inhibitor, SC-236, was very effective in blocking FGF-induced corneal angiogenesis at doses between 1–6 mg/kg/day. Stomach and platelet PGE_2 and TXB_2 were not affected in SC-236 animals, indicating COX-1 was not inhibited in these animals. These pharmacologic data strongly imply that COX-2-derived prostaglandins play a critical role in FGF-induced angiogenesis in this model. Finally, in several tumor models, SC-236 consistently and effectively inhibited tumor growth and angiogenesis. This novel antiangiogenic activity of COX-2 inhibitors may partially explain the chemopreventive and antitumor activities observed for this new class of drugs and suggests their potential therapeutic utility in several types of cancer.[7]

REFERENCES

1. HANAHAN, D. & J. FOLKMAN. 1996. Patterns and emerging mechanisms of the angiogenic switch during tumorigenesis. Cell **86:** 353–364.
2. NEEDLEMAN, P., J. TURK, B.A. JAKSCHIK *et al.* 1986. Arachidonic acid metabolism. Annu. Rev. Biochem. **55:** 69–102.
3. LEVY, G.N. 1997. Prostaglandin H synthases, nonsteroidal anti-inflammatory drugs and colon cancer. FASEB J. **11:** 234–247.

4. CROFFORD, L.J., R.L. WILDER, A.P. RISTIMAKI *et al.* 1994. Cyclooxygenase-1 and -2 expression in rheumatoid synovial tissues. Effects of interleukin-1 beta, phorbol ester and corticosteroids. J. Clin.Invest. **93:** 1095–1101.
5. FORM, D.M. & R. AUERBACH. 1983. PGE2 and angiogenesis. Proc. Soc. Exp. Biol. Med. **172:** 214–218.
6. KOKI, A.T., D.A. EDWARDS, A.J. DANNENBERGH *et al.* 1998. Cyclooxygenase-2 is expressed in animal and human cancers. Proc. Annu. Meet. Am. Assoc. Cancer Res. **39:** Abstr. 1022.
7. REDDY, B.S., C.V. RAO & K. SEIBERT. 1996. Evaluation of cyclooxygenase-2 inhibitor for potential chemopreventive properties in colon carcinogenesis. Cancer Res. **56:** 4566–4569.

Micronutrient Deficiencies

A Major Cause of DNA Damage

BRUCE N. AMES[a]

University of California, Berkeley, California 94720-3202, USA

ABSTRACT: Deficiencies of the vitamins B_{12}, B_6, C, E, folate, or niacin, or of iron or zinc mimic radiation in damaging DNA by causing single- and double-strand breaks, oxidative lesions, or both. The percentage of the population of the United States that has a low intake (<50% of the RDA) for each of these eight micronutrients ranges from 2% to 20+ percent. A level of folate deficiency causing chromosome breaks occurred in approximately 10% of the population of the United States, and in a much higher percentage of the poor. Folate deficiency causes extensive incorporation of uracil into human DNA (4 million/ cell), leading to chromosomal breaks. This mechanism is the likely cause of the increased colon cancer risk associated with low folate intake. Some evidence, and mechanistic considerations, suggest that vitamin B_{12} and B_6 deficiencies also cause high uracil and chromosome breaks. Micronutrient deficiency may explain, in good part, why the quarter of the population that eats the fewest fruits and vegetables (five portions a day is advised) has about double the cancer rate for most types of cancer when compared to the quarter with the highest intake. Eighty percent of American children and adolescents and 68% of adults do not eat five portions a day. Common micronutrient deficiencies are likely to damage DNA by the same mechanism as radiation and many chemicals, appear to be orders of magnitude more important, and should be compared for perspective. Remedying micronutrient deficiencies is likely to lead to a major improvement in health and an increase in longevity at low cost.

INTRODUCTION

Approximately 40 micronutrients (the vitamins, essential minerals, and other compounds required in small amounts for normal metabolism) are required in the human diet.[1] For each micronutrient, metabolic harmony requires an optimal intake (i.e., to give maximal life span); deficiency distorts metabolism in numerous and complicated ways, many of which may lead to DNA damage. The recommended dietary allowance (RDA)[2–4] of a micronutrient is mainly based on information on acute effects, because the optimum amount for long-term health is generally not known. For many micronutrients, a sizable percentage of the population is deficient relative to the current RDA.[5] Remedying these deficiencies, which can be done at low cost, is likely to lead to a major improvement in health and an increase in longevity. The optimum intake of a micronutrient can vary with age and genetic constitution and be influenced by other aspects of diet. Determining these optima, and

[a]Address for correspondence: 401 Barker Hall MCB/BMB, Berkeley, CA. Voice: 510-642-5165; fax: 510-643-7935.

e-mail: bnames@uclink4.berkeley.edu

remedying deficiencies, and in some cases excesses, will be a major public health project for the coming decades. Long-term health is also influenced by many other aspects of diet.

Micronutrient deficiency can mimic radiation (or chemicals) in damaging DNA by causing single- and double-strand breaks, or oxidative lesions, or both. Those micronutrients whose deficiency mimics radiation are folic acid, B_{12}, B_6, niacin, C, E, iron, and zinc, with the laboratory evidence ranging from likely to compelling. The percentage of the population that is deficient for each of these eight micronutrients ranges from 2% to 20+%, and may constitute *in toto* a considerable percentage of the population of the United States. Micronutrient deficiency is a plausible explanation for the strong epidemiological evidence that shows an association between low consumption of fruits and vegetables and cancer at most sites.

DIETARY FRUITS AND VEGETABLES AND CANCER PREVENTION

Greater consumption of fruits and vegetables is associated with a lower risk of degenerative diseases, including cancer, cardiovascular disease, cataracts, and brain dysfunction.[6] More than 200 studies in the epidemiological literature have been reviewed and show, with great consistency, an association between low consumption of fruits and vegetables and the incidence of cancer.[7–9] The quarter of the population with the lowest dietary intake of fruits and vegetables has roughly twice the cancer rate for most types of cancer (lung, larynx, oral cavity, esophagus, stomach, colon and rectum, bladder, pancreas, cervix, and ovary[7]) when compared to the quarter with the highest intake. In a different survey the lowest quartile of adults consumed 2.7 portions or less and the highest quartile 5.6 portions or more (Krebs-Smith, personal communication). These observations are consistent with data on the Seventh Day Adventists, who are nonsmokers and mostly vegetarians, and have about half the cancer mortality rate and a longer life span, than the average American.[10] Eighty percent of American children and adolescents[11] and 68% of adults[12] did not meet the intake recommended by the National Cancer Institute and the National Research Council: five servings of fruits and vegetables per day. Publicity about hundreds of minor hypothetical risks, such as that from pesticide residues in the diet,[13] has contributed to a lack of perspective on disease prevention. Half of the American population does not list fruit and vegetable consumption as a protective factor against cancer,[14] and two-thirds think that for good health only two servings per day need to be consumed.[15] Fruit and vegetable consumption is lowest among the poor, particularly African-Americans.[12,16]

Many components of fruits and vegetables may be responsible for their protective effect, such as micronutrients, plant phenolics, and fiber. This paper argues that inadequate intake of many micronutrients, such as folic acid and vitamins C and B_6 contributes to DNA damage, cancer, and degenerative disease. A major part of the protective effect of fruits and vegetables may be due to their micronutrient content. In addition, dietary deficiencies of micronutrients whose sources are not primarily fruits and vegetables, such as zinc, iron, niacin, vitamin E, and vitamin B_{12}, also appear to contribute to DNA damage and are also common in the United States. Other micronutrients are likely to be added to this list in the coming years.

Table 1. Micronutrient deficiency and DNA Damage

Micronutrient	Percent[a] U.S. Deficient	DNA Damage	Health Effects
Folic acid	10%	Chromosome breaks (Radiation mimic)	Cancer: colon Heart disease Brain dysfunction Birth defects
Vitamin B_{12}	4% (<half RDA)	Chromosome breaks?	(see Folic acid) Neuronal damage
Vitamin B_6	10% (<half RDA)	Chromosome breaks?	(see Folic acid)
Vitamin C	15% (<half RDA)	Radiation mimic (DNA oxidation)	Cataract 4× Cancer Heart disease
Vitamin E	20% (<half RDA) (RDA may be too low)	Radiation mimic (DNA oxidation)	Cancer: Colon 2× Heart disease 1.5× Immune dysfunction
Iron	7% (<half RDA) (19% women 12–50 yr)	DNA breaks Radiation mimic	Brain dysfunction Immune dysfunction Cancer
Zinc	18% (<half RDA)	Chromosome breaks Radiation mimic	Brain dysfunction Immune dysfunction Cancer
Niacin	2% (<half RDA)	Disables DNA repair (poly-ADP-ribose)	Neurological symptoms Memory loss
Selenium		Radiation mimic (DNA oxidation)	Cancer: Prostate

[a]1% = 2.7 million people

FOLIC ACID

Folate deficiency, a common vitamin deficiency in people who eat few fruits and vegetables, causes chromosome breaks in human genes.[17] Approximately 10% of the U.S. population[18,19] are deficient at the level causing chromosome breaks. In two small studies of low-income (mainly African-American) elderly[20] and adolescents[21] done nearly 20 years ago, about half had a folate deficiency at this level, though the issue should be reexamined. The mechanism of chromosome breaks has now been shown to be deficient methylation of uracil to thymine, and subsequent incorporation of uracil into human DNA (4 million/cell).[17] Uracil in DNA is excised by a repair glycosylase with the formation of a transient single-strand break in the DNA; two opposing single-strand breaks cause a double-strand chromosome break, which is difficult to repair. Both high DNA uracil levels and chromosome breaks in humans are reversed by folate administration.[17] Folate supplementation above the RDA minimized chromosome breakage.[22] Folate deficiency has been associated with increased risk of colon cancer,[23,24] and the 15-year use of a multivitamin supplement containing folate lowered colon cancer risk by about 75 percent.[25] Folate and B_{12}

deficiencies are associated with cognitive defects in humans,[17] and neurotoxicity in children is caused by methotrexate, which lowers folate pools if folate is not replenished.[26] Chromosome breaks could contribute to the increased risk of cancer, and possibly cognitive defects, associated with folate deficiency in humans.[17] Folate deficiency causes increased homocysteine accumulation, which has been associated with neural tube defects in the fetus and an estimated 10% of heart disease in the United States, both of which could be eliminated by folate supplements, food fortification, or better diets.[27–32] Homocysteine damages endothelial cells in culture and is a risk factor for arterial endothelial dysfunction in humans.[33]

A polymorphism (a common, alternate, form of a gene) in the gene for methylene-tetrahydrofolate (THF) reductase, the enzyme responsible for reducing methylene-THF to methyl-THF, results in homozygotes having a decreased activity and a twofold increase in plasma homocysteine. Homozygotes, 5–25% of individuals, depending on the ethnicity,[34,35] have an increased risk of heart disease,[30] stroke, [28,36] and neural tube defects.[35,37] This polymorphism increases the methylene-THF pool at the expense of the methyl-THF pool, resulting in decreased DNA uracil levels and increased serum homocysteine. The potential role in human carcinogenesis of uracil misincorporation is supported by two studies that show a two- to fourfold lower risk of colon cancer for individuals who are homozygous for the mutant alleles of methylene-THF reductase compared to controls.[32,38]

VITAMIN B_{12}

The main dietary source of B_{12} is meat. About 4% of the U.S. population consumes below half of the RDA of vitamin B_{12}.[5] About 14% of elderly Americans and about 24% of elderly Dutch have mild B_{12} deficiency, in part accountable by the Americans taking more vitamin supplements.[39] Vitamin B_{12} would be expected to cause chromosome breaks by the same mechanism as folate deficiency. Both B_{12} and methyl-THF are required for the methylation of homocysteine to methionine. If either folate or B_{12} is deficient, then homocysteine, a major risk factor for heart disease,[28,29] accumulates. When B_{12} is deficient, then tetrahydrofolate is trapped as methyl-THF; the methylene-THF pool, which is required for methylation of dUMP to dTMP, is consequently diminished. Therefore, B_{12} deficiency, like folate deficiency, should cause uracil to accumulate in DNA, and there is accumulating evidence for this [Ingersoll et al., unpublished and ref. 40]. The two deficiencies may act synergistically. In a study of healthy elderly men,[22] or young adults,[41] increased chromosome breakage was associated with either a deficiency in folate, or B_{12}, or with elevated levels of homocysteine. B_{12} supplementation above the RDA was necessary to minimize chromosome breakage.[41] B_{12} deficiency is known to cause neuropathy due to demyelination and loss of peripheral neurons (reviewed in ref. 17).

VITAMIN B_6

About 10% of the U.S. population consumes less than half of the RDA (1.6 mg/day) of vitamin B_6.[5] Vitamin B_6 deficiency causes a decrease in the enzyme activity of serine hydroxymethyl transferase, which supplies the methylene group for methylene-THF.[42] If the methylene-THF pool is decreased in B_6 deficiency, then uracil incorporation, with associated chromosome breaks, would be expected. Evidence for this has been found in women at a level of 32 nmol/L of vitamin B_6 in blood (0.5 mg/day intake) (Ingersoll, Shultz, and Ames, unpublished). In a case-control study of diet and cancer, vitamin B_6 intake was inversely associated with prostate cancer.[43] Vitamin B_6 deficiency appears to contribute to heart disease and supplementation reduces risk;[44] levels above the RDA may be necessary to minimize risk.[31] A level of vitamin B_6 in blood below 23 nmol/L is a risk factor for stroke and atherosclerosis.[45] Diets low in vitamin B_6 are associated with brain dysfunction in children and adults.[46] Good sources of vitamin B_6 are whole grain bread and cereal, liver, bananas, and green beans. A major source in the United States is fortified breakfast cereal.

ANTIOXIDANTS

The beneficial effects of fruits and vegetables may be due, in part, to antioxidants and other micronutrients.[6,7,47–51] Oxidant by-products of normal energy metabolism—superoxide, hydrogen peroxide, and hydroxyl radical—are the same mutagens produced by radiation. Ingesting inadequate amounts of dietary antioxidants, such as vitamins C and E, mimics radiation exposure.[6,52–54] Oxidative damage to DNA and other macromolecules appears to have a major role in aging and degenerative diseases associated with aging, such as cancer.[6,55–57] Oxidative lesions accumulate with age in DNA[58] and protein.[59] A young rat has about 24,000 oxidative DNA lesions per cell and an old rat has about 66,000.[58] DNA is oxidized in normal metabolism because antioxidant defenses, though numerous, are not perfect. When lipid is oxidized, aldehydes are produced,[60,61] some of which are mutagenic.[62–64] Aldehydes, such as malondialdehyde, bind to protein and accumulate with age.[65]

White cells and other phagocytic cells of the immune system combat bacteria, parasites, and virus-infected cells by destroying them with the mutagenic oxidizing agents NO, HOCl, and H_2O_2.[66,67] The burst of oxidants, and consequent inflammation, from phagocytic cells is a major source of NOx (a mixture of reactive nitrogen oxides) and contributes to both cancer and heart disease.[66] These oxidants protect humans from immediate death from infection, but they also cause oxidative damage to DNA, chronic cell killing with compensatory cell division, and mutation,[68,69] thus contributing to the carcinogenic process and perhaps to aging.[70] Chronic infections cause about 21% of new cancer cases in developing countries and 9% in developed countries.[71]

Antioxidants may explain much of the protective effect of fruit and vegetable intake against the stomach and lung cancer caused by chronic inflammation.[7,8] NOx is the main oxidative mutagen in cigarette smoke; it depletes the antioxidants ascorbate and α-tocopherol in smokers. Smokers in the bottom quartile of fruit and vegetable intake have about double the risk of lung cancer compared to smokers in the top quartile of intake,[7,8] probably because of decreased antioxidant intake.[72] The risk of bladder cancer is increased by smoking and decreased by supplementation with multivitamins or ascorbate.[73] Supplementation of the diet with a mixture of the antioxidant vitamins C, E, and β-carotene significantly lowered oxidative DNA damage in lymphocytes of both smokers and nonsmokers, as measured by the comet assay.[74] In a randomized trial in China in a poorly nourished population, cancer mortality was significantly decreased by a supplement of vitamin E, selenium, and β-carotene.[75] Antioxidant defenses against oxidative damage involve ascorbate (vitamin C), α-tocopherol (vitamin E), such carotenoids as β-carotene and lycopene, glutathione, lipoic acid, and selenium, zinc, and copper.

VITAMIN E

Vitamin E, the major fat-soluble antioxidant, is consumed primarily from dietary vegetable oils and nuts: 20% of the population consumes less than half of the RDA.[5] Evidence is accumulating that the optimum intake may be higher, as discussed below. Studies on vitamin E supplementation have all been done with α-tocopherol, but γ-tocopherol, the main form in the U.S. diet, has a different function than α-tocopherol, and the two complement each other.[76] γ-Tocopherol is a powerful nucleophile and thus traps electrophilic mutagens that reach the membrane. In the soluble part of the cell, glutathione acts as both an antioxidant and a nucleophile. In the membrane α-tocopherol is the antioxidant and γ-tocopherol (or lycopene) can act as a nucleophile. An important electrophilic mutagen destroyed by γ-tocopherol is NOx. γ-Tocopherol reacts with NOx to form nitro-γ-tocopherol, thus protecting lipids, DNA, and protein.[76–78]

People taking vitamin E supplements (200 IU/day) for 10 years reduced their risk of colon cancer by about half,[79] and evidence suggests a marked protective effect of a supplement (50 IU/day) on prostate cancer.[80,81] Vitamin E appears to protect against brain dysfunction,[82,83] and deficiency leads to various neuropathologies.[84]

Vitamin E supplements (100 IU–400 IU) also reduced the risk of coronary heart disease by about 40%,[85–90] as well as mortality from all causes.[87] The role of oxidants and the protective role of antioxidants in heart disease have recently been reviewed.[49,50] In a study of a population with low levels of vitamin C and E, doses of vitamin E from 70 to 560 IU lowered lipid peroxidation, whereas a dose of 1050 IU increased it,[91] emphasizing that information on the toxic level, as well as the optimum level, of each micronutrient is desirable.

Both vitamin E and selenium enhance the immune system in animals,[92] and vitamin E supplementation (200–400 units/day) enhances human immunity.[93] Vitamin E[94] or vitamin C[95] reduced oxidative stress and malformations in offspring of diabetic rats.

VITAMIN C

Fifteen percent of the U.S. population consumes less than half the RDA (60 mg/day) of ascorbate,[5] which comes from dietary fruits and vegetables.

There is a large literature on supplementation studies with vitamin C in humans using biomarkers of oxidative damage to DNA, lipids (lipid oxidation releases mutagenic aldehydes), and protein. Though there are positive and negative studies, if the fact that the blood cell saturation occurs at about 100 mg/day[96,97] is taken into consideration, then the evidence suggests that this level minimizes DNA damage.[74,98,99]

Cataracts appear to be due to oxidation of lens protein, and such antioxidants as vitamins C and E, and carotenoids appear to protect against cataracts and macular degeneration of the eye in rodents and humans.[100–102] The use of vitamin C supplements for 10 years or more reduced lens opacities by about 80 percent.[103]

Spontaneous oxidative damage in the DNA of an old rat is about 66,000 adducts per diploid cell[58] and, unlike uracil misincorporation, is likely to be equally frequent on both strands. Glycosylase repair of oxidative adducts also results in transient single-strand breaks in DNA. Therefore, increased oxidative damage, together with elevated levels of uracil in DNA, would be expected to lead to more double-strand (chromosome) breaks in individuals who are deficient in both folate and antioxidants. There is some evidence for this synergy,[104,105] which may be important, because 10–15% of men in the United States had serum ascorbate levels (< 0.3 mg/dL) close to the scurvy threshold.[5,106]

Some studies suggest that vitamin C protects against cancer, which would be plausible based on the mechanistic data, though other studies show no effect. The variable of tissue saturation again is critical. A significant protective effect was observed for renal cancer in nonsmokers, though not in smokers.[107] In a review of nutrition and pancreatic cancer, fruit and vegetable intake and vitamin C were protective, though it is difficult to rule out that vitamin C is a surrogate for some other compounds in fruits and vegetables.[108] Both experimental and epidemiological data suggest that vitamin C protects against stomach cancer,[109] a result that is plausible because of the role of oxidative damage from inflammation by *Helicobacter pylori* infection, which is the main risk factor for stomach cancer. The role of vitamin C in inhibiting oral cancer has recently been reviewed.[110] Vitamin C improves endothelial dysfunction, an early stage of atherosclerosis, in heavy smokers.[111] Vitamin C supplementation was associated with a reduction in overall mortality, and in cardiovascular disease, in a follow up of the NHANES I study.[112]

Men with low consumption of antioxidants, or who smoke, oxidize the DNA of their sperm as well as their somatic DNA. When the level of dietary vitamin C is insufficient to maintain seminal fluid vitamin C, the oxidative lesions in sperm DNA are more than doubled.[98,113] Oxidative lesions in sperm DNA are higher in smokers than nonsmokers.[53] Smoking is a severe oxidative stress, and the NOx in cigarette smoke depletes both vitamin C and vitamin E.[114] Thus, smokers must ingest two to three times more vitamin C than nonsmokers to achieve the same level in blood. They rarely do, however. Inadequate vitamin C levels are more common among the poor and smokers. Smokers also have more chromosomal abnormalities in their sperm than nonsmokers.[115]

Germ line mutations, and their associated cancer and genetic abnormalities, are predominately of paternal origin.[116] Smoking by fathers, therefore, may plausibly increase the risk of childhood cancer and birth defects, a thesis supported by epidemiological evidence.[113,114] The evidence on smoking fathers' offspring having an increased rate of childhood cancer is becoming more persuasive.[117–120] A new epidemiological study from China makes the case stronger; acute lymphocytic leukemia, lymphoma, and brain cancer are each increased three- to fourfold in offspring of male smokers.[117] The studies on paternal smoking and childhood cancer did not examine the effect of diet. It seems likely, given the above evidence, that the cancer risk to offspring of male smokers would be higher when dietary antioxidant intake is low. Maternal use of multivitamins lowers the risk of childhood cancer in offspring.[121] In one study the maternal use of vitamins throughout the pregnancy lowered the risk of brain tumors in the offspring by about half.[122] In a study of children with childhood cancer, serum levels of β-carotene, vitamin E, and zinc were significantly lower than controls.[123] Thus a multivitamin supplement (or a better diet) for both parents might markedly lower childhood cancer. In addition, several studies suggest an increased rate of birth defects in offspring of smoking fathers (reviewed in refs. 113 and 114).

Diets deficient in fruits and vegetables are commonly low in folate, antioxidants, (e.g., vitamin C) and many other micronutrients, and it seems plausible that the higher cancer rates associated with consuming deficient diets are due, in good part, to increased DNA damage.[7,17,66]

SELENIUM

Selenium is important in enzymatic defenses against oxidants, and deficiency would be expected to lead to oxidative DNA damage.[124] An RDA of 70 μg/day of selenium and an upper limit of 350 μg/day has been proposed.[125] The average intake in the United States is about 100 μg/day, though different areas of the country have different selenium levels in the soil, and the bioavailability depends on the selenium form in foods.[124]

A growing body of evidence suggests that selenium plays an important role in the prevention of cancer in a variety of organs and species.[126,127] Prostate cancer incidence was reduced by two-thirds in the selenium-supplemented group (200 μg/day) compared to the placebo group in a randomized, double-blind, cancer-prevention trial; total cancer mortality, lung, and colorectal cancer were also significantly reduced.[128,129] In a cohort study,[130] men in the highest selenium quintile of intake had only one-half the odds ratio of prostate cancer as men in the lowest quintile. In a nested, case-control prospective study on ovarian cancer, serum selenium was associated with decreased risk.[131] In a study of postmenopausal breast cancer patients, a strong inverse relationship was observed between triiodothyronine (T3) levels and cancer (OR=0.17; CI95%=0.08–0.36) between the highest and lowest tertiles.[132] Toenail selenium was positively associated with T3 levels in both cases and controls; the selenoenzyme, iodothyronine deiodinase, synthesizes T3. Prostate and breast cancer cells were about 25 times more sensitive than normal cells to selenomethionine, a major form of selenium in cells.[133] In a study of selenium intake and colorectal cancer that adjusted for possible confounders, the individuals in the lowest quartile of plasma selenium had four times the risk of colorectal adenomas compared to those in the highest quartile.[134] Selenium and glutathione peroxidase levels were found to be lowered in patients with uterine cervical carcinoma.[135] In a Chinese study, cervical cancer mortality was inversely associated with several factors, including serum selenium levels.[136]

Several hypotheses have been proposed to explain the protection against carcinogenesis by supplemental selenium.[124] One of these is its protection against oxidative damage involving selenium as an essential component of the antioxidant enzyme glutathione peroxidase,[137] or selenoprotein-P.[138–140]

Excess selenium intake appears to cause oxidative damage and cancer in rodents.[141] The case for selenium supplementation is becoming stronger, though the toxicity of high selenium levels must be taken into account.

IRON

A major dietary source of iron is meat. The United Nations Food and Agriculture Organization has estimated that the world has about 2 billion people at risk for iron deficiency, mainly women and children. In the United States about 7% of the population and about 19% of women, aged 12–50, ingest below 50% of the RDA;[5] about nine million people have been estimated to be clinically deficient.[142] Iron deficiency appears to lead to oxidative DNA damage.[143] Iron deficiency in children is associated with cognitive dysfunction.[144,145] Low iron intake results in anemia, immune dysfunction, and adverse pregnancy outcomes, such as prematurity.[145]

Excess iron appears to also lead to oxidative DNA damage in rats that is reversed by vitamin E.[146] Increased risk of human cancer[145,147] and heart disease[148,149] has been associated with excess iron.

ZINC

Major sources of zinc are meat, eggs, nuts, and whole grains. Zinc deficiency causes a variety of health effects that have been reviewed in depth.[150] Eighteen percent of the U.S. population consumes less than half the RDA for zinc (12 mg women, 15 mg men).[5] Mean daily intakes reported for poor children (5 mg), middle income children (6.3 mg), and vegetarians (6.4 mg) in the United States appear insufficient.[150] Zinc is a component of over 300 proteins, over 100 DNA-binding proteins with zinc fingers, Cu/Zn superoxide dismutase, the estrogen receptor, and the synaptic transmission protein.[150] Functioning of p53, a zinc protein that is mutated in half of human tumors, is disrupted on loss of zinc.[151] P53 prevents mutation by inhibiting cell division and inducing apoptosis in response to DNA lesions.[152]

Chromosome breaks in rats have been reported with a zinc-deficient diet.[153] The offspring of zinc-deficient rhesus monkeys also have increased chromosome breaks.[154] The chromosome breaks might be due to increased oxidative damage,[154,155] perhaps due to loss of activity of Cu/Zn superoxide dismutase or the zinc-containing DNA-repair enzyme, Fapy glycosylase, which repairs oxidized guanine.[156] Zinc deficiency has been suggested as a contributor to esophageal cancer in humans and has been shown to cause esophageal tumors in rats in conjunction with a single low dose of a nitrosamine.[157–159] Severe zinc deficiency by itself can cause esophageal tumors in rats.[159]

Zinc is known to be an essential trace element for testicular development and spermatogenesis.[160] Zinc concentrations in seminal plasma are hundreds of times greater than that in blood plasma, which suggests a specific function for this trace element in spermatogenesis and stability of spermatozoa.[150] Zinc concentrations are correlated positively with sperm cell density, and lower zinc concentrations are found in infertile men compared with fertile men.[161] Zinc deficiency leads to increased oxidative damage to testicular cell DNA (as measured by oxo^8dG) and increased protein carbonyl content.[162]

A considerable literature in experimental animals and humans suggests that zinc deficiency slows growth and development of the neonate. Severe deficiency in animals is teratogenic.[154] In a pair-matched, double-blind, study in Chile of preschool boys of low socioeconomic status, those supplemented with 10 mg zinc/day grew significantly more rapidly than the placebo group.[163] This is consistent with earlier reports in the United States and other countries on growth stimulation of poor children supplemented with zinc.[150]

Zinc deficiency leads to alterations in brain development and growth.[144] Zinc deficiency in pregnant rats, at a level that does not impair the pregnancy or the growth of the pups, impairs cognitive function in adult offspring.[150] Zinc deficiency in adult rats impairs hippocampal and behavioral functions.[150] Several studies on monkeys show that maternal zinc deficiency leads to learning and behavioral disabilities in offspring.[150] Six studies in humans suggest that zinc deficiency leads to cognitive defects.[150]

Several animal and human studies indicate that mild zinc deficiency impairs the immune system.[150,164] The incidence of respiratory infections in a group of institutionalized elderly was decreased by over twofold ($p = <0.01$) when they were given a supplement of zinc (20 mg) plus selenium (100 mg) in a double-blind placebo study; in other studies very high doses of zinc (100–150 mg/day) had an adverse effect on the immune system.[165]

NIACIN

In the United States, 2.3% of the population consumes less than half the RDA for niacin.[5] The main dietary sources of niacin include meat and beans. Tryptophan from protein can also provide niacin equivalents.[166] Fifteen percent of some populations have been reported to be severely deficient.[167] Niacin contributes to the repair of DNA breaks by maintaining nicotinamide adenine dinucleotide levels for the poly-ADP ribose protective response to DNA damage;[168–170] deficiency compromises repair of DNA nicks and breaks and thus is expected to act synergistically with folate and antioxidant deficiencies in causing DNA damage and cancer.[171]

[NOTE ADDED IN PROOF: Several recent references that were added (173–175) are relevant to folate/B_{12}/B_6 deficiency.]

ACKNOWLEDGMENTS

This work was supported by the National Cancer Institute Outstanding Investigator Grant CA39910, the National Institute of Environmental Health Sciences Center Grant ESO1896, and a National Foundation for Cancer Research Grant. This paper was adapted, in part, from Ames.[172] We are indebted to A. Huang and T. Nufert for critiques.

REFERENCES

1. SALTMAN, P., J. GURIN & I. MOTHNER. 1993. The University of California San Diego Nutrition Book. Little, Brown & Company. Boston.
2. INSTITUTE OF MEDICINE. 1997. Dietary Reference Intakes: Calcium, Phosphorus, Magnesium, Vitamin D, and Fluoride. Committee on the Scientific Evaluation of Dietary Reference Intakes, Food and Nutrition Board, National Academy of Sciences, Washington, D. C. National Academy Press.
3. INSTITUTE OF MEDICINE. 1998. Dietary Reference Intakes for Thiamin, Riboflavin, Niacin, Vitamin B_6, Folate, Vitamin B_{12}, Pantothenic Acid, Biotin, and Choline. Committee on the Scientific Evaluation of Dietary Reference Intakes, Food and Nutrition Board, National Academy of Sciences, Washington, D. C. National Academy Press.
4. NATIONAL RESEARCH COUNCIL. 1989. Recommended Dietary Allowances. Subcommittee on the Tenth Edition of the RDAs, Food and Nutrition Board. Commission on Life Sciences, National Academy of Sciences, Washington D.C. National Academy Press.
5. WILSON, J.W., C.W. ENNS, J.D. GOLDMAN, K.S. TIPPETT, S.J. MICKLE, L.E. CLEVELAND & P.S. CHAHIL. 1997. Data tables: Combined results from USDA's 1994 and 1995 continuing survey of food intakes by individuals and 1994 and 1995 diet and health knowledge survey. USDA/ARS Food Surveys Research Group, Beltsville Human Nutrition Research Center. Riverdale, MD.
6. AMES, B.N., M.K. SHIGENAGA & T.M. HAGEN. 1993. Oxidants, antioxidants, and the degenerative diseases of aging. Proc. Natl. Acad. Sci. USA **90:** 7915–7922.
7. BLOCK, G., B. PATTERSON & A. SUBAR. 1992. Fruit, vegetables and cancer prevention: A review of the epidemiologic evidence. Nutr. Cancer **18:** 1–29.
8. STEINMETZ, K.A. & J.D. POTTER. 1996. Vegetables, fruit, and cancer prevention: A review. J. Am. Diet. Assoc. **96:** 1027–1039.
9. WILLETT, W.C. & D. TRICHOPOULOS. 1996. Nutrition and cancer: A summary of the evidence. Cancer Causes & Control **7:** 178–180.
10. MILLS, P.K., W.L. BEESON, R.L. PHILLIPS & G.E. FRASER. 1994. Cancer incidence among California Seventh-day Adventists. Am. J. Clin. Nutr. **59** (Suppl.): 1136S–1142S.
11. KREBS-SMITH, S.M., A. COOK, A.F. SUBAR, L. CLEVELAND, J. FRIDAY & L.L. KAHLE. 1996. Fruit and vegetable intakes of children and adolescents in the United States. Arch. Pediatr. Adolesc. Med. **150:** 81–86.
12. KREBS-SMITH, S.M., A. COOK, A.F. SUBAR, L. CLEVELAND & J. FRIDAY. 1995. US adults' fruit and vegetable intakes, 1989 to 1991: A revised baseline for the *healthy people 2000* objective. Am. J. Public Health **85:** 1623–1629.
13. AMES, B.N. & L.S. GOLD. 1997. Environmental pollution, pesticides, and the prevention of cancer: Misconceptions. FASEB J. **11:** 1041–1052.
14. NATIONAL CANCER INSTITUTE GRAPHIC. 1996. Why eat five? J. Natl. Cancer Inst. **88:** 1314.
15. KREBS-SMITH, S., J. HEIMENDINGER, B. PATTERSON, A. SUBAR, R. KESSLER & E. PIVONKA. 1995. Psychosocial factors associated with fruit and vegetables consumption. Am. J. Health Promot. **10:** 98–104.
16. POPKIN, B.M., A.M. SIEGA-RIZ & P.S. HAINES. 1997. Correction and revision of conclusions—Dietary trends in the United States. N. Engl. J. Med. **337:** 1846–1848.
17. BLOUNT, B.C., M.M. MACK, C. WEHR, J. MACGREGOR, R. HIATT, G. WANG, S.N. WICKRAMASINGHE, R.B. EVERSON & B.N. AMES. 1997. Folate deficiency causes uracil misincorporation into human DNA and chromosome breakage: Implications for cancer and neuronal damage. Proc. Natl. Acad. Sci. USA **94:** 3290–3295.
18. SENTI, F.R. & S.M. PILCH. 1985. Analysis of folate data from the second National Health and Nutrition Examination Survey (NHANES II). J. Nutr. **115:** 1398–1402.

19. SUBAR, A.F., G. BLOCK & L.D. JAMES. 1989. Folate intake and food sources in the US population. Am. J. Clin. Nutr. **50:** 508–516.
20. BAILEY, L.B., P.A. WAGNER, G.J. CHRISTAKIS, P.E. ARAUJO, H. APPLEDORF, C.G. DAVIS, J. MASTERYANNI & J.S. DINNING. 1979. Folacin and iron status and hematological findings in predominately black elderly persons from urban low-income households. Am. J. Clin. Nutr. **32:** 2346–2353.
21. BAILEY, L.B., P.A. WAGNER, G.J. CHRISTAKIS, C.G. DAVIS, H. APPLEDORF, P.E. ARAUJO, E. DORSEY & J.S. DINNING. 1982. Folacin and iron status and hematological findings in black and Spanish-American adolescents from urban low-income households. Am. J. Clin. Nutr. **35:** 1023–1032.
22. FENECH, M.F., I.E. DREOSTI & J.R. RINALDI. 1997. Folate, vitamin B12, homocysteine status and chromosome damage rate in lymphocytes of older men. Carcinogenesis **18:** 1329–1336.
23. GIOVANNUCCI, E., M.J. STAMPFER, G.A. COLDITZ, E.B. RIMM, D. TRICHOPOULOS, B.A. ROSNER, F.E. SPEIZER & W.C. WILLETT. 1993. Folate, methionine, and alcohol intake and risk of colorectal adenoma. J. Natl. Cancer Inst. **85:** 875–884.
24. MASON, J.B. 1994. Folate and colonic carcinogenesis: Searching for a mechanistic understanding. J. Nutr. Biochem. **5:** 170–175.
25. GIOVANNUCCI, E., M. J. STAMPFER, G. A. COLDITZ, D. J. HUNGER, C. FUCHS, B.A. ROSNER, F.E. SPEIZER & W.C. WILLETT. 1998. Multivitamin use, folate, and colon cancer in women in the nurses' health study. Ann. Intern. Med. **129:** 517–524.
26. QUINN, C.T., J.C. GRIENER, T. BOTTIGLIERI, K. HYLAND, A. FARROW & B.A. KAMEN. 1997. Elevation of homocysteine and excitatory amino acid neurotransmitters in the CSF of children who receive methotrexate for the treatment of cancer. J. Clin. Oncol. **15:** 2800–2806.
27. BERESFORD, S.A.A. & C.J. BOUSHEY. 1997. Homocysteine, folic acid, and cardiovascular disease risk. *In* Preventive Nutrition: The Comprehensive Guide for Health Professionals. A. Bendich & R.J. Deckelbaum, Eds.: 193–224. Humana Press, Inc. Totowa, NJ.
28. BOUSHEY, C.J., S.A. BERESFORD, G.S. OMENN & A.G. MOTULSKY. 1995. A quantitative assessment of plasma homocysteine as a risk factor for vascular disease. Probable benefits of increasing folic acid intakes. J. Am. Med. Assoc. **274:** 1049–1057.
29. OAKLEY, G.P., JR., M.J. ADAMS & C.M. DICKINSON. 1996. More folic acid for everyone, now. J. Nutr. **126:** 751S–755S.
30. REFSUM, H., P.M. UELAND, O. NYGÅRD & S.E. VOLLSET. 1998. Homocysteine and cardiovascular disease. Annu. Rev. Med. **49:** 31–62.
31. RIMM, E.B., W.C. WILLETT, F.B. HU, L. SAMPSON, G.A. COLDITZ, J.E. MANSON, C. HENNEKENS & M.J. STAMPFER. 1998. Folate and vitamin B_6 from diet and supplements in relation to risk of coronary heart disease among women. J. Am. Med. Assoc. **279:** 359–364.
32. TUCKER, K.L., B. MAHNKEN, P.W. WILSON, P. JACQUES & J. SELHUB. 1996. Folic acid fortification of the food supply: Potential benefits and risks for the elderly population. J. Am. Med. Assoc. **276:** 1879–1885.
33. WOO, K.S., P. CHOOK, Y.I. LOLIN, A.S.P. CHEUNG, L.T. CHAN, Y.Y. SUN, J.E. SANDERSON, C. METREWELI & D.S. CELERMAJER. 1997. Hyperhomocyst(e)inemia is a risk factor for arterial endothelial dysfunction in humans. Circulation **96:** 2542–2544.
34. FROSST, P., H.J. BLOM, R. MILOS, P. GOYETTE, C.A. SHEPPARD, R.G. MATTHEWS, G.J. BOERS, M. DEN HEIJER, L.A. KLUIJTMANS, L.P. VAN DEN HEUVEL & R. ROZEN. 1995. A candidate genetic risk factor for vascular disease: A common mutation in methylenetetrahydrofolate reductase [letter]. Nat. Genet. **10:** 111–113.

35. WHITEHEAD, A.S., P. GALLAGHER, J.L. MILLS, P.N. KIRKE, H. BURKE, A.M. MOLLOY, D.G. WEIR, D.C. SHIELDS & J.M. SCOTT. 1995. A genetic defect in 5,10 methylene-tetrahydrofolate reductase in neural tube defects. Q. J. Med. **88:** 763–766.
36. MORRISON, H.I., D. SCHAUBEL, M. DESMEULES & D.T. WIGLE. 1996. Serum folate and risk of fatal coronary heart disease [see comments]. J. Am. Med. Assoc. **275:** 1893–1896.
37. POSEY, D.L., M.J. KOURY, J. MULINARE, M.J. ADAMS, JR. & C.Y. OU. 1996. Is mutated MTHFR a risk factor for neural tube defects? Lancet **347:** 686–687.
38. CHEN, J., E. GIOVANNUCCI, K. KELSEY, E.B. RIMM, M.J. STAMPFER, G.A. COLDITZ, D. SPIEGELMEN, W.C. WILLETT & D.J. HUNTER. 1996. A methylenetetrahydrofolate reductase polymorphism and the risk of colorectal cancer. Cancer Res. **56:** 4862–4864.
39. VAN ASSELT, D.Z., L.C. DE GROOT, W.A. VAN STAVEREN, B.H. J, R.A. WEVERS, I. BIEMOND & W.H. HOEFNAGELS. 1998. Role of cobalamin intake and atrophic gastritis in mild cobalamin deficiency in older Dutch subjects. Am. J. Clin. Nutr. **68:** 328–334.
40. WICKRAMASINGHE, S.N. & S. FIDA. 1994. Bone marrow cells from vitamin B_{12}- and folate-deficient patients misincorporate uracil into DNA. Blood **83:** 1656–1661.
41. FENECH, M., C. AITKEN & J. RINALDI. 1998. Folate, vitamin B_{12}, homocysteine status and DNA damage in young Australian adults. Carcinogenesis **19:** 1163–1171.
42. STABLER, S.P., D.A. SAMPSON, L.P. WANG & R.H. ALLEN. 1997. Elevations of serum cystathionine and total homocysteine in pyridoxine-, folate-, and cobalamin-deficient rats. J. Nutr. Biochem. **8:** 279–289.
43. KEY, T.J., P.B. SILCOCKS, G.K. DAVEY, P.N. APPLEBY & D.T. BISHOP. 1997. A case-control study of diet and prostate cancer. Br. J. Cancer **76:** 678–687.
44. RIMM, E., W. WILLETT, J. MANSON, F. SPEIZER, C. HENNEKENS & M. STAMPFER. 1996. Folate and vitamin B_6 intake and risk of myocardial infarction among U.S. women (abstract). Am. J. Epidemiol. **143** (Suppl): S36.
45. ROBINSON, K., K. ARHEART, H. REFSUM, L. BRATTSTROM, G. BOERS, P. UELAND, P. RUBBA, R. PALMA-REIS, R. MELEADY, L. DALY, J. WITTEMAN & I. GRAHAM. 1998. Low circulating folate and vitamin B_6 concentrations: Risk factors for stroke, peripheral vascular disease, and coronary artery disease. European COMAC Group. Circulation **97:** 437–443.
46. LEKLEM, J.E. 1996. Vitamin B-6. *In* Present Knowledge in Nutrition. E.E. Ziegler & L.J. Filer, Jr., Eds.: 174–183. ILSI Press. Washington, D.C.
47. BLOCK, G. 1992. The data support a role for antioxidants in reducing cancer risk. Nutr. Rev. **50:** 207–213.
48. BYERS, T. & N. GUERRERO. 1995. Epidemiologic evidence for vitamin C and vitamin E in cancer prevention. Am. J. Clin. Nutr. **62:** 13855–13925.
49. DIAZ, M.N., B. FREI, J.A. VITA & J.F. KEANEY, JR. 1997. Antioxidants and atherosclerotic heart disease. N. Engl. J. Med. **337:** 408–416.
50. DIPLOCK, A.T. 1997. Commentary. Will the 'Good Fairies' please prove to us that vitamin E lessens human degenerative disease? Free Radical Res. **27:** 511–532.
51. HERCBERG, S., P. GALAN, P. PREZIOSI, M.J. ALFAREZ & C. VAZQUEZ. 1998. The potential role of antioxidant vitamins in preventing cardiovascular diseases and cancers. Nutrition **14:** 513–520.
52. BECKMAN, K.B. & B.N. AMES. 1997. Oxidative decay of DNA. J. Biol. Chem. **272:** 19633–19636.
53. FRAGA, C.G., P.A. MOTCHNIK, A.J. WYROBEK, D.M. REMPEL & B.N. AMES. 1996. Smoking and low antioxidant levels increase oxidative damage to sperm DNA. Mutat. Res. **351:** 199–203.

54. GERSTER, H. 1995. Beta-carotene, vitamin E and vitamin C in different stages of experimental carcinogenesis. Eur. J. Clin. Nutr. **49:** 155–168.
55. BECKMAN, K.B. & B.N. AMES. 1998. The free radical theory of aging matures. Physiol. Rev. **78:** 547–581.
56. HAGEN, T.M., D.L. YOWE, J.C. BARTHOLOMEW, C.M. WEHR, K.L. DO, J.-Y. PARK AND B.N. AMES. 1997. Mitochondrial decay in hepatocytes from old rats: Membrane potential declines, heterogeneity and oxidants increase. Proc. Natl. Acad. Sci. USA **94:** 3064–3069.
57. HAGEN, T.M., R.T. INGERSOLL, C.M. WEHR, J. LYKKESFELDT, V. VINARSKY, J.C. BARTHOLOMEW, M.-H. SONG & B.N. AMES. 1998. Acetyl-L-Carnitine fed to old rats partially restores mitochondrial function and ambulatory activity. Proc. Natl. Acad. Sci. USA **95:** 9562–9566.
58. HELBOCK, H.J., K.B. BECKMAN, M.K. SHIGENAGA, P. WALTER, A.A. WOODALL, H.C. YEO & B.N. AMES. 1998. DNA oxidation matters: The HPLC-EC assay of 8-oxo-deoxyguanosine and 8-oxo-guanine. Proc. Natl. Acad. Sci. USA **95:** 288–293.
59. BERLETT, B.S. & E.R. STADTMAN. 1997. Protein oxidation in aging, disease, and oxidative stress. J. Biol. Chem. **272:** 20313–20316.
60. LIU, J., H.C. YEO, S.J. DONIGER & B.N. AMES. 1997. Assay of aldehydes from lipid peroxidation: Gas chromatography—mass spectrometry compared to thiobarbituric acid. Anal. Biochem. **245:** 161–166.
61. YEO, H.C., H.J. HELBOCK, D.W. CHYU & B.N. AMES. 1994. Assay of malondialdehyde in biological fluids by gas chromatography-mass spectrometry. Anal. Biochem. **220:** 391–396.
62. BURCHAM, P.C. 1998. Genotoxic lipid peroxidation products: Their DNA damaging properties and role in formation of endogenous DNA adducts. Mutagenesis **13:** 287–305.
63. DEDON, P.C., J.P. PLASTARAS, C.A. ROUZER & L.J. MARNET. 1998. Indirect mutagenesis by oxidative DNA damage: Formation of the pyrimidopurinone adduct of deoxyguanosine by base propenal. Proc. Natl. Acad. Sci. USA **95:** 11113–11116.
64. MARNETT, L.J., H. HURD, M.C. HOLLSTEIN, D.E. ESTERBAUER & B.N. AMES. 1985. Naturally occurring carbonyl compounds are mutagens in *Salmonella* tester strain TA104. Mutat. Res. **148:** 25–34.
65. HAGEN, T.M., R.T. INGERSOLL, J. LIU, J. LYKKESFELDT, C.M. WEHR, V. VINARSKY, J.C. BARTHOLOMEW & B.N. AMES. 1998. (R)-α-Lipoic acid-supplemented old rats have improved mitochondrial function, decreased oxidative damage, and increased metabolic rate. FASEB J. **13:** 411–418.
66. AMES, B.N., L.S. GOLD & W.C. WILLETT. 1995. The causes and prevention of cancer. Proc. Natl. Acad. Sci. USA **92:** 5258–5265.
67. CHRISTEN, S., T.M. HAGEN, M.K. SHIGENAGA & B.N. AMES. 1999. Chronic infection and inflammation lead to mutation and cancer. *In* Microbes and Malignancy: Infection as a Cause of Cancer. J. Parsonnet & S. Horning, Eds.: 35–88. Oxford University Press. Oxford.
68. SHACTER, E., E.J. BEECHAM, J.M. COVEY, K.W. KOHN & M. POTTER. 1988. Activated neutrophils induce prolonged DNA damage in neighboring cells [published erratum appears in Carcinogenesis 1989 **10**(3):628]. Carcinogenesis **9:** 2297–2304.
69. YAMASHINA, K., B.E. MILLER & G.H. HEPPNER. 1986. Macrophage-mediated induction of drug-resistant variants in a mouse mammary tumor cell line. Cancer Res. **46:** 2396–2401.
70. KUKOVETZ, E.M., G. BRATSCHITSCH, H.P. HOFER, G. EGGER & R.J. SCHAUR. 1997. Influence of age on the release of reactive oxygen species by phagocytes as measured by a whole blood chemiluminescence assay. Free Rad. Biol. Med. **22:** 433–438.

71. PISANI, P., D.M. PARKIN, N. MUÑOZ & J. FERLAY. 1997. Cancer and infection: Estimates of the attributable fraction in 1990. Cancer Epidemiol. Biomarkers Prev. **6:** 387–400.

72. YONG, L.C., C.C. BROWN, A. SCHATZKIN, C.M. DRESSER, M.J. SLESINSKI, C.S. COX & P.R. TAYLOR. 1997. Intake of vitamins E, C and A and risk of lung cancer—The NHANES I Epidemiologic Followup Study. Am. J. Epidemiol. **146:** 231–243.

73. BRUEMMER, B., E. WHITE, T.L. VAUGHAN & C.L. CHENEY. 1996. Nutrient intake in relation to bladder cancer among middle-aged men and women. Am. J. Epidemiol. **144:** 485–495.

74. DUTHIE, S.J., A. MA, M.A. ROSS & A.R. COLLINS. 1996. Antioxidant supplementation decreases oxidative DNA damage in human lymphocytes. Cancer Res. **56:** 1291–1295.

75. BLOT, W.J. 1997. Vitamin/mineral supplementation and cancer risk: International chemoprevention trials. Proc. Soc. Exp. Biol. Med. **216:** 291–296.

76. CHRISTEN, S., A.A. WOODALL, M.K. SHIGENAGA, P.T. SOUTHWELL-KEELY, M.W. DUNCAN & B.N. AMES. 1997. γ-Tocopherol traps mutagenic electrophiles such as NOx and complements α-tocopherol: Physiological implications. Proc. Natl. Acad. Sci. USA **94:** 3217–3222.

77. COONEY, R.V., P.J. HARWOOD, A.A. FRANKE, K. NARALA, A.K. SUNDSTROM, P.-O. BERGGREN & L.J. MORDAN. 1995. Products of gamma-tocopherol reaction with NO2 and their formation in rat insulinoma (RINm5F) cells. Free Rad. Biol. Med. **19:** 259–269.

78. SHIGENAGA, M.K., H. LEE, B. BLOUNT, S. CHRISTEN, E.T. SHIGENO, H. YIP & B.N. AMES. 1997. Inflammation and NOX-induced nitration: Assay for 3-nitrotyrosine by HPLC with electrochemical detection. Proc. Natl. Acad. Sci. USA **94:** 3211–3216.

79. WHITE, E., J.S. SHANNON & R.E. PATTERSON. 1997. Relationship between vitamin and calcium supplement use and colon cancer. Cancer Epidemiol. Biomarkers Prev. **6:** 769–774.

80. HARTMAN, T.J., D. ALBANES, P. PIETINEN, A.M. HARTMAN, M. RAUTALAHTI, J.A. TANGREA & P.R. TAYLOR. 1998. The association between baseline vitamin E, selenium, and prostate cancer in the alpha-tocopherol, beta-carotene cancer prevention study. Cancer Epidemiol. Biomarkers Prev. **7:** 335–340.

81. HEINONEN, O.P., D. ALBANES, J. VIRTAMO, P.R. TAYLOR, J.K. HUTTUNEN, A.M. HARTMAN, J. HAAPAKOSKI, N. MALILA, M. RAUTALAHTI, S. RIPATTI, H. MAENPAA, L. TEERENHOVI, L. KOSS, M. VIROLAINEN & B.K. EDWARDS. 1998. Prostate cancer and supplementation with alpha-tocopherol and beta-carotene: Incidence and mortality in a controlled trial [see comments]. J. Natl. Cancer Inst. **90:** 440–446.

82. LETHEM, R. & M. ORRELL. 1997. Antioxidants and dementia. Lancet **349:** 1189–1189.

83. SANO, M., C. ERNESTO, R.G. THOMAS, M.R. KLAUBER, K. SCHAFER, M. GRUNDMAN, P. WOODBURY, J. GROWDON, C.W. COTMAN, E. PFEIFFER, L.S. SCHNEIDER & L.J. THAL. 1997. A controlled trial of selegiline, alpha-tocopherol, or both as treatment for Alzheimer's disease. The Alzheimer's Disease Cooperative Study. N. Engl. J. Med. **336:** 1216–1222.

84. SOKOL, R.J. 1996. Vitamin E. *In* Present Knowledge in Nutrition. E.E. Ziegler & L.J. Filer, Jr., Eds.: 130–136. ILSI Press. Washington, D. C.

85. BURING, J.E. & J.M. GAZIANO. 1997. Antioxidant vitamins and cardiovascular disease. *In* Preventive Nutrition: The Comprehensive Guide for Health Professionals. A. Bendich & R.J. Deckelbaum, Eds.: 171–180. Humana Press, Inc. Totowa, NJ.

86. KUSHI, L.H., A.R. FOLSOM, R.J. PRINEAS, P.J. MINK, Y. WU & R.M. BOSTICK. 1996. Dietary antioxidant vitamins and death from coronary heart disease in postmenopausal women. N. Engl. J. Med. **334:** 1156–1162.

87. LOSONCZY, K.G., T.B. HARRIS & R.J. HAVLIK. 1996. Vitamin E and vitamin C supplement use and risk of all-cause and coronary heart disease mortality in older persons: The established populations for epidemiologic studies of the elderly. Am. J. Clin. Nutr. **64:** 190–196.
88. RIMM, E.B., M.J. STAMPFER, A. ASCHERIO, E. GIOVANNUCCI, G.A. COLDITZ & W.C. WILLETT. 1993. Vitamin E consumption and the risk of coronary heart disease in men. N. Engl. J. Med. **328:** 1450–1456.
89. STAMPFER, M.J. & E.B. RIMM. 1995. Epidemiologic evidence for vitamin E in prevention of cardiovascular disease. Am. J. Clin. Nutr. **62** (Suppl): 1365S–1369S.
90. STEPHENS, N.G., A. PARSONS, P.M. SCHOFIELD, F. KELLY, K. CHEESEMAN, M.J. MITCHINSON & M.J. BROWN. 1996. Randomised controlled trial of vitamin E in patients with coronary disease: Cambridge Heart Antioxidant Study (CHAOS). Lancet **347:** 781–786.
91. BROWN, K.M., P.C. MORRICE & G.G. DUTHIE. 1997. Erythrocyte vitamin E and plasma ascorbate concentrations in relation to erythrocyte peroxidation in smoker and nonsmokers: Dose response to vitamin E supplementation. Am. J. Clin. Nutr. **65:** 496–502.
92. FINCH, J.M. & R.J. TURNER. 1996. Effects of selenium and vitamin E on the immune responses of domestic animals. Res. Vet. Sci. **60:** 97–106.
93. MEYDANI, S.N., M. MEYDANI, J.B. BLUMBERG, L.S. LEKA, G. SIBER, R. LOSZEWSKI, C. THOMPSON, M.C. PEDROSA, R.D. DIAMOND & B.D. STOLLAR. 1997. Vitamin E supplementation and *in vivo* immune response in healthy elderly subjects: A randomized controlled trial. J. Am. Med. Assoc. **277:** 1380–1386.
94. SIMÁN, C.M. & U.J. ERIKSSON. 1997. Vitamin E decreases the occurrence of malformations in the offspring of diabetic rats. Diabetes **46:** 1054–1061.
95. SIMÁN, C.M. & U.J. ERIKSSON. 1997. Vitamin C supplementation of the maternal diet reduces the rate of malformation in the offspring of diabetic rats. Diabetologia **40:** 1416–1424.
96. KALLNER, A., D. HARTMANN & D. HORNIG. 1979. Steady-state turnover and body pool of ascorbic acid in man. Am. J. Clin. Nutr. **32:** 530–539.
97. LEVINE, M., C. CONRY-CANTILENA, Y. WANG, R.W. WELCH, P.W. WASHKO, K.R. DHARIWAL, J.B. PARK, A. LAZAREV, J.F. GRAUMLICH, J. KING & L.R. CANTILENA. 1996. Vitamin C pharmacokinetics in healthy volunteers: Evidence for a recommended dietary allowance. Proc. Natl. Acad. Sci. USA **93:** 3704–3709.
98. FRAGA, C.G., P.A. MOTCHNIK, M.K. SHIGENAGA, H.J. HELBOCK, R.A. JACOB & B.N. AMES. 1991. Ascorbic acid protects against endogenous oxidative damage in human sperm. Proc. Natl. Acad. Sci. USA **88:** 11003–11006.
99. HARATS, D., S. CHEVION, M. NAHIR, Y. NORMAN, O. SAGEE & E.M. BERRY. 1998. Citrus fruit supplementation reduces lipoprotein oxidation in young men ingesting a diet high in saturated fat: Presumptive evidence for an interaction between vitamins C and E *in vivo*. Am. J. Clin. Nutr. **67:** 240–245.
100. HANKINSON, S.E., M.J. STAMPFER, J.M. SEDDON, G.A. COLDITZ, B. ROSNER, F.E. SPEIZER & W.C. WILLETT. 1992. Nutrient intake and cataract extraction in women: A prospective study. Br. Med. J. **305:** 335–339.
101. HUNG, S. & J.M. SEDDON. 1997. The relationship between nutritional factors and age-related macular degeneration. *In* Preventive Nutrition: The Comprehensive Guide for Health Professionals. A. Bendich & R.J. Deckelbaum, Eds.: 245–265. Human Press, Inc. Totowa, NJ.
102. TAYLOR, A. & P.F. JACQUES. 1997. Antioxidant status and risk for cataract. *In* Preventive Nutrition: The Comprehensive Guide for Health Professionals. A. Bendich & R.J. Deckelbaum, Eds.: 267–283. Humana Press, Inc. Totowa, NJ.
103. JACQUES, P.F., A. TAYLOR, S.E. HANKINSON, W.C. WILLETT, B. MAHNKEN, Y. LEE, K. VAID & M. LAHAV. 1997. Long-term vitamin C supplement use and prevalence of early age-related lens opacities. Am. J. Clin. Nutr. **66:** 911–916.
104. MACGREGOR, J.T., C.M. WEHR, R.A. HIATT, B. PETERS, J.D. TUCKER, R. LANGLOIS, R.A. JACOB, R.H. JENSEN, J.W. YAGER, M.K. SHIGENAGA, B. FREI, B.P. EYNON &

B.N. AMES. 1997. "Spontaneous" genetic damage in man: Evaluation of interindividual variability, relationship among markers of damage, and influence of nutritional status. Mutat. Res. **377:** 125–135.

105. WALLOCK, L., A. WOODALL, R. JACOB & B. AMES. 1997. Nutritional status and positive relation of plasma folate to fertility indices in nonsmoking men [abstract]. FASEB J. **11:** A184 –1068.

106. NATIONAL CENTER FOR HEALTH STATISTICS. 1982. Hematological and nutritional biochemistry reference data for persons 6 months-74 years of age: United States 1976-1980. Vital and Health Statistics. U.S. Government Printing Office. Washington, DC.

107. WOLK, A., P. LINDBLAD & H.-O. ADAMI. 1996. Nutrition and renal cell cancer. Cancer Causes & Control **7:** 5–18.

108. HOWE, G.R. & J.D. BURCH. 1996. Nutrition and pancreatic cancer. Cancer Causes & Control **7:** 69–82.

109. KONO, S. & T. HIROHATA. 1996. Nutrition and stomach cancer. Cancer Causes & Control **7:** 41–55.

110. CHAN, S.W.Y. & P.C. READE. 1998. The role of ascorbic acid in oral cancer and carcinogenesis. Oral Dis. **4:** 120–129.

111. HEITZER, T., H. JUST & T. MÜNZEL. 1996. Antioxidant vitamin C improves endothelial dysfunction in chronic smokers. Circulation **94:** 6–9.

112. ENSTROM, J.E., L.E. KANIM & M.A. KLEIN. 1992. Vitamin C intake and mortality among a sample of the United States population. Epidemiology **3:** 194–202.

113. AMES, B.N., P.A. MOTCHNIK, C.G. FRAGA, M.K. SHIGENAGA & T.M. HAGEN. 1994. Antioxidant prevention of birth defects and cancer. *In* Male-Mediated Developmental Toxicity. D.R. Mattison & A. Olshan, Eds.: 243–259. Plenum Publishing Corporation. New York.

114. MAYR, C.A., A.A. WOODALL & B.N. AMES. 1999. DNA damage to sperm from micronutrient deficiency may increase the risk of birth defects and cancer in offspring. *In* Preventative Nutrition: The Comprehensive Guide for Health Professionals. A. Bendich & R. Deckelbaum, Eds. Humana Press. Totowa, NJ. In press.

115. WYROBEK, A.J., J. RUBES, M. CASSEL, D. MOORE, S. PERRAULT, V. SLOTT, D. EVENSON, Z. ZUDOVA, L. BORKOVEC, S. SELEVAN & X. LOWE. 1995. Smokers produce more aneuploid sperm than non-smokers. Am. J. Hum. Genet. **57:** 737.

116. CROW, J. 1993. How much do we know about spontaneous human mutation rates? Environ. Mol. Mutagen. **21:** 122–129.

117. JI, B.-T., X.-O. SHU, M.S. LINET, W. ZHENG, S. WACHOLDER, Y.-T. GAO, D.-M. YING & F. JIN. 1997. Paternal cigarette smoking and the risk of childhood cancer among offspring of nonsmoking mothers. J. Natl. Cancer Inst. **89:** 238–244.

118. SORAHAN, T., R.J. LANCASHIRE, P. PRIOR, I. PECK & A.M. STEWART. 1995. Childhood cancer and parental use of alcohol and tobacco. Ann. Epidemiol. **5:** 354–359.

119. SORAHAN, T., R.J. LANCASHIRE, M.A. HULTEN, I. PECK & A.M. STEWART. 1997. Childhood cancer and parental use of tobacco—deaths from 1953 to 1955. Br. J. Cancer **75:** 134–138.

120. SORAHAN, T., P. PRIOR, R.J. LANCASHIRE, S.P. FAUX, M.A. HULTEN, I. PECK & A.M. STEWART. 1997. Childhood cancer and parental use of tobacco: Deaths from 1971 to 1976. Br. J. Cancer **76:** 1525–1531.

121. BUNIN, G.R. & J.M. CARY. 1997. Diet and childhood cancer. *In* Preventive Nutrition: The Comprehensive Guide for Health Professionals. A. Bendich & R.J. Deckelbaum, Eds.: 17–32. Humana Press, Inc. Totowa, NJ.

122. PRESTON-MARTIN, S., J.M. POGODA, B.A. MUELLER, E.A. HOLLY, W. LIJINSKY & R.L. DAVIS. 1996. Maternal consumption of cured meats and vitamins in relation to pediatric brain tumors. Cancer Epidemiol. Biomarkers Prev. **5:** 599–605.

123. MALVY, D.J., J. ARNAUD, B. BURTSCHY, D. SOMMELET, G. LEVERGER, L. DOSTA-
     LOVA & O. AMEDEE-MANESME. 1997. Antioxidant micronutrients and childhood
     malignancy during oncological treatment. Med. Pediatr. Oncol. **29:** 213–217.
124. LEVANDER, O.A. & R.F. BURK. 1996. Selenium. *In* Present Knowledge in Nutrition.
     E.E. Ziegler & L.J. Filer, Eds.: 320–328. ILSI Press. Washington, D.C.
125. LEVANDER, O.A. & P.D. WHANGER. 1996. Deliberations and evaluations of the
     approaches, endpoints and paradigms for selenium and iodine dietary recommen-
     dations. J. Nutr. **126:** 2427S–2434S.
126. GIOVANNUCCI, E. 1998. Selenium and risk of prostate cancer. Lancet **352:** 755–756.
127. HARRISON, P.R., J. LANFEAR, L. WU, J. FLEMING, L. MCGARRY & L. BLOWER. 1997.
     Chemopreventive and growth inhibitory effects of selenium. Biomed. Environ. Sci.
     10: 235–245.
128. CLARK, L.C., G.F. COMBS, JR., B.W. TURNBULL, E.H. SLATE, D.K. CHALKER, J.
     CHOW, L.S. DAVIS, R.A. GLOVER, G.F. GRAHAM & E.G. GROSS. 1996. Effects of
     selenium supplementation for cancer prevention in patients with carcinoma of the
     skin: A randomized controlled trial. J. Am. Med. Assoc. **276:** 1957–1963.
129. CLARK, L.C., B. DALKIN, A. KRONGRAD, G.F. COMBS, JR., B.W. TURNBULL, E.H.
     SLATE, R. WITHERINGTON, J.H. HERLONG, E. JANOSKO, D. CARPENTER, C. BOROSSO,
     S. FALK & J. ROUNDER. 1998. Decreased incidence of prostate cancer with sele-
     nium supplementation: Results of a double-blind cancer prevention trial. Br. J.
     Urol. **81:** 730–734.
130. YOSHIZAWA, K., W.C. WILLETT, S.J. MORRIS, M.J. STAMPFER, D. SPIEGELMAN, E.B.
     RIMM & E. GIOVANNUCCI. 1998. Study of prediagnostic selenium level in toenails
     and the risk of advanced prostate cancer. J. Natl. Cancer Inst. **90:** 1219–1224.
131. HELZLSOUER, K.J., A.J. ALBERG, E.P. NORKUS, J.S. MORRIS, S.C. HOFFMAN & G.W.
     COMSTOCK. 1996. Prospective study of serum micronutrients and ovarian cancer. J.
     Natl. Cancer Inst. **88:** 32–37.
132. STRAIN, J.J., E. BOKJE, P. VAN'T VEER, J. COULTER, C. STEWART, H. LOGAN, W.
     ODLING-SMEE, R.A. SPENCE & K. STEELE. 1997. Thyroid hormones and selenium
     status in breast cancer. Nutr. Cancer **27:** 48–52.
133. REDMAN, C., J.A. SCOTT, A.T. BAINES, J.L. BASYE, L.C. CLARK, C. CALLEY, D. ROE,
     C.M. PAYNE & M.A. NELSON. 1998. Inhibitory effect of selenomethionine on the
     growth of three selected human tumor cell lines. Cancer Lett. **125:** 103–110.
134. RUSSO, M.W., S.C. MURRAY, J.I. WURZELMANN, J.T. WOOSLEY & R.S. SANDLER.
     1997. Plasma selenium levels and the risk of colorectal adenomas. Nutr. Cancer
     28: 125–129.
135. BHUVARAHAMURTHY, V., N. BALASUBRAMANIAN & S. GOVINDASAMY. 1996. Effect
     of radiotherapy and chemoradiotherapy on circulating antioxidant system of
     human uterine cervical carcinoma. Mol. Cell. Biochem. **158:** 17–23.
136. GUO, W.D., A.W. HSING, J.Y. LI, J.S. CHEN, W.H. CHOW & W.J. BLOT. 1994. Cor-
     relation of cervical cancer mortality with reproductive and dietary factors, and
     serum markers in China. Int. J. Epidemiol. **23:** 1127–1132.
137. ROTRUCK, J.T., A.L. POPE, H.E. GANTHER, A.B. SWANSON, D.G. HAFEMAN & W.G.
     HOEKSTRA. 1973. Selenium: Biochemical role as a component of glutathione per-
     oxidase. Science **179:** 588–590.
138. BURK, R.F., R.A. LAWRENCE & J.M. LANE. 1980. Liver necrosis and lipid peroxida-
     tion in the rat as the result of paraquat and diquat administration. Effect of sele-
     nium deficiency. J. Clin. Invest. **65:** 1024–1031.
139. HILL, K.E. & R.F. BURK. 1997. Selenoprotein P: Recent studies in rats and in
     humans. Biomed. Environ. Sci. **10:** 198–208.
140. YANG, J.G., K.E. HILL & R.F. BURK. 1989. Dietary selenium intake controls rat
     plasma selenoprotein P concentration. J. Nutr. **119:** 1010–1012.

141. GOLD, L.S., T.H. SLONE & B.N. AMES. 1997. Overview and update analyses of the carcinogenic potency database. *In* Handbook of Carcinogenic Potency and Genotoxicity Databases. L.S. Gold & E. Zeiger, Eds.: 661–685. CRC Press. Boca Raton, FL.

142. LOOKER, A.C., P.R. DALLMAN, M.D. CARROLL, E.W. GUNTER & C.L. JOHNSON. 1997. Prevalence of iron deficiency in the United States. J. Am. Med. Assoc. **277:** 973–976.

143. WALTER, P.B., M.D. KNUTSON, Y. XU, F.E. VITERI & B.N. AMES. 1997. Iron supplements, mitochondrial function, and DNA damage in iron-normal and deficient rats [abstract]. *In* Oxygen 97: The 4th Annual Meeting of the Oxygen Society, 1997. Nov. 20–24, San Francisco, CA. The Oxygen Society: 106 (abstr. no. 3–34).

144. BEARD, J. 1996. Nutrient status and central nervous system function. *In* Present Knowledge in Nutrition. E.E. Ziegler & L.J. Filer, Jr., Eds.: 612–622. ILSI Press. Washington, D.C.

145. YIP, R. & P.R. DALLMAN. 1996. Iron. *In* Present Knowledge in Nutrition. E.E. Ziegler & L.J. Filer, Jr., Eds.: 277–292. ILSI Press. Washington, D C.

146. ZHANG, D., S. OKADA, Y.Y. YU, P. ZHENG, R. YAMAGUCHI & H. KASAI. 1997. Vitamin E inhibits apoptosis, DNA modification, and cancer incidence induced by iron-mediated peroxidation in Wistar rat kidney. Cancer Res. **57:** 2410–2414.

147. TOYOKUNI, S. 1996. Iron-induced carcinogenesis: The role of redox regulation. Free Rad. Biol. Med. **20:** 553–566.

148. SEMPOS, C.T., R.F. GILLUM & A.C. LOOKER. 1997. Iron and heart disease. *In* Preventive Nutrition: The Comprehensive Guide for Health Professionals. A. Bendich & R.J. Deckelbaum, Eds.: 181–192. Humana Press Inc. Totowa, NJ.

149. TUOMAINEN, T.-P., K. PUNNONEN, K. NYYSSLÖNEN & J.T. SALONEN. 1998. Association between body iron stores and the risk of acute myocardial infarction in men. Circulation **97:** 1461–1466.

150. WALSH, C.T., H.H. SANDSTEAD, A.S. PRASAD, P.M. NEWBERNE & P.J. FRAKER. 1994. Zinc: Health effects and research priorities for the 1990s. Environ. Health Perspect. **102** (Suppl 2): 5–46.

151. PAVLETICH, N.P., K.A. CHAMBERS & C.O. PABO. 1993. The DNA-binding domain of p53 contains the four conserved regions and the major mutation hot spots. Genes & Dev. **7:** 2556–2564.

152. SARKAR, B. 1995. Metal replacement in DNA-binding zinc finger proteins and its relevance to mutagenicity and carcinogenicity through free radical generation. Nutrition **11:** 646–649.

153. CASTRO, C.E., L.C. KASPIN, S.-S. CHEN & S.G. NOLKER. 1992. Zinc deficiency increases the frequency of single-strand DNA breaks in rat liver. Nutr. Res. **12:** 721–736.

154. OLIN, K.L., M.K. SHIGENAGA, B.N. AMES, M.S. GOLUB, M.E. GERSHWIN, A.G. HENDRICKX & C.L. KEEN. 1993. Maternal dietary zinc influences DNA strand break and 8-hydroxy-2′-deoxyguanosine levels in infant rhesus monkey liver. Proc. Soc. Exp. Biol. Med. **203:** 461–466.

155. OTEIZA, P.L., K.L. OLIN, C.E. FRAGA & C.L. KEEN. 1996. Oxidant defense systems in testes from zinc-deficient rats (44040). Proc. Soc. Exp. Biol. Med. **213:** 85–91.

156. O'CONNOR, T.R., R.J. GRAVES, G. DE MURCIA, B. CASTAING & J. LAVAL. 1993. Fpg protein of *Escherichia coli* is a zinc finger protein whose cysteine residues have a structural and/or functional role. J. Biol. Chem. **268:** 9063–9070.

157. FONG, L.Y.Y., J. LI, J.L. FARBER & P.N. MAGEE. 1996. Cell proliferation and esophageal carcinogenesis in the zinc-deficient rat. Carcinogenesis **17:** 1841–1848.

158. FONG, L.Y.Y., K.-M. LAU, K. HUEBNER & P.N. MAGEE. 1997. Induction of esophageal tumors in zinc-deficient rats by single low doses of *N*-nitrosomethylbenzy-

lamine (NMBA): Analysis of cell proliferation, and mutations in H-*ras* and *p53* genes. Carcinogenesis **18:** 1477–1484.

159. NEWBERNE, P.M., S. BROITMAN & T.F. SCHRAGER. 1997. Esophageal carcinogenesis in the rat: Zinc deficiency, DNA methylation and alkyltransferase activity. Pathobiology **65:** 253–263.

160. ANDERSON, M.B., K. LEPAK, V. FARINAS & W.J. GEROGE. 1993. Protective action of zinc against cobalt-induced testicular damage in the mouse. Reprod. Toxicol. **7:** 49–54.

161. XU, B., S.E. CHIA & C.H. ONG. 1994. Concentrations of cadmium, lead, selenium and zinc in human blood and seminal plasma. Biol. Trace Element Res. **40:** 49–57.

162. OTEIZA, P.I., K.L. OLIN, C.G. FRAGA & C.L. KEEN. 1995. Zinc deficiency causes oxidative damage to proteins, lipids and DNA in rat testes. J. Nutr. **125:** 823–829.

163. RUZ, M., C. CASTILLO-DURAN, X. LARA, J. CODOCEO, A. REBOLLEDO & E. ATALAH. 1997. A 14-mo zinc-supplementation trial in apparently healthy Chilean preschool children. Am. J. Clin. Nutr. **66:** 1406–1413.

164. SOLOMONS, N.W. 1998. Mild human zinc deficiency produces an imbalance between cell-mediated and humoral immunity. Nutr. Rev. **56:** 27–28.

165. JOHNSON, M.A. & K.H. PORTER. 1997. Micronutrient supplementation and infection in institutionalized elders. Nutr. Rev. **55:** 400–404.

166. MCCREANOR, G.M. & D.A. BENDER. 1986. The metabolism of high intakes of tryptophan, nicotinamide and nicotinic acid in the rat. Br. J. Nutr. **5:** 577–586.

167. JACOBSON, E.L. 1993. Niacin deficiency and cancer in women. J. Am. Coll. Nutr. **12:** 412–416.

168. JACOBSON, E.L., W.M. SHIEH & A.C. HUANG. 1999. Mapping the role of NAD metabolism in prevention and treatment of carcinogenesis. Mol. Cell. Biochem. **193:** 69–74.

169. RAWLING, J.M., T.M. JACKSON, E.R. DRISCOLL & J.B. KIRKLAND. 1994. Dietary niacin deficiency lowers tissue poly(ADP-ribose) and NAD+ concentrations in Fischer-344 rats. J. Nutr. **124:** 1597–1603.

170. ZHANG, J.Z., S.M. HENNING & M.E. SWENDSEID. 1993. Poly(ADP-ribose) polymerase activity and DNA strand breaks are affected in tissues of niacin-deficient rats. J. Nutr. **123:** 1349–55.

171. HENNING, S.M., M.E. SWENDSEID & W.F. COULSON. 1997. Male rats fed methyl- and folate-deficient diets with or without niacin develop hepatic carcinomas associated with decreased tissue NAD concentrations and altered poly(ADP-ribose) polymerase activity. J. Nutr. **127:** 30–36.

172. AMES, B.N. 1998. Micronutrients prevent cancer and delay aging. Toxicol. Lett. **102–103:** 5–18.

173. FENECH, M. 1999. Micronucleus frequency in human lymphocytes is related to plasma vitamin B_{12} and homocysteine. Mutat. Res. **428:** 299–304.

174. SKIBOLA, C.F., M.T. SMITH, E. KANE, E. ROMAN, S. ROLLINSON, R.A. CARTWRIGHT & G. MORGAN. 1999. Polymorphisms in the methylenetetrahydrofolate reductase gene are associated with susceptibility to acute leukemia in adults. Proc. Natl. Acad. Sci. USA **96:** 12810–12815.

175. AMES, B.N. 1999. Cancer prevention and diet: Help from single nucleotide polymorphisms [commentary]. Proc. Natl. Acad. Sci. USA **96:** 12216–12218.

Calcium and Vitamin D

Their Potential Roles in Colon and Breast Cancer Prevention

CEDRIC F. GARLAND,[a,c] FRANK C. GARLAND,[a,b] AND EDWARD D. GORHAM[a,b,d]

[a]Department of Family and Preventive Medicine, University of California, San Diego, California 92093, USA

[b]Naval Health Research Center, San Diego, California, USA

ABSTRACT: The geographic distribution of colon cancer is similar to the historical geographic distribution of rickets. The highest death rates from colon cancer occur in areas that had high prevalence rates of rickets—regions with winter ultraviolet radiation deficiency, generally due to a combination of high or moderately high latitude, high-sulfur content air pollution (acid haze), higher than average stratospheric ozone thickness, and persistently thick winter cloud cover. The geographic distribution of colon cancer mortality rates reveals significantly low death rates at low latitudes in the United States and significantly high rates in the industrialized Northeast. The Northeast has a combination of latitude, climate, and air pollution that prevents any synthesis of vitamin D during a five-month vitamin D winter. Breast cancer death rates in white women also rise with distance from the equator and are highest in areas with long vitamin D winters. Colon cancer incidence rates also have been shown to be inversely proportional to intake of calcium. These findings, which are consistent with laboratory results, indicate that most cases of colon cancer may be prevented with regular intake of calcium in the range of 1,800 mg per day, in a dietary context that includes 800 IU per day (20 μg) of vitamin D_3. (In women, an intake of approximately 1,000 mg of calcium per 1,000 kcal of energy with 800 IU of vitamin D would be sufficient.) In observational studies, the source of approximately 90% of the calcium intake was vitamin D–fortified milk. Vitamin D may also be obtained from fatty fish. In addition to reduction of incidence and mortality rates from colon cancer, epidemiological data suggest that intake of 800 IU/day of vitamin D may be associated with enhanced survival rates among breast cancer cases.

The essential roles of calcium and vitamin D in human health have been recognized since the 1920s.[1] The earliest known example of a disease due to deficiency of

[c]Address for communication: Department of Family and Preventive Medicine, University of California, San Diego, 9500 Gilman Drive, Dept. 0631C, La Jolla, CA 92093. Voice: 858-558-0796; fax: 858-558-0797.

e-mail: cgarland@ucsd.edu

[d]The views expressed in this paper are those of the authors and do not reflect the official policy or position of the Navy, Department of Defense, or the United States Government.

calcium and vitamin D is rickets. The disease was once common in children who received virtually no solar ultraviolet radiation, an observation made by the epidemiologist Palm, based on the worldwide geographic epidemiology of the disease.[2] Rickets was first described nearly 350 years earlier, as a distinct disease, mainly of the poor of London.[3] It was assumed that rickets was hereditary, because it clustered in the poor families of London's tenement alleys. Progression from the epidemiological observation to discovery of a reliable means of preventing and curing rickets (using vitamin D or calcium) took approximately 30 years.[4]

The global geographic epidemiology of several other diseases, including colon cancer, is similar to that of rickets. The highest death rates from colon cancer occur in areas that had high prevalence rates of rickets—regions with winter ultraviolet radiation deficiency, generally due to a combination of high or moderately high latitude, high-sulfur content types of air pollution (acid haze), higher than average stratospheric ozone thickness, and winter cloud cover.[5–10] The geographic distribution of colon cancer mortality rates among white men reveals significantly low death rates at low latitudes in the United States and significantly high rates in the northeastern United States (FIG. 1).[5,11] The northeastern United States has a combination of latitude, climate, and sulfur-based air pollution that prevents any synthesis of vitamin D during a five-month duration vitamin D winter, beginning in November and continuing through March.[7] All areas in the United States south of 37° north latitude, which tend to have short or absent vitamin D winters, had significantly low death rates from colon cancer. The pattern was nearly identical in white women and was similar for rectal cancer.[5,11]

The emergence of rickets as a previously unrecognized disease in the mid 1450s corresponded with burning in London[12] of high-sulfur content coal, from the port of Newcastle, following destruction of forests surrounding the city that previously provided wood, a fuel that contained only traces of sulfur. Although it was not then known that air pollution from high-sulfur coal could indirectly cause rickets by absorbing ultraviolet energy, proclamations were issued that attempted (without much long-term success) to limit the discharge of high-sulfur air pollution.[12] Air pollution with a high sulfur content (termed acid haze[13]) has persisted in some regions into the new millennium,[12] particularly in the northeastern coal belts and in eastern Canada, where high-sulfur coal is used in smelting. Acid haze consists of a persistent aerosol consisting of sulfuric acid droplets, ammonium sulfate particles, and sulfur dioxide gas.[13,14] Acid haze removes ultraviolet light from sunlight through a photochemical mechanism that shares some features with the effects of stratospheric ozone.[15]

Although rickets may be induced by sunlight deficiency, it can be prevented or cured by administration of adequate amounts of absorbable forms of vitamin D with calcium. The geographic distribution of colon cancer; epidemiological studies of diet;[16,17] clinical and laboratory studies of the influence of calcium supplementation on markers of colonic epithelial proliferation[18] and of vitamin D on calcium metabolism in the colonic crypts;[19] and epidemiological analyses of serum levels of vitamin D compounds (specifically 25(OH)D)[20,21] have indicated that calcium, vitamin D, and 25-hydroxyvitamin D (25(OH)D) may reduce the risk of several types of cancer. Epidemiologic findings, coupled with increased understanding of the physiological roles of vitamin D and calcium, have indicated that vitamin D and calcium may

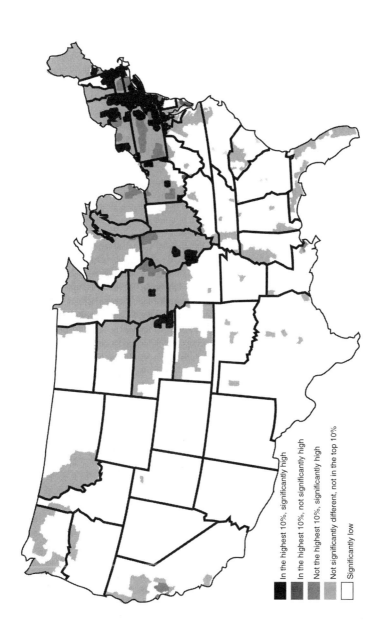

FIGURE 1. Age-adjusted colon cancer mortality rates, white men, United States, 1970–1980. Source: National Cancer Institute.[11]

be important in prevention of colon cancer. Vitamin D metabolites promote cellular differentiation, which is important in cancer prevention.[22–26] The strength of the evidence from epidemiological studies, clinical studies, and laboratory research has provided sufficient rationale for including a calcium and vitamin D intervention as one of the sthree arms of the Women's Health Initiative, in addition to studying the roles of calcium and vitamin D in forestalling bone disease. The other interventions are an estrogen-progestin regimen and a low-fat diet. The epidemiological and laboratory research in calcium and vitamin D has also stimulated research on analogues of vitamin D metabolites that might be useful in chemoprevention of cancer.[27,28] This review will examine the potential role of vitamin D metabolites and calcium in the prevention of colon and breast cancer.

The main storage and circulating form of vitamin D is (25(OH)D), whose concentration is the standard measure of vitamin D status.[29–32] Rickets and osteomalacia typically occur when there is chronic severe deficiency in the circulating levels of 25(OH)D, generally in the range from 0 to 5 ng/mL, although rickets is unrelated to deficiency in circulating levels of $1,25(OH)_2D$, a metabolite that is synthesized in the kidney and locally in some tissues.[33] Rickets also occurs in individuals lacking enzymes needed for metabolism of vitamin D to 25(OH)D, even when sunlight exposure is adequate,[34] and, importantly, in individuals with extremely low intakes of calcium.

In contrast to the severe level of vitamin D deficiency that is the main factor in most cases of rickets, there is evidence to suggest that the incidence rate of colon cancer is elevated in persons whose circulating 25(OH)D levels are much higher than those associated with rickets and other bone diseases, potentially as high as 30 ng per milliliter.[20,21] The threshold of vitamin D deficiency for elevating the risk of colon cancer appears to be approximately six times higher than the threshold for induction of rickets. This suggests that levels of vitamin D intake (or solar ultraviolet exposure) sufficient to prevent rickets are not sufficient for prevention of colon cancer.

Age-adjusted mortality rates of colorectal cancer[5] and breast cancer[35,36] rise with increasing distance from the equator and are highest in areas with the least winter sunlight and longest vitamin D winters (periods when no detectable vitamin D can be synthesized in the skin).[7] Apparent exceptions, such as breast cancer in Los Angeles, probably represent migration to the region of women from the urbanized and heavily polluted northeastern United States. Risk of breast cancer in association with latitude may be established early in life.[37]

Sulfate air pollution is considerably more concentrated in atmosphere of the northeastern United States and other high-sulfur coal-burning areas of the United States, where death rates of colon cancer and breast cancer are higher than in other regions.[38] The consistency of the geographic distribution suggests a common etiology of these malignancies, despite the well-recognized historical risk factors that are believed to be unique to each. It also suggests that there is an association between the environmental and dietary circumstances that were once associated with rickets and incidence of these diseases.

Circulating levels of 25(OH)D are far higher in populations living at sunny lower latitudes (such as Florida, at 26°N) compared to those at higher latitudes (such as

Finland, at 61°N).[39] Vitamin D levels are also low in regions distant from the equator in the Southern Hemisphere, where little or no vitamin D can be synthesized during late fall through early spring at 55° South.[40] The mean springtime concentration of 25(OH)D in healthy women is 36 ng/mL in Florida but only 15 ng/mL in Finland.[39] The median winter value in normal adults in Middlesex, England, historically in the rickets belt, is 10 ng/mL.[41]

Like sulfur-based air pollution, stratospheric ozone plays a well-known role in absorption of solar ultraviolet radiation.[42,43] Within North America, the industrialized Northeast is the region where the stratospheric ozone thickness is greatest, typically 400 mm compared to a worldwide average of 300 millimeters.[15,44] Effects of stratospheric ozone thickness and sulfate-based acid haze tend to be exponential and multiplicative with thickness and concentration, respectively.[42,43] So areas that have both an unusually thick ozone layer and a high concentration of sulfate acid haze, such as the industrialized northeastern United States, are at a great disadvantage with respect to the ultraviolet radiation needed for synthesis of vitamin D during the winter and early spring.[7] Apart from effects associated with acid haze, age-adjusted annual mortality rates from colon cancer tend, in general, to rise by approximately three per 100,000 population per ten degrees of latitude within the United States.[11] There are few exceptions, the most notable of which is Japan, where intake of fish containing vitamin D is high, and colon cancer death rates are historically low despite its moderately high latitude (36° N).[45]

Geographic differences in age-adjusted colon and breast cancer mortality rates that exist by latitude in the United States cannot be readily accounted for by differences in regional per capita intake of fruits, vegetables, red meat, or fish, according to food intake (disappearance) surveys performed by the U.S. Department of Agriculture.[5] North–south differences in dietary intake of fat, for example, could not account for the strong association between latitude and these disorders, because slightly more fat was consumed per person in the southern than in the northern United States.[5] Furthermore, no association of overall intake of fiber with incidence of colon cancer or adenomas was found in a recent cohort study that studied 88,757 subjects, although there were mildly favorable associations with certain kinds of soluble fiber, such as pectins that are contained in fruits and vegetables.[46]

Migration southward from New York to Florida is associated with a decline in the risk of colon cancer,[47] whereas migration northward from Mexico and Puerto Rico to the northern United States is associated with a twofold increase in risk of death from colon cancer.[48] There have been nine epidemiological observational studies of the association of dietary vitamin D intake with estimated risk of colon cancer.[16,49–56] Eight of the nine studies indicated that daily intake of 160 IU per day or more of vitamin D was associated with a reduced risk of colon cancer.[16,49,50,52–56] The median reduction in risk of colon cancer associated with dietary vitamin D intake at this level was 32% (odds ratio = 0.68, 95% confidence interval, 0.5–0.7).[57,58]

A similar effect of vitamin D has been reported in two prospective studies of circulating 25(OH)D, the long-lived metabolite of vitamin D most appropriate for use as a biomarker for vitamin D status.[29–31] A nested case-control study was conducted in a cohort of 25,620 healthy adult resident volunteers in Washington County, Maryland.[20] Each volunteer provided samples of serum in 1974–1975, and the specimens were frozen at −70°C and stored for a median of eight years. Serum samples were then thawed for cases of colon cancer and two controls per case, and matched on age, race, sex, county of residence, and date of serum collection. They were analyzed blindly for 25(OH) concentration. Serum levels of 25(OH)D greater than 20 ng/mL were associated with reduction by half in colon cancer incidence.[20] Most of the association of serum 25(OH)D with risk of colon cancer occurred during the first decade of follow-up, suggesting that the main role of vitamin D in prevention of colon cancer is during the promotional phase.[59]

Factors other than calcium and vitamin D also have been of major interest in understanding the risk of colorectal cancer, including well-known associations with genetic predisposition.[60–62,63] In one of the longest cohort studies to date, however, baseline dietary intake of fat (42% of energy) and carbohydrates was approximately identical in participants who developed colon cancer and those who did not during a 19-year period of follow-up.[16] Whereas some cases of colorectal cancer are of established genetic etiology, the overwhelming majority (approximately 90%) appear to be of mainly environmental rather than genetic origin.[60]

New impetus for studies of the role of calcium in cancer prevention emerged when Lipkin and Newmark reported that intake of 2,000 mg/day of calcium markedly reduced the rate of colonic epithelial proliferation in subjects at high risk of colon cancer.[18,64,65] Their research supported a hypothesis, previously described by Newmark et al., stating that the role of calcium in prevention of colon cancer may be due, at least in part, to its ability to complex and inactivate potentially carcinogenic bile acids.[66]

Davies and associates recently reported that vitamin D deficiency interferes with calcium-mediated apoptosis of colonocytes at the mouths of the crypts, allowing colonocytes to persist for abnormally long periods of time.[67] Colonocytes of vitamin-D-deficient animals failed to undergo differentiation and apoptosis because basal surges in intracellular calcium were of insufficient magnitude to take the cell out of the proliferating pool. This resulted in an unusually proliferative colonocyte population. Although the approach used by Davies was very different to that used by Lipkin and Newmark,[18] it helped to confirm that both calcium and vitamin D may affect the rate of colonic epithelial proliferation and further strengthened the linkages among calcium, vitamin D, and prevention of colon cancer.

Breast cancer mortality rates follow a geographic gradient in the United States that is similar to those of colon cancer,[35] with highest rates in the Northeast (FIG. 4); the pattern was similar in Canada[13] and the Soviet Union.[68] In the broad geographic regions with the highest death rates, ultraviolet B radiation levels are insufficient to allow synthesis of vitamin D during nearly half the year.[7] Age-adjusted mortality rates from breast cancer tend to be approximately 40% higher in these areas than in Hawaii, which has no vitamin D winter, and considerably higher than in the sunniest regions of the southwest (Arizona and New Mexico).[35] As with colon cancer, higher than average stratospheric ozone thickness and high levels of sulfate air pollution also are associated with elevated breast cancer mortality rates.[13,35] Regional difference in reproductive factors could possibly account for some proportion of the latitudinal variation in breast cancer death rates but cannot account for any of the latitudinal variation in colon cancer, which is similar in men and women.

VITAMIN D AND SURVIVAL IN COLON AND BREAST CANCER

Serum 25(OH)D levels remain high throughout the year in areas with no vitamin D winter, such as Florida and Hawaii, but usually plummet during the winter in regions at higher latitudes or in persons using sunscreens on a chronic basis. In addition to the geographic distribution of colon cancer mortality rates shown in FIGURES 1–3, there is variation in survival rates following diagnosis of colon cancer. Currently the only uniform source for colon cancer survival rates over a large geographic range is the SEER registry of the National Cancer Institute.[69] There are nine cancer registries in the United States reporting survival rates to SEER. Hawaii is at the lowest latitude of any SEER cancer registry (18°N). Consistent with its latitude, the five-year relative case-fatality rate from colon cancer in whites was lowest in Hawaii (32%) of the nine cancer registries reporting survival rates to SEER (overall mean for all registries, 38%).[69] The colon cancer case-fatality rate for all races combined was also lowest in Hawaii.[69]

The association of high latitude with high mortality rates of breast cancer mainly is due to higher case-fatality rates from breast cancer at higher latitudes. The five-year relative case-fatality rate from breast cancer in whites was lowest in Hawaii (9%) of all cancer registries reporting survival rates to SEER (overall mean 16%).[69]

According to research summarized by Newmark, the influence of vitamin D on mammary carcinogenesis is particularly strong early in life, suggesting that low circulating levels of 25(OH)D in adolescence may be an important predisposing factor for breast cancer risk later in life.[70] The roles of vitamin D, calcium, and fats may be linked by a mechanism suggested by Newmark and associates.[66]

It is well known that vitamin D is stored in tissues and therefore can potentially have toxic effects at high doses.[71] The National Academy of Sciences, Institute of Medicine, has suggested 5,000 IU per day as the safe upper limit of vitamin D intake.[72] Such potential toxic effects as bone demineralization, hypercalcemia, hypercalciuria, or nephrocalcinosis are seen rarely, and only when the daily dose exceeds 10,000 IU on a chronic basis.[74] Most concerns about vitamin D toxicity have been due to massive overdoses in the range of 50,000–150,000 IU per day, on a relatively long-term basis.

Theoretical risks associated with dosages of vitamin D in the pharmacological range (up to 2,000 IU per day) have been shown to be largely unfounded. For example, the serum concentration of several vitamin D metabolites did not differ between renal stone formers and healthy controls.[75–77] In the Tromsø Health Study, higher serum levels of 25(OH)D did not predispose to heart disease and were significantly associated with reduced incidence of myocardial infarction.[78] Similar protective effects for heart disease and for mortality rates from all causes were observed for calcium intake equal to or higher than 1,245 mg per day in a large cohort study.[79] Intake of 800 IU per day of vitamin D_3 does not induce hypercalcemia or other known adverse effects,[80] and this dosage is consistent with reduced risk of heart disease and mortality from all causes combined.[78]

Vitamin D from sources other than solar exposure is needed during November through March in northeastern United States and other high-latitude industrialized regions to maintain adequate circulating levels of 25(OH)D. Cutaneous synthesis of vitamin D is re-

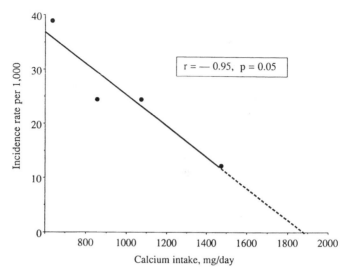

FIGURE 2. Dose-response relationship of calcium intake with incidence rates of colon cancer; 19-year cohort study of men.[16]

duced by 60–70% in the elderly, due to lower concentration of the 7-dehydrocholesterol substrate in aging skin.[33,81] Vitamin D deficiency has been reported in approximately 40% of adults in the general population.[82]

IMPLICATIONS FOR PREVENTION OF COLON AND BREAST CANCER

Colon cancer incidence rates have, in general, been shown to be inversely proportional to dietary intake of calcium.[16,17] The association follows a dose-response gradient (FIG. 2) and is present in both genders (FIGURES 3 and 4) (dashed lines are linear extrapolations of the least squares line). These findings, which are consistent with well-established laboratory findings,[18] indicate that colon cancer may be prevented with adequate intake of calcium in the range of 1,800 mg per day, in a dietary context that includes appropriate amounts of vitamin D. In the epidemiological studies that yielded this finding, the source of approximately 90% of the calcium intake was milk. Milk also contains vitamin D (in the United States, Canada, and some other countries) and other compounds (such as short-chain fatty acids and conjugated linoleic acid) that might influence the effect of calcium and vitamin D on the risk of colon cancer. Until the possible contributions of various components of milk to cancer prevention have been isolated, the main recommended source of calcium for cancer prevention should be milk.

A logical target, based on existing evidence,[10,16,18,70] for minimizing the risk of colon cancer throughout the lifetime would be an intake of 1,800 IU of calcium and 800 IU (20 μg) of vitamin D_3 per day, preferably from such foods as milk, or from fatty fish, such as tuna, mackerel, herring, and sardines. (In women, an intake of ap-

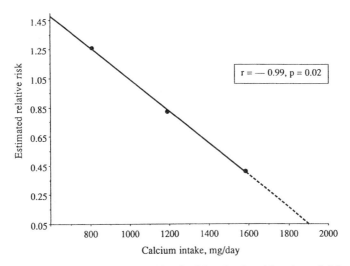

FIGURE 3. Dose-response relationship of calcium intake with estimated risk of colon cancer in men.[17]

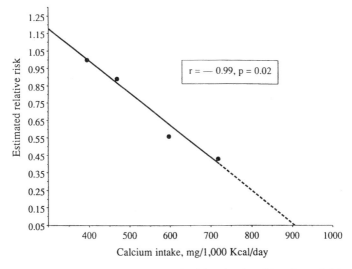

FIGURE 4. Dose-response relationship of calcium intake with estimated risk of colon cancer in women.[17]

proximately 1,000 mg per day per 1,000 kcal of energy, with 800 IU per day of vitamin D_3 would be appropriate, although higher intakes of calcium may be needed to meet nutritional guidelines for prevention of osteoporosis.) Some degree of supplementation of both calcium and vitamin D may be required if these targets cannot be achieved solely with food.

REFERENCES

1. PARK, E. 1923. The etiology of rickets. Physiol. Rev. (Baltimore) **iii:** 106–163.
2. PALM, T. Rickets. 1890. The Practitioner.
3. GLISSON, F. 1542. Treatise on rickets (Tractatus de Rachitide). London.
4. MELLANBY, E. 1918. The part played by an 'accessory factor' in the production of experimental rickets. J. Physiol. 52 (xi).
5. GARLAND, C. & F. GARLAND. 1980. Do sunlight and vitamin D reduce the likelihood of colon cancer? Int. J. Epidemiol. **9:** 227–231.
6. GARLAND, C. & F. GARLAND. 1986. Calcium and colon cancer. Clin. Nutr. **5:** 162–166.
7. WEBB, A., L. KLINE & M. HOLICK. 1988. Influence of season and latitude on the cutaneous synthesis of vitamin D_3: Exposure to winter sunlight in Boston and Edmonton will not promote vitamin D_3 synthesis in human skin. J. Clin. Endocrinol. Metab. **67:** 373–378.
8. FREDERICK, J. & D. LUBIN. 1988. The budget of biologically active ultraviolet radiation in the earth-atmosphere system. J. Geophys. Res. **93:** 3825–3832.
9. GARLAND, C., F. GARLAND & E. GORHAM. 1991. Colon cancer parallels rickets. *In* Calcium, vitamin D, and prevention of colon cancer. M. Lipkin, H. Newmark & G. Kelloff, Ed.: 81–111. CRC Press. Boca Raton.
10. GARLAND, C., F. GARLAND & E. GORHAM. 1999. Epidemiology of cancer risk and Vitamin D. *In* Vitamin D: Molecular Biology, Physiology, and Clinical Applications. M. Holick, Ed.: 375–409. Humana. New Jersey.
11. PICKLE, L., T. MASON, N. HOWARD, R. HOOVER & J. FRAUMENI JR. 1987. Atlas of U.S. cancer mortality among whites: 1950–1980. (DHHS Publication No. (NIH) 87-2900): 52–56. National Cancer Institute. Bethesda, MD.
12. BRIMBLECOMBE, P. 1987. The big smoke: A history of air pollution in London since medieval times. Methuen. London. pp. 22–38.
13. GORHAM, E., C. GARLAND & F. GARLAND. 1989. Acid haze air pollution and breast and colon cancer in 20 Canadian cities. Can. J. Public Health **80:** 96–100.
14. WAGGONER, A., A. VANDERPOOL, R. CHARLSON *et al.* 1976. Sulfate light scattering as an index of the role of sulfur in tropospheric optics. Nature **261:** 120–122.
15. LABITZKE, K., A. MILLER, J. ANGELL, J. DELUISI, J. FREDERICK *et al.* 1985. Ozone and temperature trends. *In* WMO Global Ozone Research and Monitoring Project. World Meteorological Organization. Geneva.
16. GARLAND, C., R. SHEKELLE & E. BARRETT-CONNOR. 1985. Dietary vitamin D and calcium and risk of colorectal cancer: A 19-year prospective study in men. Lancet **1:** 307–309.
17. SLATTERY, M., A. SORENSON & M. FORD. 1988. Dietary calcium intake as a mitigating factor in colon cancer. Am. J. Epidemiol. **128:** 504–114.
18. LIPKIN, M., & H. NEWMARK. 1985. Effect of added dietary calcium on colonic epithelial cell proliferation in subjects at high risk for familial colon cancer. N. Engl. J. Med. **313:** 1381–1384.
19. BRENNER, B., N. RUSSELL, S. ALBRECHT & R. DAVIES. 1998. The effect of dietary vitamin D3 on the intracellular calcium gradient in mammalian colonic crypts. Cancer Lett. **12**(7): 43–53.
20. GARLAND, C., G. COMSTOCK, F. GARLAND, K. HELSING, E. SHAW & E. GORHAM. 1989. Serum 25-hydroxyvitamin D and colon cancer: Eight-year prospective study. Lancet **2:** 1176–1178.
21. TANGREA, J., K. HELZLSOUER, P. PIETINEN *et al.* 1997. Serum levels of vitamin D metabolites and the subsequent risk of colon and rectal cancer in Finnish men. Cancer Causes & Control **8**(4): 615–625.
22. EISMAN, J., D. BARKLA & P. TUTTON. 1987. Suppression of *in vivo* growth of human cancer solid tumor xenografts by 1,25-dihydroxyvitamin D3. Cancer Res. **47:** 21–25.
23. FRANCESCHI, R., C. LINSON, T. PETRER & P. ROMANO. 1987. Regulation of cellular adhesion and fibronectin synthesis by 1-alpha,25-dihydroxyvitamin D3. J. Biol. Chem. **262:** 4165–4171.

24. COLSTON, K., U. BERGER, P. WILSON *et al.* 1988. Mammary gland 1,25-dihydroxyvitamin D3 receptor content during pregnancy and lactation. Mol. Cell. Endocrinol. **60:** 15–22.
25. COLSTON, K., U. BERGER & R. COOMBES. 1989. Possible role for vitamin D in controlling breast cancer cell proliferation. Lancet **1:** 188–191.
26. FRAPPART, L., N. FALETTE, M. LEFEBRE, A. BREMOND, J. VAUZELLE & S. SAEZ. 1989. *In vitro* study of the effects of 1,25 dihydroxyvitamin D3 on the morphology of human breast cancer cell line BT-20. Differentiation **40:** 63–69.
27. KELLOFF, G., C. BOONE, J. CROWELL *et al.* 1996. New agents for cancer chemoprevention. J. Cell. Biochem. **26** (Suppl): 1–28.
28. OGATA, E. 1997. The potential use of vitamin D analogs in the treatment of cancer. Calcif. Tissue Int. **60:** 130–133.
29. HOLICK, M., L. MATSUOKA & J. WORTSMAN. 1989. Age, vitamin D and solar ultraviolet radiation. Lancet **4:** 1104–1105.
30. LIPS, P., F. VAN GINKEL, M. JONGEN, F. RUBERTUS, W. VAN DER VIGH & J. NETELENBOS. 1987. Determinants of vitamin D status in patients with hip fracture and in elderly control subjects. Am. J. Clin. Nutr. **46:** 1005–1010.
31. CHEN, T. 1999. Photobiology of vitamin D. Humana. Totowa, NJ. pp. 17–37.
32. LAMBERG-ALLARD, T. 1984. Vitamin D intake, sunlight exposure and 25-hydroxyvitamin D levels in elderly during one year. Ann. Nutr. Metab. **28:** 144–50.
33. HOLICK, M. 1995. Vitamin D photobiology, metabolism and clinical applications. *In* Endocrinology, 3rd ed. L. DeGroot, Ed.: 990–1013. Saunders. Philadelphia.
34. KRANE, S. & M. HOLICK. 1998. Metabolic bone disease. *In* Harrison's Principles of Internal Medicine. A. Fauci, E. Braunwald, K. Isselbacher *et al.*, Eds.: 2247–2259. New York: McGraw-Hill.
35. GARLAND, F., C. GARLAND, E. GORHAM & J. YOUNG JR. 1990. Geographic variation in breast cancer mortality in the United States: A hypothesis involving exposure to solar radiation. Prev. Med. **19:** 614–622.
36. GORHAM, E., F. GARLAND & C. GARLAND. 1990. Sunlight and breast cancer incidence in the USSR. Int. J. Epidemiol. **19:** 820–824.
37. BERRINO, F. & G. GATTA. 1989. Energy-rich diet and breast cancer risk. Int. J. Cancer **44:** 186–187.
38. LEADERER, B., R. TANNER, P. LIOY & J. STOLWIJK. 1981. Seasonal variations in light scattering in the New York region and their relation to sources. Atmos. Environ. **15:** 2407–2420.
39. PUNNONEN, R., M. GILLESPY, M. HAHL *et al.* 1988. Serum 25-OHD, vitamin A and vitamin E concentrations in healthy Finnish and Floridian Women. Int. J. Vitam. Nutr. Res. **58:** 37–39.
40. LU, Z., T. CHEN, L. KLINE *et al.* 1992. Photosynthesis of previtamin D$_3$ in cities around the world. *In* Biologic Effects of Light. M. Holick & A. Kligman, Eds.: 48–52. Walter de Gruyter. New York.
41. PREECE, M., J. O'RIORDAN, D. LAWSON & E. KODICEK. 1974. A competitive protein-binding assay for 25-hydroxycholecalciferol and 25-hydroxyergocalciferol in serum. Clin. Chim. Acta **54:** 235–242.
42. WAGGONER, A., R. WEISS, R. AHLQUIST, D. COVERT, S. WILL & R. CHARLSON. 1981. Optical characteristics of atmospheric aerosols. Atmos. Environ. **15:** 1891–1909.
43. GREEN, A., T. SAWADA & E. SHETTLE. 1974. The middle ultraviolet reaching the ground. Photochem. Photobiol. **19:** 251–259.
44. BOWMAN, K. 1984. A global climatology of total ozone from the Nimbus-7 total ozone mapping spectrometer. *In* Ozone Symposium. C. Zerefos, Ed. Ozone Symposium. Athens.
45. PARKIN, D., S. WHELAN, J. FERLAY, L. RAYMOND & J. YOUNG, Eds. 1997. Cancer incidence in five continents. Volume VII (IARC Publication No. 143). International Agency for Research on Cancer. Lyon.

46. FUCHS, C., E. GIOVANNUCCI, G. COLDITZ et al. 1999. Dietary fiber and the risk of colorectal cancer and adenoma in women. N. Engl. J. Med. **340:** 169–176.
47. ZIEGLER, R. 1986. Epidemiologic patterns of colorectal cancer. In Important Advances in Oncology. V.T.H.S. DeVita & S.A. Rosenberg, Ed.: 209–232. Lippincott. Philadelphia.
48. MALLIN, K. & K. ANDERSON. 1988. Cancer mortality in Illinois, Mexican, and Puerto Rican immigrants, 1979–1984. Int. J. Cancer **41:** 670–676.
49. HEILBRUN, L., A. NOMURA, J. HANKIN et al. 1985. Dietary vitamin D and calcium and risk of colorectal cancer. Lancet **1:** 925.
50. BENITO, E., A. OBRADOR, A. STIGGELBOUT et al. 1990. A population-based case-control study of colorectal cancer in Majorca. I. Dietary factors. Int. J. Cancer **45:** 69–76.
51. PETERS, R., M. PIKE, D. GARABRANT & T. MACK. 1992. Diet and colon cancer in Los Angeles County, California. Cancer Causes & Control **3:** 457–473.
52. BOSTICK, R., J. POTTER, T. SELLERS, D. MCKENZIE, L. KUSHI & A. FOLSOM. 1993. Relation of calcium, vitamin D, and dairy food intake to incidence of colon cancer among older women. Am. J. Epidemiol. **137:** 1302–1317.
53. FERRARONI, M., C. LA VECCHIA, B. D'AVANZO et al. 1994. Selected micronutrient intake and the risk of colorectal cancer. Br. J. Cancer **70:** 1150–1155.
54. KEARNEY, J., E. GIOVANUCCI, E. RIMM et al. 1996. Calcium, vitamin D, and dairy foods and the occurrence of colon cancer in men. Am. J. Epidemmiol. **143**(9)**:** 907–917.
55. PRITCHARD, R., J. BARON & M. GERHARDSSON DE VERDIER. 1996. Dietary calcium, vitamin D, and the risk of colorectal cancer in Stockholm, Sweden. Cancer Epidemiol. Biomarkers Prev. **5:** 897–900.
56. MARTINEZ, M., E. GIOVANNUCCI, G. COLDITZ et al. 1996. Calcium, vitamin D, and the occurrence of colorectal cancer among women. J. Natl. Cancer Inst. **88:** 1375–1382.
57. GARLAND, F., E. GORHAM & C. GARLAND. 1998. Meta-analysis of the role of vitamin D in epidemiological studies of cancer (abstract). Photodermatol. Photoimmunol. & Photomed. **14:** 183.
58. MANTEL, N. & W. HAENSZEL. 1959. Statistical analysis of the data from retrospective studies of disease. J. Natl. Cancer Inst. **22:** 719–748.
59. BRAUN, M., K. HELZLSOUER, B. HOLLIS & G. COMSTOCK. 1995. Colon cancer and serum vitamin D metabolite levels 10–17 years prior to diagnosis. Am. J. Epidemiol. **142:** 608–611.
60. RUSTGI, A. 1994. Hereditary gastrointestinal polyposis and nonpolyposis syndromes. N. Engl. J. Med. **331:** 1694–1702.
61. BISGAARD, M., K. FENGER, S. BULOW, E. NIEBUHR & J. MOHR. 1994. Familial adenomatous polyposis (FAP): Frequency, penetrance, and mutation. Hum. Mutat. **3:** 121–125.
62. MAHER, E., D. BARTON, R. SLATTER et al. 1993. Evaluation of molecular genetic diagnosis in the management of familial adenomatous polyposis coli: A population based study. J. Med. Genet. **30:** 675–678.
63. KONISHI, M., R. KIKUCHI-YANOSHITA, K. TANAKA et al. 1996. Molecular nature of colon tumors in hereditary nonpolyposis colon cancer, familial polyposis, and sporadic colon cancer. Gastroenterology **111:** 307–317.
64. LIPKIN, M., E. FRIEDMAN, S. WINAWER & H. NEWMARK. 1989. Colonic epithelial cell proliferation in responders and nonresponders to supplemental dietary calcium. Cancer Res. **49:** 248–254.
65. LIPKIN, M., H. NEWMARK & G. KELLOFF. 1990. Calcium, vitamin D, and prevention of colon cancer. National Cancer Institute and CRC Press. Bethesda, MD and Boca Raton, FL.

66. NEWMARK, H., M. WARGOVICH & W. BRUCE. 1984. Colon cancer, and dietary fat, phosphate, and calcium: A hypothesis. J. Natl. Cancer Inst. **72:** 1321–1325.
67. BRENNER, B., N. RUSSELL, S. ALBRECHT & R. DAVIES. 1998. The effect of dietary vitamin D_3 on the intracellular calcium gradient in mammalian colonic crypts. Cancer Lett. **127:** 43–53.
68. GORHAM, E., F. GARLAND & C. GARLAND. 1990. Sunlight and breast cancer incidence in the USSR. Int. J. Epidemiol. **19:** 820–824.
69. KOSARY, C. *et al.* 1996. SEER cancer statistics review, 1973–1992. (Publication No. 96-2798): 131,168. National Cancer Institute. Bethesda.
70. NEWMARK, H. 1994. Vitamin D adequacy: A possible relationship to breast cancer. *In* Diet and Breast Cancer. 109–114. Plenum. New York.
71. PARFITT, A., J. GALLAGHER, R. HEANEY, C. JOHNSON, R. NEER & G. WHEDON. 1982. Vitamin D and bone health in the elderly. Am. J. Clin. Nutr. **36:** 1014–1031.
72. NATIONAL ACADEMY OF SCIENCES–INSTITUTE OF MEDICINE. 1997. Vitamin intake recommendations. National Academy of Sciences. Washington, DC.
73. JEANS, P. & G. STEARNS. 1938. The human requirement of vitamin D. J. Am. Med. Assoc. **111:** 703–711.
74. SMITH, E., R. HILL, R. LEHMAN *et al.* 1983. Principles of Biochemistry, 7th ed. McGraw-Hill. New York.
75. NETELENBOS, J., M. JONGEN, W. VAN DER VIGH, P. LIPS & F. VAN GINKEL. 1985. Vitamin D status in urinary calcium stone formation. Arch. Intern. Med. **145:** 681–684.
76. NIAZI, M., A. KHANUM, M. SHEIKH & A. NAQVI. 1987. Study of 25-hydroxyvitamin D3, calcium, and phosphorus in normal subjects and patients with renal calculi. J. Pakist. Med. Assoc. **37:** 198–199.
77. CALDAS, A., R. GRAY & J. LEMANN JR. 1978. The simultaneous measurement of vitamin D metabolites in plasma: Studies of healthy adults and in patients with calcium nephrolithiasis. J. Lab. Clin. Med. **91:** 840–849.
78. VIK, T., K. TRY, D. THELLE & O. FØRDE. 1979. Tromsø Heart Study: Vitamin D metabolism and myocardial infarction. Br. Med. J. **21:** 176.
79. VAN DER VIJVER, L., M. VAN DER WAAL, K. WETERINGS, J. DEKKER, E. SCHOUTEN & F. KOK. 1992. Calcium intake and 28-year cardiovascular disease mortality in Dutch civil servants. Int. J. Epidemiol. **21:** 36–39.
80. MCKENNA, M., R. FREANEY, A. MEADE & F. MULDOWNEY. 1985. Prevention of hypovitaminosis D in the elderly. Calcif. Tissue Int. **37:** 112–116.
81. RECIHEL, H., H. KOEFFLER & A. NORMAN. 1989. The vitamin D systenm in health and disease. N. Engl. J. Med. **320:** 981–991.
82. MALABANAN, A., I. VERONIKIS & M. HOLICK. 1998. Redefining vitamin D deficiency. Lancet **351:** 805–806.

Preclinical and Early Human Studies of Calcium and Colon Cancer Prevention

MARTIN LIPKIN[a]

Strang Cancer Research Laboratory at The Rockefeller University, New York, New York 10021, USA

ABSTRACT: Colorectal cancer continues to be a major cause of tumor mortality in the United States and other countries; despite attempts to improve the screening of high-risk populations, the incidence of this disease is still very high. Therefore, chemoprevention continues to be an important goal for the primary prevention of colorectal cancer. Among recent chemopreventive approaches, the administration of calcium and vitamin D continue to be evaluated in both preclinical and clinical studies. Many experimental findings described below have indicated associations between high calcium and vitamin D intake and decreased risk for colorectal cancer.

BASIC STUDIES OF CALCIUM METABOLISM

Calcium is both an essential structural body component and a critical functional element in living cells. It is a key component for maintaining cell structure, membrane viscosity or rigidity, and the related membrane permeability is partly dependent on local calcium concentration. Calcium is also a pivotal regulator of a wide variety of cell functions in its role as a major second messenger.[1]

Among the numerous cell properties modulated by calcium, its participation in cell division and the regulation of cell proliferation and differentiation are particularly important.[2] Low levels of intracellular ionized calcium contribute to cell proliferation, and increasing calcium concentration in cell and organ culture media decreased cell proliferation and induced cell differentiation in rat esophageal epithelial cells,[3] murine epidermal cells,[4] mammary cells,[5,6] and colon cells.[7]

The absorption and metabolism of calcium are carefully regulated; 1,25 dihydroxy vitamin D_3 is an important calcium modulator that can become deficient as a consequence of inappropriate diet or inadequate exposure to sunlight. Therefore vitamin D_3 also may have a role in the regulation of cell proliferation and differentiation while modulating calcium metabolism. It has also been shown to directly inhibit the proliferation of several malignant cell lines *in vitro*,[8–10] and to induce the differentiation of human colonic cells,[11] human myeloid leukemia cells,[12] and other cell lines *in vitro*.[13,14] A role for vitamin D as a chemopreventive agent has also been studied in rodent models,[15–19] and the tumor growth and promotional stage of chemical carcinogenesis has been inhibited by vitamin D. On the other hand, vitamin D_3

[a]Address for communication: Strang Cancer Prevention Center, Box 287, The Rockefeller University, 1230 York Avenue, New York, NY 10021. Voice: 212-734-0567 ext. 206; fax: 212-570-6995.

e-mail: lipkin@rockvax.rockefeller.edu

TABLE 1. Summary of studies on calcium and colon cancer

- Majority of epidemiologic studies suggest protective effect
- *In vitro* studies: decreased proliferation and increased differentiation and maturation of many types of epithelial cells
- *In vivo* rodent studies: numerous studies demonstrated inhibition of colonic tumor development preceded by decreased hyperproliferation, ODC and ras mutations, binding of bile and fatty acids into insoluble complexes reducing irritant and hyperproliferative effects, reduced cytotoxicity of fecal water
- Human studies: decreased hyperproliferation in most studies, increased differentiation and maturation of colonic epithelial cells, binding of bile and fatty acids into insoluble complexes, decreased cytotoxcity of fecal water
- Decreased recurrence of human adenomas

enhanced chemically induced transformation of cultured cells *in vitro*[20,21] and promoted skin tumor formation in mice.[22]

PRECLINICAL AND EARLY HUMAN INTERVENTION STUDIES OF EFFECTS OF INCREASED DIETARY CALCIUM

Preclinical Studies

The results of direct experimental studies of calcium intake and colon cancer development are summarized in TABLE 1. The results of the many individual studies are further described in TABLES 2–5. In many different preclinical experimental models, calcium effects on colon cancer development and on cellular processes associated with colon cancer have been remarkably consistent: (1) decreasing and normalizing excessive proliferation of colonic epithelial cells, reducing the susceptibility of proliferating epithelial cells to accumulate abnormalities in nuclear DNA; (2) reducing the cytotoxicity of fecal water; (3) increasing the differentiation and maturation of colonic epithelial cells; and (4) decreasing the ultimate end-stage development of colon cancer itself.

In animal models (TABLES 2 and 3), oral calcium supplementation was shown to decrease epithelial cell hyperproliferation when it was induced by several factors that stimulate tumor promotion: the administration of bile acids and fatty acids, dietary fat, a Western-style diet, and partial enteric resection. Of further importance, colonic carcinogenesis itself, when induced by chemical carcinogens was decreased by increasing dietary calcium intake, with almost all studies showing a decrease in the number of tumors induced, the percent of invasive carcinomas, or the numbers of animals with multiple tumors.

Thus, a wide variety of rodent studies (TABLES 1–3 with references) demonstrated that increasing the intake of dietary calcium reduced colonic tumor formation, and mechanisms involved included decreased epithelial cell hyperproliferation; decreased ornithine decarboxylase activity; decreased ras mutations in colonic epithelial cells; and calcium-binding of bile acids, fatty acids, and phosphate into insoluble complexes, reducing their direct irritant and hyperproliferative effects on colonic epithelial cells and reducing the cytotoxicity of fecal water.

TABLE 2. Dietary calcium effects on epithelial cells in the colon and other organs of rodents

Cell Proliferation	References[a]
Calcium decreased hyperproliferation	Govers et al. 1994
Calcium: decreased hyperproliferation when induced by deoxycholic acid	Wargovich et al. 1983
Decreased hyperproliferation when induced by fatty acids	Wargovich et al. 1984
Decreased hyperproliferation when induced by cholic acid	Bird et al. 1986
Decreased hyperproliferation induced by partial enteric resection	Appleton et al. 1986
Decreased deoxycholic acid–induced hyperproliferation	Hu et al. 1989
Decreased MNNG-induced hyperproliferation on diet low in fat and calcium	Reshef et al. 1990
Decreased hyperproliferation induced by Western-style diet	Newmark et al. 1991
Decreased AOM[b]-induced ODC and Tyr K	Arlow et al. 1989
Decreased ODC[c] induced by bile acids	Baer et al. 1989
Decreased hyperproliferation when induced by Western-style diet	Richter et al.[24]
Decreased hyperproliferation in other organs when induced by Western-style diet	Xue et al.[25]

[a]Studies without reference numbers are found in ref. 23.
[b]AOM, azoxymethane.
[c]ODC, ornithine decarboxylase.

TABLE 3. Dietary calcium effects on colonic epithelial cells of rodents

Tumor Development	References[a]
Calcium: decreased tumors induced by partial enteric resection and carcinogen	Appleton et al. 1987
Decreased proliferation and tumor formation induced by dietary fat and carcinogen	Pence et al. 1988
Decreased intestinal tumors after AOM	Skrypec et al. 1988
Decreased colonic tumors induced by AOM	Wargovich et al. 1990
Decreased invasive carcinomas after MNU and cholic acid	McSherry et al. 1989
Decreased the number of rats with multiple tumors after DMH	Sitrin et al. 1991
Decreased K-ras mutations	Llor et al. 1990
Unchanged tumor incidence after DMH	Karkara et al. 1989
Unchanged tumor incidence after DMH	Kaup et al. 1989
Decreased late-stage precancerous lesion of whole colonic crypt dysplasia	Risio et al.[26]

[a]Studies without reference numbers are found in ref. 23.

Two recent series of preclinical studies also have evaluated the effects of calcium and vitamin D on colonic tumor development when these nutrients were fed to rodents on Western-style diets. The first series of studies used models with normal mice. In the colonic crypts of these normal mice, hyperproliferation, hyperplasia, abnormal differentiation and maturation of colonic crypt epithelial cells, and the late-

TABLE 4. Calcium effects on colonic cell proliferation, differentiation, and cytotoxicity in human subjects

In vitro	References[a]
Decreased proliferation (2 mM)	Buset *et al.* 1986
Decreased proliferation (2–4 mM)	Appleton *et al.* 1988
Decreased proliferation (2 mM)	Arlow *et al.* 1988
Decreased proliferation (2 mM)	Buset *et al.* 1987
Decreased proliferation (2 mM)	Friedman *et al.* 1989
Protected colonic cells against toxicity of bile acids and fatty acids (5 mM)	Buset *et al.* 1989
Decreased growth of human colon cancer cell lines	Guo *et al.*[27]
Increased histone acetylation: cell differentiation (1–2 mM)	Boffa *et al.* 1989

[a]Studies without reference numbers are found in ref. 23.

stage preneoplastic lesion of whole-colonic-crypt dysplasia developed when the mice were fed Western-style diets containing low calcium and vitamin D.[26,33,34]

The second series of studies used mice having targeted mutations that are relevant to human colon cancer, the targeted mutations causing adenomas and carcinomas to develop in the mice.[35,36] Recent studies demonstrated that Western-style diets increased the development of the neoplastic colonic lesions that were initiated by several mutations; and the neoplasms, including carcinomas, were decreased by (a) increasing calcium and vitamin D, together with lowering the fat content of the diet,[37] or (b) increasing dietary calcium and vitamin D alone (Yang *et al.*, unpublished data).

In other organs, Western-style diets also have induced epithelial cell hyperproliferation and hyperplasia in mammary gland,[38,39] and hyperproliferation in pancreas[40] and prostate gland[41] in short-term studies; increasing dietary calcium and vitamin D alone also inhibited the development of those lesions.[25]

EARLY HUMAN CLINICAL TRIALS OF CALCIUM AND COLON CANCER CHEMOPREVENTION

Prior to most of the preclinical studies noted above, a first human study was carried out[28] that began to evaluate calcium's chemopreventive effects on the human colon. That first study, and a majority of the human studies that followed, demonstrated that increased dietary calcium could decrease hyperproliferation of colonic epithelial cells in human subjects; and several studies further demonstrated calcium's binding of bile acids and fatty acids into insoluble complexes in the colon, decreasing the cytotoxicity of fecal water, the latter contributing to the decreased colonic epithelial cell hyperproliferation observed in human subjects (TABLES 4 and 5).

The first pilot study of this human series[28] noted above, and several others that followed, demonstrated significant reductions of excessive colonic epithelial cell proliferation, or reduced size of the proliferative compartment in colonic crypts. However, other human studies of supplemental calcium administration did not show this effect.[42] Several of those studies were accompanied by experimental techniques

TABLE 5. Calcium effects on colonic cell proliferation, differentiation and cytotoxicity of fecal water in human subjects

In vivo	References[a]
Decreased hyperproliferation	Lipkin et al.[28]
Decreased hyperproliferation	Lipkin et al. 1989
Decreased hyperproliferation	Rozen et al. 1989
Decreased proliferation	Lynch et al. 1991
Decreased proliferation	Berger et al. 1991
Decreased proliferation	Wargovich et al. 1992
Decreased proliferation	Barsoum et al. 1992
Decreased proliferation	O'Sullivan et al. 1993
Decreased proliferation	Bostick et al. 1995
Unchanged proliferation	Gregoire et al. 1989
Unchanged proliferation	Cats et al. 1995
Decreased ODC	Lans et al.[29]
Normalized differentiation-associated lectin binding	Yang et al.[30]
Decreased cytotoxicity of fecal water	Govers et al.[31]
Decreased adenoma recurrence	Baron et al.[32]

[a]Studies without reference numbers are found in ref. 23.

that included extremely low initial baseline levels of colonic cell proliferation measured before calcium administration, very high amounts of calcium intake by subjects before calcium was given, and enemas given prior to colonic biopsies that likely perturbed the mucosa.[42] Because early positive results were found in humans where calcium reduced colonic epithelial cell proliferation,[28] a further large randomized adenoma-recurrence clinical trial was developed and carried out, recently verifying that increased calcium intake caused a significant reduction in the development of actual tumors (recurrent adenomas) in the human colon.[32] The following two papers in this volume (Holt and Baron) will describe the two most recent clinical trials of calcium's effect in the human colon, the first describing increased maturation of colonic epithelial cells following increased dietary calcium intake,[43] and the second demonstrating the inhibition of colonic adenoma recurrence.[32]

REFERENCES

1. RASMUSSEN, H. The calcium messenger system (in 2 parts). 1986. N. Engl. J. Med. **314:** 1094, 1164.
2. WHITFIELD, J.F., A.L. BOYNTON, J.P. MACMANUS, M. SIKORSKA & B.K. TSANG. 1979. The regulation of cell proliferation by calcium and cyclic AMP. Mol. Cell. Biochem. **27:** 155–179.
3. BABCOCK, M.S., M.R. MARINO, W.T. GUNNING III & G.D. STONER. 1983. Clonal growth and serial propagation of rat esophageal epithelial cells. In Vitro **19:** 403–415.
4. HENNINGS, H., D. MICHAEL, C. CHENG, P. STEINHART, K. HOLBROOK & S.H. YUSPA. 1980. Calcium regulation of growth and differentiation of mouse epidermal cells in culture. Cell **19:** 245–254.

5. McGrath, C.M. & H.D. Soule. 1984. Calcium regulation of normal mammary epithelial cell growth in culture. In Vitro **20**: 652–662.
6. Soule, H.D. & C.M. McGrath. 1985. A simplified method for passage and long-term growth of human mammary epithelial cell. In Vitro **22**: 6–12.
7. Boffa, L.C., M.R. Mariani, H. Newmark & M. Lipkin. 1989. Calcium as modulator of nucleosomal histones acetylation in cultured cells. Proc. Am. Assoc. Cancer Res. **30**: 8.
8. Niendorf, A., H. Arps & M. Dietel. 1987. Effect of 1,25-dihydroxyvitamin D_3 on human colon cancer in vitro. J. Steroid Biochem. **27**: 825–828.
9. Colston, K., M.J. Colston & D. Feldman. 1981. 1,25-Dihydroxyvitamin D_3 and malignant melanoma: The presence of receptors and inhibition of cell growth in culture. Endocrinology **108**: 1083–1086.
10. Lointier, P., M.J. Wargovich, S. Saez, B. Levin, D.M. Wildrick & B. M. Boman. 1987. The role of vitamin D_3 in the proliferation of a human colon cancer cell line in vitro. Anticancer Res. **7**: 817–822.
11. Higgins, P.J. & Y. Tanaka. 1991. Cytoarchitectural response and expression of c-fos/p52 genes during enhancement of butyrate-initiated differentiation of human colon carcinoma cells by 1,25-dihydroxyvitamin D_3 and its analogs. In Calcium, Vitamin D, and Prevention of Colon Cancer. M. Lipkin, H.L. Newmark & G. Kelloff, Eds.: 305–326. CRC Press. Boca Raton.
12. Miyaura, C., E. Abe, T. Kuribayashi, H. Tanaka, K. Konno, Y. Nishii & T. Suda. 1981. $1\alpha,25$-Dihydroxyvitamin D_3 induces differentiation of human myeloid leukemia cells. Biochem. Biophys. Res. Commun. **102**: 937–943.
13. Kuroki, T., K. Chida, H. Hashiba, J. Hosoi, J. Hosomi, K. Sasaki, E. Abe & T. Suda. 1985. Regulation of cell differentiation and tumor promotion by $1\alpha,25$-dihydroxyvitamin D_3. In Carcinogenesis—A Comprehensive Survey. E. Humberman & S.H. Barr, Eds.: 275–286. Raven Press. New York. .
14. Suda, T., C. Miyaura, E. Abe E & T. Kuroki. 1986. Modulation of cell differentiation, immune responses and tumor promotion by vitamin D compounds. Bone Min. Res. **4**: 1–48.
15. Eisman, J.A., D.H. Barkla & P.J.M. Tutton. 1987. Suppression of in vivo growth of human cancer solid tumor xenografts by $1\alpha,25$-dihydroxyvitamin D_3. Cancer Res. **47**: 21–25.
16. Honma, Y., M. Hozumi, E. Abe, K. Konna, M. Fukushima, S. Hata, Y. Nishji, H.F. DeLuca & T. Suda. 1983. $1\alpha,25$-Dihydroxyvitamin D_3 and 1α-hydroxyvitamin D_3 prolong survival time of mice inoculated with myeloid leukemia cells. Proc. Natl. Acad. Sci. USA **80**: 201–204.
17. Chida, K., H. Hashiba, M. Fukushim, T. Suda & T. Kuroki. 1985. Inhibition of tumor promotion in mouse skin by $1\alpha,25$-dihydroxyvitamin D_3. Cancer Res. **45**: 5426–5430.
18. Kawaura, A., N. Tanida, K. Sawada, M. Oda & T. Shimoyama. 1989. Supplemental administration of 1-hydroxyvitamin D_3 inhibits promotion by intrarectal instillation of lithocholic acid in N-methyl-N-nitrosourea-induced colonic tumorigenesis in rats. Carcinogenesis **10**: 647–649.
19. Hashiba, H., M. Fukushima, K. Chida & T. Kuroki. 1987. Systemic inhibition of tumor promoter-induced ornithine decarboxylase in 1α-hydroxyvitamin D_3-treated animals. Cancer Res. **47**: 5031–5035.
20. Kuroki, T., K. Sasaki, K. Chida, E. Abe & T. Suda. 1983. $1\alpha,25$-Dihydroxyvitamin D_3 markedly enhances chemically-induced transformation in BALB 3T3 cells. GANN **74**: 611–614.
21. Jones, C.A., M.F. Callaham & E. Huberman. 1984. Enhancement of chemical-carcinogen-induced cell transformation in hamster embryo cells by $1\alpha,25$-dihydroxycholecalciferol, the biologically active metabolite of vitamin D_3. Carcinogenesis **5**: 1155–1159.

22. WOOD, A.W., R.L. CHANG, M-T. HUANG, E. BAGGIOLINI, J.J. PARTRIDGE, M. USKOK-OVIC & A.H. CONNEY. 1985. Stimulatory effect of 1α,25-dihydroxyvitamin D_3 on the formation of skin tumors in mice treated chronically with 7,12-dimethyl-benz[a]anthracene. Biochem. Biophys. Res. Commun. 130: 924–931.

23. LIPKIN, M. & H. NEWMARK. 1995. Calcium and the prevention of colon cancer. J. Cell. Biochem. (Suppl.) 22: 65–73.

24. RICHTER, F., H. NEWMARK, A. RICHTER, D. LEUNG & M. LIPKIN. 1995. Inhibition of Western diet induced hyperproliferation and hyperplasia in mouse colon by two sources of calcium. Carcinogenesis 16: 2685–2689.

25. XUE, L., M. LIPKIN, H. NEWMARK & J. WANG. 1999. Influence of dietary calcium and vitamin D on diet-induced epithelial cell hyperproliferation in mice. J. Natl. Cancer Inst. 91: 176–181.

26. RISIO, M., M. LIPKIN, H. NEWMARK, K. YANG, F. ROSSINI, V. STEELE, C. BOONE & G. KELLOFF. 1996. Apoptosis, cell replication, and Western-style diet-induced tumorigenesis in mouse colon. Cancer Res. 56: 4910–4916.

27. GUO, Y.S., E. DRAVIAM, C.M. TOWNSEND JR. & P. SINGH. 1990. Differential effects of Ca^{2+} on proliferation of stomach, colonic, and pancreatic cancer lines in vitro. Nutr. Cancer 14: 149.

28. LIPKIN, M. & H. NEWMARK. 1985. Effect of added dietary calcium on colonic epithelial-cell proliferation in subjects at high risk for familial colonic cancer. N. Engl. J. Med. 313(22): 1381–1384.

29. LANS, J.I., R. JASZEWSKI, F.L. ARLOW, J. TUREAUD, G.D. LUK & A.P. MAJUMDAR. 1991. Supplemental calcium suppresses colonic mucosal ornithine decarboxylase activity in elderly patients with adenomatous polyps. Cancer Res. 51(13): 3416–3419.

30. YANG, K., L. COHEN & M. LIPKIN. 1991. Lectin soybean agglutinin: Measurements in colonic epithelial cells of human subjects following supplemental dietary calcium. Cancer Lett. 56: 65–69.

31. GOVERS, M.J., D.S. TREMONT, J.A. LAPRE, J.H. KLEIBEUKER, R.J. VONK & R. VAN DER MEER. 1996. Calcium in milk products precipitates intestinal fatty acids and secondary bile acids and thus inhibits colonic cytotoxicity in humans. Cancer Res. 56: 3270–3275.

32. BARON, J.A., M. BEACH, J.S. MANDEL et al. 1999. Calcium supplements for the prevention of colorectal adenomas. N. Engl. J. Med. 340: 101–107.

33. NEWMARK, H., M. LIPKIN & N. MAHESHWARI. 1990. Colonic hyperplasia and hyperproliferation induced by a nutritional stress diet with four components of Western-style diet. J. Natl. Cancer Inst. 82: 491–496.

34. NEWMARK, H., M. LIPKIN & N. MAHESHWARI. 1991. Colonic hyperproliferation induced in rats and mice by nutritional stress diets containing four components of human Western-style diet (Series 2). Am. J. Clin. Nutr. 54: 209s–214s.

35. FODDE, R., W. EDELMANN, K. YANG, C. VAN LEEUWEN, C. CARLSON, B. RENAULT, C. BREUKEL, E. ALT, M. LIPKIN & P. KHAN. 1994. A targeted chain-termination mutation in the mouse Apc gene results in multiple intestinal tumors. Proc. Natl. Acad. Sci. USA 91: 8969–8973.

36. YANG, K., W. EDELMANN, K. FAN, K. LAU, V.R. KOLLI, R. FODDE, M. KHAN, R. KUCHERLAPTI & M. LIPKIN. 1997. A mouse model of human familial adenomatous polyposis. J. Exp. Zool. 277: 245–254.

37. YANG, K., W. EDELMANN, K.H. FAN, K. LAU, D. LEUNG, H. NEWMARK, R. KUCHERLAPATI & M. LIPKIN. 1998. Dietary influences on neoplasms in a mouse model for human familial adenomatous polyposis. Cancer Res. 58: 5713–5717.

38. KHAN, N., K. YANG, H. NEWMARK, G. WONG, N. TELANG, R. RIVLIN & M. LIPKIN. 1994. Mammary duct epithelial cell hyperproliferation and hyperplasia induced by

a nutritional stress diet containing four components of a Western-style diet. Carcinogenesis **15:** 2645–2648.

39. XUE, L., H. NEWMARK, K. YANG & M. LIPKIN. 1996. Model of mouse mammary gland hyperproliferation and hyperplasia induced by a Western-style diet. Nutr. Cancer **26:** 281–287.

40. XUE, L., K. YANG, H. NEWMARK, D. LEUNG & M. LIPKIN. 1996. Epithelial cell hyperproliferation induced in the exocrine pancreas of mice by a Western-style diet. J. Natl. Cancer Inst. **88**(21)**:** 1586–1590.

41. XUE, L., K. YANG, H. NEWMARK & M. LIPKIN. 1993. Induced hyperproliferation in epithelial cells of mouse prostate by a Western-style diet. Carcinogenesis **18:** 995–999.

42. LIPKIN, M. & H. NEWMARK. 1993. Chemoprevention studies: Controlling effects of initial nutrient levels. J. Natl. Cancer Inst. **85:** 1870–1871.

43. HOLT, P., E. ATALLASOY, J. GELMAN, J. GUSS, S. MOSS, H. NEWMARK, K. FAN, K. YANG & M. LIPKIN. 1998. Modulation of abnormal colonic epithelial cell proliferation and differentiation by low fat dairy foods. J. Am. Med. Assoc. **280:** 1074–1079.

Studies of Calcium in Food Supplements in Humans

PETER R. HOLT[a]

Division of Gastroenterology, St. Lukes-Roosevelt Hospital Center,
New York, New York 10025, USA

ABSTRACT: Colon cancer is one of the commonest cancers in the Western world. Environmental factors appear to predominate as exemplified by a change in incidence in colon cancer within 20 years when people emigrate from a low- to a high-incidence country. It had been suggested that a diet high in energy, fat, and meat content and low in fiber content is most likely responsible. Epidemiologic observations have pointed to a potential effect of calcium or/and vitamin D in reducing the incidence of colon cancer. Other studies have shown a reduction in preneoplastic colon adenomas with increased calcium or/and vitamin D intake. High fat diets were shown to be accompanied by an increase in fecal fatty acids and bile acids or a change in bile acid composition. Soluble fatty acids and bile acids then could interact with the colonic epithelium inducing cell damage and increased proliferation. A hypothesis was developed suggesting that calcium supplementation and increased calcium in the colonic lumen would precipitate these bile acids and fatty acids. Examination of the effect of supplemental calcium or calcium in dairy foods showed a major reduction in fecal bile acids and fatty acids in solution in volunteers and accompanied by a reduction in cytolytic activity. Studies then were performed in patients at risk for colon cancer seeking a change in proliferative biomarkers of risk from a high-risk to a low-risk pattern with supplemental calcium administration. These studies generally have shown a beneficial effect of the addition of calcium at 1.2–2 gm per day in addition to a regular diet for periods of 2 to 6 months. A recently published study also demonstrated that a diet, in which low-fat dairy foods containing an average of about 825 mg of calcium, significantly improved proliferative biomarkers as well as two differentiation biomarkers of risk for colon cancer from a high- to a low-risk pattern. These observations, together with recent studies showing reduced adenomatous polyp recurrence when supplemental calcium was provided, demonstrate the potential of calcium and perhaps vitamin D as chemopreventive agents for colorectal neoplasia.

Colorectal cancer is extremely common in the Western world. In the United States, colon cancer represents the second leading cause of cancer deaths. The disease occurs both in men and women and increases dramatically with advancing age. Present recommendations for prevention include annual testing of stool samples for occult

[a]Address for communication: Division of Gastroenterology, St. Lukes-Roosevelt Hospital Center, Amsterdam Ave. at 114 Street, New York, NY 10025. Voice: 212-523-3679; fax: 212-523-3683.
e-mail: pholt@slrhc.org

blood as well as sigmoidoscopies performed every five years if no occult blood is found in the feces. These methods of detection of colorectal cancer and adenomatous polyps are standard after the age of 50 years in subjects at average risk. If a polyp is found at sigmoidoscopy or if fecal occult blood testing shows a positive result, then fiberoptic colonoscopy of the whole colon is advised. Removal of colorectal adenomas has been shown to reduce the subsequent risk of colorectal cancer.[1] The recommendations for prevention are modified for subjects with a strong family history of colorectal cancer.[2]

The past decade has led to a remarkable explosion of data focused upon changes in genes during the process of colorectal carcinogenesis. The now classic study of Vogelstein and his colleagues resulted in the description of a schema of progressive accumulation of genetic damage during colorectal cancer formation.[3] At the same time, many aspects of the two major hereditary diseases leading to colon cancer, that is familial adenomatous polyposis and hereditary nonpolyposis colon cancer, have been elucidated. Although we have come to learn so much about changes in colonic epithelial cell genes during carcinogenesis, it is important to recognize that much of the available epidemiologic data points to the overwhelming effect of the environment in colorectal cancer formation. First, there are large variations in the incidence of such cancers worldwide, so that there are "high-risk" and "low-risk" nations. Second, when populations move from a low-risk to a high-risk country, the migrants develop the incidence of their new environment within the same generation, that is within 20 years of the migration. Similar data have been shown for individuals who have moved from a high- to a low-risk area. These data overwhelmingly emphasized that major environmental factors must be responsible for the rate of colorectal cancer incidence in the high-risk westernized nations. Subsequent epidemiologic data focused upon changes in the diet as paramount. There has been much argument about which individual dietary factor has the greatest impact for this increase in colorectal cancer incidence. When all the results are examined together, it is most accurate to state that a diet that is high in energy, high in meat intake and fat, and low in fiber intake is the combination that is responsible. It is hypothesized that excess dietary fat results in the passage of lipids (and bile salts) into the colon that may be major factors in initiating tumorigenesis and promoting the cancer process during subsequent years.

Colorectal neoplasia should be particularly susceptible to chemoprevention. Chemoprevention is based upon the principle that the cancer under study results mainly from environmental factors, that it takes a long time to progress, and that identified environmental factors may be modified or interrupted by extraneous agents. The development of colonic adenomatous polyps takes a considerable amount of time (even in familial adenomatous polyposis patients), and progression from adenoma to cancer takes a further 10 to 20 years. In addition, the data of Vogelstein indicate that multiple identified steps occur between initiation in the flat colorectal mucosa of an "at-risk" subject and the aberrant crypt foci formation, colorectal adenomas (polyps), and then to colorectal cancer.

This review focuses on the effect of calcium and dairy foods in the prevention of colorectal carcinogenesis. The epidemiologic studies described by Cedric Garland elsewhere in this volume focuses on the relationship between the dietary intake of calcium and dairy foods, and colorectal neoplasia. Overall, an increasing intake of

Table 1. Dairy food components that may be protective against colon cancer

Calcium
Vitamin D
Conjugated linoleic acid
Sphingolipids
Butyric acid
Bacterial cultures

dietary calcium has shown benefit in reducing colorectal tumors, and this increase consisted predominantly of dairy foods. In addition to the calcium content of the dairy foods, several other components are present that could play a role in altering the process of colorectal neoplasia (TABLE 1). In whole dairy foods, calcium and vitamin D have been demonstrated to have some beneficial effect; in addition, conjugated linoleic acid, sphingolipids, butyric acid, and even bacterial cultures have shown some possible beneficial effect in *in vitro* or in animal studies.

Several lines of evidence have pointed to changes in colonic contents as mainly responsible for increasing the risk of colon cancer. As a result of epidemiologic data suggesting that an excess of dietary fat is an important component of colon cancer risk, several studies measured changes in human fecal components during high-fat diet intake.[4] The feces of such subjects were shown to contain an excess of fat as well as bile salts when compared to the feces from individuals taking low-fat diets.[5] As a result of these observations, Harold Newmark and coworkers developed a hypothesis that fatty acids and bile acids are the colonic components most responsible for inducing epithelial cells in the direction of carcinogenesis. They also emphasized that colonic fatty acids and bile acids would need to be in the aqueous phase of colonic contents in order to interact with the colonic mucosa and to stimulate pathogenic changes.[6] They then postulated that if an excess of calcium entered the colon, then soluble bile acids and fatty acids would be precipitated and therefore no longer be able to alter the epithelium. Calcium principally precipitates deoxycholic and lithocholic acids that can stimulate colorectal proliferation.[7] This initial hypothesis has been successfully tested in animal studies as described by Martin Lipkin elsewhere in this volume.

In studies of human feces during the ingestion of varying amounts of calcium, the accuracy of the original hypothesis of Newmark *et al.* was confirmed. A series of experiments by a group of investigators, headed by Van der Meer in Holland, demonstrated that the provision of supplemental calcium[8] or a regular high-calcium milk diet[9] increased the amount of calcium appearing in the stool when compared to volunteers not taking supplemental calcium or a placebo milk low in calcium content. This was associated with an increase in total bile acid and lipid excretion.[10] However, when the bile and fatty acid content in the aqueous portion of the stool was examined, there was a dramatic reduction in these components (FIG. 1). Because the original hypothesis implied a degree of cytotoxicity of soluble bile acids and fatty acids that might be reversed by calcium, Van der Meer's group then directly examined cytotoxicity of fecal aqueous solutions of subjects taking a low- and high-calcium diet using as test components either red cells or colon cancer cells *in vitro*. In these studies these investigators clearly demonstrated reduced cytotoxicity during

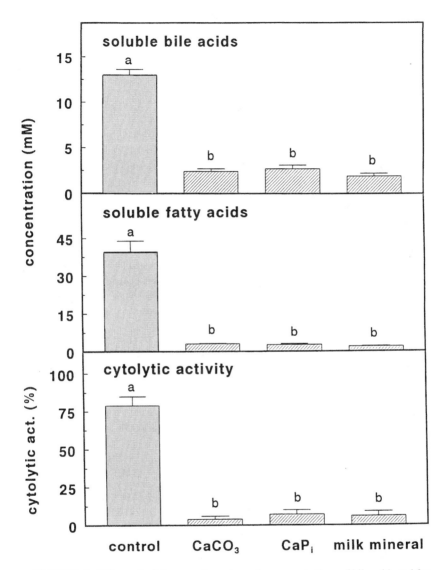

FIGURE 1. Effects of calcium supplements on the concentrations of bile acids and fatty acids in fecal water and on the cytolytic activity of fecal water. The control diet contains 30 mmol calcium/kg, whereas the other diets contain 180 mmol calcium/kg diet. Bars not sharing the same superscript are significantly different ($p < 0.05$).

the dietary administration of calcium or a high-calcium milk diet.[11,12] Bile acids also may stimulate proliferation directly. Calcium also has been shown to reduce the colonic content of diacylglycerol,[13] formed by bacteria, which may activate cellular signal transduction pathways,[14] and has been postulated as increasing proliferation in the colonic epithelium.[15] Whether diacylglycerol plays any role in colon carcinogenesis is unclear at the present time.

For studies of chemoprevention, two major different end points have been used as intermediate biomarkers of risk in colorectal neoplasia. A late intermediate biomarker of risk is the formation of adenomatous polyps, which usually have been investigated in volunteers who have previously had adenomatous polyps and therefore are at risk for recurrence. Early intermediate biomarkers of risk have been detected in the flat normal-appearing mucosa of similar subjects at risk for the development of colon adenomas and cancer. Studies of recurrence of adenomatous polyps as a late intermediate end point for chemoprevention requires a considerable amount of time and are very expensive. J.A. Baron will describe one important study of calcium prevention of adenomatous polyp recurrence elsewhere in this volume. Early intermediate biomarkers generally have been used for pilot studies to indicate what experimental approaches might be used for subsequent evaluation in this field. The most common early intermediate biomarker that has been used in this field has been a change in cell proliferation. This was based upon the observations of Lipkin and coworkers of a progressive change in the number of crypt-proliferating cells and an upward shift of such proliferating cells in the crypt in at-risk patients with colon cancer, colon adenomas, familial colon cancer, as well as other conditions that have an increased risk of colon cancer, such as ulcerative colitis[16] and has been confirmed by others.[17–19] Polyp recurrence has also been reported more frequently in patients who demonstrate a shift in crypt-proliferating cells toward the colonic surface.[20] Following the concept of using supplemental calcium to reduce the risk of colorectal neoplasia, studies were performed to determine the relationship between dietary calcium intake and colorectal proliferation and to measure the effects of calcium supplementation upon proliferation. The original studies of Lipkin, Newmark, and associates all pointed to a dramatic improvement in several parameters of proliferation when calcium was provided in doses of about 1.2 to 1.5 gms per day.[21] This group carefully validated their short-term organ culture technique.[22] Other investigators appeared to confirm these studies using similar or differing methods of detection.[23–25] However, later authors have questioned the reproducibility of data that demonstrate changes in proliferation during calcium supplementation.[26,27] Thus it is important to review the data that have been published that included such determinations. Some studies have been performed in at-risk patients who have had colon cancer surgery, yet it does not seem appropriate to study subjects in whom surgical reaction clearly would alter the colonic content of putative pathogenic compounds. Subjects with such familial syndromes as familial adenomatous polyposis (FAP) have genetic changes that cannot be generalized to the at-risk population at large. Furthermore, it is important to recognize that no "improvement" in proliferation can be expected if the baseline proliferative rate is extremely low. Evaluations of differences in studies that have shown a beneficial effect or no beneficial effect indicate that no benefit was shown when rates of proliferation (i.e., labeling indices) were extremely low, much lower than those of "positive studies" (TABLE 2). Clearly, if proliferation is already low, it hardly can be expected that the addition of a chemopreventive agent will reduce proliferation further.

Recent publications commenting on the vagaries of proliferative markers for the study of chemoprevention illustrate the pitfalls of such evaluations. The study by McShane and coworkers was performed in several separate centers, the endoscopic

TABLE 2. Effects of calcium supplementation upon total labeling index[a]

Authors	Method	Change in Labeling Index (%)
	Positive Results	
Lipkin and Newmark[21]	[³H]dThd	16.7 → 10.0
Buset et al.[35]	[³H]dThd	Responder 16.1 → 7.9
		Nonresponder 7.4 → 6.9
Lipkin et al.[36]	[³H]dThd	Responder 14.1 → 8.7
		Nonresponder 9.1 → 8.8
Rozen et al.[23]	[³H]dThd	6.6 → 4.4
Wargovich et al.[24]	[³H]dThd	7.2 → 6.5
O'Sullivan et al.[25]	BrdU	8.8 → 4.7
	Negative Results	
Baron et al.[26]	PCNA	3.9 → 3.9
Bostick et al.[27]	[³H]dThd	4.7 → 5.3
Bostick et al.[37]	PCNA	3.6 → 4.0[b]
Weisgerber et al.[38]	BrdU	13.5 → 11.4
Alberts et al.[39]	[³H]dThd	7.4 → 6.7

[a]Restricted to studies in patients postpolypectomy for adenomatous polyps with an intact colon and without evidence of inflammatory bowel disease or colon cancer. Also excluded are studies using measurements of crypt cell production rate.
[b]Significant shift in proliferating cells to crypt basal positions.

procedures were performed for clinical reasons, and preparation of patients was not standardized. Incubations were not performed by verified original methods, and a description of how the slides were read indicates that scoring was based on individual judgement[28] (TABLE 3). Another, much quoted, summary of issues with proliferation data also suffered from similar problems.[29] The studies performed by Lipkin's group and our own were performed with tight control of all of the steps, as is necessary in any pilot study using small numbers of subjects (TABLE 4).

Our group, together with that of Martin Lipkin, recently has completed a study of the effect of a diet high in dairy foods upon proliferation, two differentiation markers, and changes in epithelial cell nuclei.[30] This study separated a group of 70 volunteers who had undergone a recent polypectomy for colonic adenomatous polyps into two groups. One group continued their individual baseline diet, and in the other we aimed to increase dairy food components by an amount containing up to 1200 mg of calcium daily. The diet of this experimental group was modified in order to keep the energy, fat, and protein content constant. Rectal biopsies were obtained twice at baseline, at 6 and at 12 months. These biopsies were analyzed for changes in proliferation (as measured by incubation and [³H]thymidine incorporation into DNA), differentiation markers, and nuclear morphometry. In fact, the dairy food supplemental study group increased their dairy food calcium intake by approximately 825 mg to a total of about 1500 mg per day of dietary calcium. The sources of dietary intake of calcium from dairy foods increased from 53% at baseline to 83% during the study.

TABLE 3. "Proliferation measures amid the noise"[28]

- Several separate centers

- Preparation of patients not standardized
  (a) Biopsies taken during colonoscopy
  (b) Many endoscopists involved

- Incubations (BrdU) not performed under increased atmospheric pressure

- Multiple scorers of immunostained slides read at differing times

- Readings of immunostained slides too personal
  (a) For BrdU, read only deepest staining crypts
  (b) For PCNA, read darkest and next darkest nuclei

TABLE 4. How proliferation studies should be done

- Subjects must be examined identically
  (a) Same endoscopist
  (b) Same technologist

- Slides must be examined identically
  (a) Same slide scorer
  (b) There must be clear differences between labeled (positive) and unlabeled (negative) cells
  (c) All specimens from the same subject should be processed and read together

- Proliferation rate (or shift in proliferating cells) must be high enough at baseline to see effect of putative chemopreventive agents

The results of the study showed that the experimental group of subjects taking an increased dairy intake had a significantly lower number of labeled cells per crypt, total labeling index, as well as labeling index in the upper crypt compartment at either 6 or 12 months or both. In addition, there was a significant change in the two major differentiation markers that we studied, cytokeratin AE1 and acidic mucins, from the direction found in high-risk subjects toward that seen in low-risk subjects. There were no consistent changes in nuclear morphometry in this study. Thus, this pilot study showed a clearly beneficial effect of low-fat dairy foods upon biomarkers of risk seen in flat mucosa of individuals at risk for colonic neoplasia. This occurred at levels of added dairy food calcium well below that previously found to have an effect in similar subjects provided supplemental calcium in pill form. This raised the possibility that the low-fat dairy foods had a greater effect upon the biomarkers studied than would be expected from the content of dairy calcium provided as a supplement. Studies are presently being conducted to explore this further.

It is important to point out that any potential chemopreventive strategy must have a very positive benefit-to-risk ratio. There are potential adverse effects of calcium that have raised some concerns in the literature. However, hypercalcemia has not been reported in any of the large number of studies of calcium supplementation that have been performed. Constipation, if it occurs, is not seen commonly, and several studies have discounted the potential effects upon kidney stone formation. Indeed epidemiologic studies appear to show that administration of calcium supplements reduces the risk of kidney stones in both men[31] and women.[32] Furthermore, the possible negative effect of calcium upon iron absorption recently has been discounted,[33] and the modest increase in fecal excretion of lipids and bile acids would tend to be beneficial rather than harmful.

In summary, for evaluation of chemopreventive agents in humans, intermediate biomarkers of risk need to be studied in order to obtain data that later might be used for public health measures.[34] Presently, adenomatous polyp regression or reduction in reappearance of such adenomas in individuals at risk is considered the best end point for chemoprevention of colon neoplasia. However, such studies require a considerable amount of time and are expensive. Pilot studies of early intermediate end points are important signposts that can determine optimal chemopreventive strategy for later polyp-prevention strategies. The data on supplemental calcium and diets high in calcium-containing dairy foods appear to show considerable promise for chemoprevention. In the future it is likely that combinations of chemopreventive agents will be used in order to amplify prevention in a way that is similar to what is done in cancer chemotherapy. Calcium or calcium-containing foods should have an important role to play in such combinations.

REFERENCES

1. WINAWER, S.J., A.G. ZAUBER, M.N. HO et al. 1993. Prevention of colorectal cancer by colonoscopic polypectomy. N. Engl. J. Med. **329:** 1977–1981.
2. WINAWER, S.J., R.H. FLETCHER, L. MILLER et al. 1997. Colorectal cancer screening: Clinical guidelines and rationale. Gastroenterology **112:** 594–642.
3. VOGELSTEIN, B., E.R. FEARON, S.R. HAMILTON et al. 1988. Genetic alterations during colorectal-tumor development. N. Engl. J. Med. **319:** 525–532.
4. WEISBURGER, J.H. 1991. Causes, relevant mechanisms, and prevention of large bowel cancer. Semin. Oncol. **18:** 316–336.
5. REDDY, B.S. 1981. Bile salts and other constituents of the colon as tumor promoters. Banbury Rep. **7:** 345–361.
6. NEWMARK, H., M. WARGOVICH & R. BRUCE. 1984. Colon cancer and dietary fat, phosphate and calcium—A hypothesis. J. Natl. Cancer Inst. **72:** 1323–1325.
7. BARTRAM, H.P., K. KASPER, G. DUSEL, E. LIEBSCHER, A. GOSTNER, C. LOGES & W. SCHEPPACH. 1997. Effects of calcium and deoxycholic acid on human colonic cell proliferation *in vitro.* Ann. Nutr. Metab. **41:** 315–323.
8. VAN DER MEER, R., J.W.M. WELBERG, F. KUIPERS et al. 1990. Effects of supplemental dietary calcium on the intestinal association of calcium, phosphate, and bile acids. Gastroenterology **99:** 1653–1659.
9. GOVERS, M.J.A.P., D.S.M.L. TERMONT, J.A. LAPRE, J.H. KLEIBEUKER, R.J. VONK & R. VAN DER MEER. 1996. Calcium in milk products precipitates intestinal fatty acids and secondary bile acids and thus inhibits colonic cytotoxicity in humans. Cancer Res. **56:** 3270–3275.
10. GOVERS, M.J.A.P., D.S.M. L. TERMONT, J.H. KLEIBEUKER, E.G.E. DE VRIES & R. VAN DER MEER. 1994. Mechanisms of the antiproliferative effect of milk mineral and other calcium supplements on colonic epithelium. Cancer Res. **54:** 95–100.
11. LAPRE, J.A., H.T. DE VRIES, D.S.M.L. TERMONT, J.H. KLEIBEUKER, E.G.E. DE VRIES & R. VAN DER MEER. 1993. Mechanism of the protective effect of supplemental dietary calcium on cytolytic activity of fecal water. Cancer Res. **53:** 248–253.
12. GOVERS, M.J.A.P., D.S.M.L. TERMONT, J.A. LAPRE, J.H. KLEIBEUKER, R.J. VONK & R. VAN DER MEER. 1996. Calcium in milk products precipitates intestinal fatty acids and secondary bile acids and thus inhibits colonic cytotoxicity in humans. Cancer Res. **56:** 3270–3275.

13. HOLT, P.R., S.F. MOSS, R. WHELAN, J. GUSS, J. GILMAN & M. LIPKIN. 1996. Fecal and rectal mucosal diacylglycerol concentrations and epithelial proliferative kinetics. Cancer Epidemiol. Biomarkers Prev. **5:** 937–940.

14. WEINSTEIN, I.B. 1993. Protein kinase C and signal transduction: A role in cancer prevention and treatment. Adv. Oncol. **9:** 3–9.

15. GUILLEM, J.G., M. MOROTOMI, S. KAHN, D.M. JOHNSON, W. JIANG & I.B. WEINSTEIN. 1991. The molecular biology of colorectal cancer. Semin. Colon & Rectal Surg. **2:** 58–63.

16. LIPKIN, M. 1998. Biomarkers of increased susceptibility to gastrointestinal cancer: New application to studies of cancer prevention in human subjects. Cancer Res. **48:** 235–245.

17. TERPSTRA, O.T., M. VAN BLANKENSTEIN, J. DEES & G.A.M. EILER. 1987. Abnormal pattern of cell proliferation in the entire colonic mucosa of patients with colon adenoma or cancer. Gastroenterology **92:** 704–708.

18. ANTI, M., G. MARRA, A. PERCESEPE, F. ARMELAO & G. GASBARRINI. 1994. Reliability of rectal epithelial kinetic patterns as an intermediate biomarker of colon cancer. J Cell. Biochem. (Suppl.) **19:** 68–75.

19. PONZ DE LEON, M., L. RONCUCCI, P.D. DONATO, L. TASSI, O. SMERIERI, G.M. AMORICO, G. MALAGOLI, D. DEMARIA, A. ANTONIOLI, J.N. CHAHIN, M. PERINI, G. RIGO, G. BARBERINI, A. MANENTI, G. BIASCO & L. BARBARA. 1988. Pattern of epithelial cell proliferation in colorectal mucosa of normal subjects and of patients with adenomatous polyps or cancer of the large bowel. Cancer Res. **48:** 4121–4126.

20. ANTI, M., G. MARRA, F. ARMELAO, A. PERCESEPE, R. FICARELLI, G.M. RICCIUTO, A. VALENTI, G.L. RAPACINI, I. DEVITIS, G. D'AGOSTINO, S. BRIGHI & F.M. VECCHIO. 1993. Rectal epithelial cell proliferation patterns as predictors of adenomatous colorectal polyp recurrence. Gut **34:** 525–530.

21. LIPKIN, M. & H. NEWMARK. 1985. Effect of added dietary calcium on colonic epithelial cell proliferation in subjects at high risk for familial colonic cancer. N. Engl. J. Med. **313:** 1381–1384.

22. LIPKIN, M., W.E. ENKER & S.J. WINAWER. 1987. Tritiated-thymidine labeling of rectal epithelial in 'non-prep' biopsies of individuals at increased risk for colonic neoplasia. Cancer Lett. **87:** 153–161.

23. ROZEN, P., A. FIREMAN, N. FINE, Y. WAX & E. RON. 1989. Oral calcium suppresses increased rectal epithelial proliferation of persons at risk for colorectal cancer. Gut **30:** 650–655.

24. WARGOVICH, M.J., G. ISBELL, M. SHABOT, R. WINN, F. LANZA, L. HOCHMAN, E. LARSON, P. LYNCH, L. ROOUBEIN & B. LEVIN. 1992. Calcium supplementation decreases rectal epithelial cell proliferation in subjects with sporadic adenoma. Gastroenterology **103:** 92–97.

25. O'SULLIVAN, K.R., P.M. MATHIAS, S. BEATTIE & C. O'MORAIN. 1993. Effect of oral calcium supplementation on colonic crypt cell proliferation in patients with adenomatous polyps of the large bowel. Eur. J. Gastroenterol. Hepatol. **5:** 85–89.

26. BARON, J.A., T.D. TOSTESON, M.J. WARGOVICH et al. 1995. Calcium supplementation and rectal mucosal proliferation: A randomized controlled trial. J. Natl. Cancer Inst. **87:** 1303–1307.

27. BOSTICK, R., J.D. POTTER, L. FOSDICK et al. 1993. Calcium and colorectal epithelial cell proliferation: A preliminary randomized, double-blinded, placebo-controlled clinical trial. J. Natl. Cancer Inst. **85:** 132–141.

28. MCSHANE, L.M., M. KULLDORFF, M.J. WARGOVICH, C. WOODS, M. PUREWAL, L.S. FREEDMAN, D.K. CORLE, R.W. BURT, D.J. MATESKI, M. LAWSON, E. LANZA, B. O'BRIEN, W.J. LAKE, J. MOLER & A. SCHATZKIN. 1998. An evaluation of rectal mucosal proliferation measure variability sources in the polyp prevention trial:

Can we detect informative differences among individuals "proliferation measures amid the noise?" Cancer Epidemiol. Biomarkers Prev. **7:** 605–612.

29. BOSTICK, R.M. 1997. Human studies of calcium supplementation and colorectal epithelial cell proliferation. Cancer Epidemiol. Biomarkers Prev. **6:** 971–980.

30. HOLT, P.R., E.O. ATTILASOY, J. GILMAN, J. GUSS, S.F. MOSS, H. NEWMARK, K. FAN, K. YANG & M. LIPKIN. 1998. Modulation of abnormal colon epithelial cell proliferation and differentiation by low-fat dairy foods: A randomized controlled trial. J. Am. Med. Assoc. **280:** 1074–1079.

31. CURHAN, G.C., W.C. WILLETT, E.B. RIMM & M.J. STAMPFER. 1993. A prospective study of dietary calcium and other nutrients and the risk of symptomatic kidney stones. N. Engl. J. Med. **328:** 833–838.

32. CURHAN, G.C., W.C. WILLETT, F.E. SPEIZER & M.J. STAMPFER. 1998. Beverage use and risk for kidney stones in women. Ann. Intern. Med. **128:** 534–540.

33. HALLBERG, L. 1998. Does calcium interfere with iron absorption? Am. J. Clin. Nutr. **68:** 3–4.

34. SCHATZKIN, A., L.S. FREEDMAN, J. DORGAN, L. MCSHANE, M. SCHIFFMAN & S.M. DAWSEY. 1996. Surrogate endpoints in cancer research: A critique. Cancer Epidemiol. Biomarkers Prev. **5:** 947–953.

35. BUSET, M., M. LIPKIN, S. WINAWER, S. SWAROOP & E. FRIEDMAN. 1986. Inhibition of human colonic epithelial cell proliferation *in vivo* and *in vitro* by calcium. Cancer Res. **46:** 5426– 5430.

36. LIPKIN, M., E. FRIEDMAN, S.J. WINAWER & H. NEWMARK. 1989. Colonic epithelial cell proliferation in responders and nonresponders to supplemental dietary calcium. Cancer Res. **49:** 248–254.

37. BOSTICK, R.M., L. FOSDICK, J.R. WOOD, P. GRAMBSCH, G.A. GRANDITS, T.J. LILLEMOE, T.A. LOUIS & J.D. POTTER. 1995. Calcium and colorectal epithelial cell proliferation in sporadic adenoma patients: A randomized, double-blinded, placebo-controlled clinical trial. J. Natl. Cancer Inst. **87:** 1307–1315.

38. WEISGERBER, U.M., H. BOEING, R.W. OWEN, R. WALDHERR, R. RAEDSCH & J. WAHRENDORF. 1996. Effect of longterm placebo controlled calcium supplementation on sigmoidal cell proliferation in patients with sporadic adenomatous polyps. Gut **38:** 396–402.

39. ALBERTS, D.S., J. EINSPAHR, C. RITENBAUGH, M. AICKIN, S. REES-MCGEE, J. ATWOOD, S. EMERSON, N. MASON-LIDDIL, L. BETTINGER, J. PATEL, S. BELLAPRAVALU, P.S. RAMANUJAM, J. PHELPS & L. CLARK. 1997. The effect of wheat bran fiber and calcium supplementation on rectal mucosal proliferation rates in patients with resected adenomatous colorectal polyps. Cancer Epidemiol. Biomarkers Prev. **6:** 161–169.

Calcium Supplements and Colorectal Adenomas

J.A. BARON,[a,b,q] M. BEACH, [c,e] J.S. MANDEL,[f] R.U. VAN STOLK,[j] R. W. HAILE,[l] R.S. SANDLER,[m] R. ROTHSTEIN,[a] R.W. SUMMERS,[n] D.C. SNOVER, [h,o] G.J. BECK,[k] H. FRANKL,[p] L. PEARSON,[b] J.H. BOND,[g,i] AND E.R. GREENBERG,[d] FOR THE POLYP PREVENTION STUDY GROUP

Departments of [a]Medicine, [b]Community and Family Medicine, [c]Anesthesia, and the [d]Norris Cotton Cancer Center, Dartmouth Hitchcock Medical Center, Lebanon, New Hampshire 03756, USA

[e]Department of Veterans Affairs, White River Junction, Vermont, USA

[f]Department of Environmental and Occupational Health, School of Public Health, Departments of [g]Medicine and [h]Pathology, School of Medicine, University of Minnesota, and [i]Minneapolis Veterans Administration Medical Center, Minneapolis, Minnesota, USA

[j]Center for Colon Polyps and Colon Cancer, Department of Gastroenterology and [k]Department of Biostatistics and Epidemiology, Cleveland Clinic Foundation, Cleveland, Ohio 44195, USA

[l]Department of Preventive Medicine, University of Southern California School of Medicine, Los Angeles, California 90033-0800, USA

[m]Department of Medicine, University of North Carolina, Chapel Hill, North Carolina 27599-7080, USA

[n]James A. Clifton Center for Digestive Diseases, Department of Internal Medicine, University of Iowa College of Medicine, Iowa City, Iowa 52242, USA

[o]Department of Pathology, Fairview Southdale Hospital, Edina, Minnesota 55435, USA

[p]Department of Internal Medicine, Southern California Permanente Medical Group, Los Angeles, California 90027, USA

ABSTRACT: Experimental and observational findings suggest that calcium intake may protect against colorectal neoplasia. To investigate this hypothesis, we conducted a randomized, double-blind trial of colorectal adenoma recurrence. Nine hundred thirty patients with a recent history of colorectal adenomas were randomly given calcium carbonate (3 gm daily; 1200 mg elemental calcium) or placebo, with follow-up colonoscopies one and four years after the qualifying examination. The main analysis focused on new adenomas found after the first follow-up endoscopy, up to (and including) the second follow-up examination. Risk ratios of at least one recurrent adenoma and ratios of the average numbers of adenomas were calculated as measures of calcium effect. There was a lower risk of recurrent adenomas in subjects assigned calcium. Eight hundred thirty-two patients had two follow-up examinations and were

[q]Address for communication: 7927 Rubin Building, Dartmouth Hitchcock Medical Center, 1 Medical Center Drive, Lebanon, New Hampshire 03756, USA. Voice: 603-650-6201; fax: 603-650-6485.
e-mail: john.baron@dartmouth.edu

138

included in the main analysis; the adjusted risk ratio of one or more adenomas was 0.81 (95% CI 0.67 to 0.99); the adjusted ratio of the average numbers of adenomas was 0.76 (95% CI 0.60 to 0.96). Among subjects who had at least one follow-up colonoscopy, the adjusted risk ratio of one or more recurrent adenomas was 0.85 (95% CI 0.74 to 0.98). The effect of calcium seemed independent of initial dietary fat and calcium intake. No toxicity was associated with supplementation. These findings indicate that calcium supplementation has a modest protective effect against colorectal adenomas, precursors of most colorectal cancers.

INTRODUCTION

Although dietary factors are widely thought to be important determinants of colorectal cancer risk, the specific constituents in diet that may explain any association are not clear. Newmark and colleagues[1] proposed that calcium can bind fat and bile acids in the lumen of the bowel and inhibit their carcinogenic effects. There are data supporting this hypothesis: animal studies have shown a protective effect of dietary calcium in experimental bowel carcinogenesis,[2,3] and some human epidemiological data have found calcium intake to be inversely related to the risk of colorectal cancer or colorectal adenomas. Other studies, however, have found no association.[4,5]

To clarify the effect of calcium intake on colorectal neoplasia, we conducted a clinical trial of the effect of supplementation with calcium carbonate on the recurrence of colorectal adenomas. We hypothesized that subjects assigned randomly to calcium would have a reduced risk of any recurrent adenoma as well as reduced numbers of adenomas.

METHODS

This clinical trial involved patients at six clinical centers: the Cleveland Clinic Foundation, Dartmouth-Hitchcock Medical Center (also the coordinating center), the University of Southern California/Southern California Permanente Medical Group, the University of Iowa, the University of Minnesota (also the pathology center), and the University of North Carolina. Human subjects committees at each center approved the study protocol; an independent safety and data monitoring committee reviewed the study semiannually.

Staff at each clinical center identified patients with at least one histologically confirmed large bowel adenoma removed within three months of recruitment, with the entire large bowel mucosa examined and judged free of remaining polyps. Eligible patients were less than 80 years old, in good health, and without polyposis syndromes, invasive large bowel cancer, malabsorption syndromes, or any condition that might be worsened by supplemental calcium.

A total of 1118 patients entered a three-month placebo run-in period to assess adherence to the study regimen of one tablet twice per day with meals. After the run-in, 930 patients were considered appropriate for randomization to calcium or placebo. Study tablets contained 3000 mg calcium carbonate (1200 mg elemental calcium) or an identical-appearing cellulose/sucrose placebo. The trial was double blind: neither subjects nor study staff were told the subjects' treatment assignments.

Subjects received two follow-up colonoscopies, the first approximately one year after the qualifying colonoscopy (about 9 months after randomization), and the second 36 months after that. Large bowel endoscopy was otherwise discouraged unless clinically necessary. After randomization, all polyps found were biopsied, removed, and reviewed by the study pathologist who classified them as neoplastic (adenoma) or nonneoplastic (e.g., hyperplastic polyp). The reviewing pathologist and the clinical center reading agreed as to presence or absence of neoplasia for 2349 (92 percent) of the 2541 specimens reviewed. If there was disagreement, we accepted the study pathologist's reading.

At enrollment, we assessed the subjects' diets with a validated food frequency questionnaire.[6] Every six months, patients were asked to complete questionnaires regarding compliance with study agents; use of medications, over-the-counter drugs, and nutritional supplements; and the occurrence of symptoms, illnesses, and hospitalizations. Recruitment began in November 1988, and the clinical phase of the study ended in December 1996.

The primary end point of the trial was the proportion of subjects having at least one adenoma detected after the first follow-up colonoscopy, up to and including the second follow-up examination (including adenomas detected during interim endoscopies). This risk period provided for the removal of adenomas overlooked at the qualifying colonoscopy (thus minimizing the numbers of prevalent polyps at the start of the main risk period) and also allowed for a latent period for calcium effect. If a subject did not have the planned follow-up examinations, we accepted two colonoscopies at least one year apart.

We compared proportions using Fisher's exact test and measured data using t-tests or rank tests.[7] We estimated the risk ratio of having at least one adenoma (using overdispersed log-linear quasilikelihood models programmed in SPlus (Seattle)) and computed the ratios of the average number of adenomas (using similar models with variance proportional to the mean).[8] Covariates included age (linear term), gender, the lifetime number of adenomas before study entry, clinical center, and the length of the surveillance interval. Possible interactions were considered using product terms. Subgroup analyses included investigation of subjects above and below the median of the calorie-adjusted intake[9] of selected nutrients. All p values were two-sided.

RESULTS

A total of 466 subjects were randomly assigned to placebo and 464 to calcium; there were no appreciable differences between the two treatment groups in demographic characteristics, dietary patterns, or adenoma history. The mean age ($\pm$SD) was 61 ± 9 years, and 72% were men. Most subjects had had only one or two adenomas removed from the large bowel. The mean estimated diameter of the largest qualifying adenoma was 0.7 ± 0.6 centimeters. The estimated mean daily dietary calcium intake at study entry (877 ± 437 mg per day) was similar in the two study groups, and less than three quarters of the amount provided the study supplements. Less than 3% of subjects were taking calcium supplements at the start of the trial; all agreed to discontinue them during the study.

TABLE 1. Cooperation of study subjects with trial examinations

	Placebo N (%)	Calcium N (%)
Randomized Subjects	466 (100)	464 (100)
Died	22 (4.7)	25 (5.4)
Dropped out: lost interest	11 (2.4)	14 (3.0)
Dropped out: ill or moved	8 (1.7)	10 (2.2)
Dropped out: other or unknown reasons	2 (0.4)	6 (1.3)
Received first follow-up colonoscopy	459 (98.5)	454 (97.8)
Received second follow-up colonoscopy	423 (90.8)	409 (88.2)

In all, 89% of subjects had two follow-up colonoscopies (TABLE 1); 47 patients died, 33 dropped out, and 18 could not be examined because they were too ill or had moved. The proportions of subjects with an inadequate study colonoscopy or with an interim endoscopy did not differ substantially between treatment groups. Compliance with the study regimen was excellent. Even during the fourth year, over 87 of living subjects took study agents 90–100% of the time, and a further 7 took them 50–89% of the time. Only 19 patients took calcium supplements on their own during the study (9 placebo, 10 calcium).

Of the 832 subjects who had two follow-up colonoscopies, one or more colorectal adenomas were diagnosed during the main risk period in 127 (31.1%) calcium patients and 159 (37.6%) placebo patients (TABLE 2). The mean size of the largest adenoma was the same in the two groups (0.4 cm; $p = 0.43$). The risk ratio for at least one adenoma was 0.83 (95% CI 0.68 to 1.00) without adjustment and 0.81 (95% CI 0.67 to 0.99) after adjustment. The ratio of the average number of adenomas was 0.75 (95% CI 0.58 to 0.97) before adjustment and 0.76 (95% CI 0.60 to 0.96) after adjustment.

A similar calcium effect was present during the first study interval. Among subjects with two follow-up colonoscopies, at least one adenoma was noted in the period up to and including the first follow-up exam in 103 calcium subjects and 138 placebo subjects (TABLE 2). The unadjusted risk ratio for at least one adenoma was 0.77 (95% CI 0.62 to 0.96); the unadjusted ratio of the average number of adenomas was 0.73 (95% CI 0.54 to 0.97). These estimates were essentially unchanged after multivariate adjustment.

A total of 913 subjects had at least one colonoscopy. The crude risk ratio of at least one postrandomization adenoma was 0.85 (95% CI 0.74 to 0.98); the ratio of the average numbers of adenomas was 0.74 (95% CI 0.59 to 0.92).

During the main study risk period, an adenoma 0.5 cm or greater was found in 120 subjects; the unadjusted risk ratio for at least one adenoma of this size versus no adenomas was 0.87 (95% CI 0.63 to 1.21); the unadjusted risk ratio for smaller adenomas was 0.75 (95% CI 0.57 to 0.98). Calcium had similar effects on adenoma recurrence in the bowel proximal to the splenic flexure and in more distal regions of the bowel (data not shown). The calcium effect was also similar in subgroups of age, gender, or baseline dietary intake of calcium, fat, or fiber (data not shown). The effect of calcium was nonsignificantly stronger among subjects who reported taking all their study agents and among those who did not report any use of aspirin or other nonsteroidal anti-inflammatory drugs (data not shown).

TABLE 2. Numbers of subjects with any adenoma recurrence, relative risks of at least one recurrence, and ratios of the average numbers of adenomas, according to treatment assignment

| | Adenomas, by Treatment Group | | | | | |
| | Placebo | | Calcium | | | |
	% with 1 or more adenomas	Mean # of adenomas	% with 1 or more adenomas	Mean # of adenomas	Relative risk of any adenoma[a]	Ratio of mean # of adenomas[a]
Subjects with two follow-up colonoscopies (423 Placebo, 409 Calcium)						
At or before the first follow-up colonoscopy	32.6%	0.60	25.2%	0.43	0.78 (0.63 to 0.96)	0.75 (0.58 to 0.96)
After the first follow-up colonoscopy, at or before the second follow-up colonoscopy	37.6%	0.73	31.1%	0.55	0.81 (0.67 to 0.99)	0.76 (0.60 to 0.96)
Any time after randomization	52.2%	1.32	44.7%	0.98	0.85 (0.74 to 0.98)	0.75 (0.62 to 0.90)
Subjects who had at least one follow-up endoscopy (459 Placebo, 454 Calcium)						
Any time after randomization	50.5%	1.26	43.2%	0.92	0.85 (0.74 to 0.98)	0.75 (0.63 to 0.90)

[a]Risk ratio of at least one adenoma and ratio of the mean numbers of adenomas. Both estimates adjusted for age, gender, clinical center, number of previous adenomas, and length of follow-up interval.

Similar proportions of calcium and placebo subjects were hospitalized for any reason (or specifically for cancer), or stopped treatment because of perceived side effects. Gastrointestinal symptoms (including constipation) did not differ materially between the two treatment groups.

DISCUSSION

In this large clinical trial, calcium supplementation conferred a moderately reduced risk of adenoma recurrence. This effect was present as early as the first colonoscopic follow-up, after approximately 9 months. The effect did not seem to be affected by baseline dietary intake of calcium or fat. The intervention did not lead to significant toxicity.

Epidemological data regarding the association between calcium intake and the risk of colorectal cancer or colorectal adenomas have varied but seem consistent with the effect we observed.[4,5,9–15] Such observational study of the effects of calcium intake is likely to be hampered by confounding by caloric intake, dietary fat, and perhaps use of vitamin/mineral supplements and aspirin. Also, the measurement errors associated with dietary assessment would tend to obscure associations between nutrients and the risk of neoplasia.[16]

Considerable animal research suggests an antineoplastic effect of calcium in the bowel. Calcium inhibits the hyperproliferation induced by bile acids or carcinogens,[2] and carcinogenesis studies in animals given high-fat diets have generally reported lower tumor incidence with supplementation.[2,3] Previous studies of calcium supplementation have supported the hypothesis that calcium may act through precipitation of bile acids or stool fatty acids, perhaps in complexes with calcium phosphate.[17] Calcium supplementation seems to reduce cytotoxicity of fecal water, reduce secondary bile acids in the bile acid pool, and lower fecal bile acid concentrations.[17–20] However, other investigations did not suggest such effects, finding no change or an increase in the concentration of water-phase fecal bile acids.[21–24] The effect of calcium on rectal mucosal proliferation is not clear.[22,23,25–29]

Our study does not directly address whether calcium affects the progression of adenomas to invasive cancer or the risk of a first adenoma. However, the similarity of risk factors for colorectal cancer, recurrent adenomas, and incident adenomas[30] supports the relevance of our finding for colorectal cancer itself. Nonetheless, the effect we observed may have been weaker for large adenomas than for small ones, implying a limited efficacy for more advanced tumors. The effect of calcium was seen less than a year after randomization and did not become stronger with time. It is possible that decreasing compliance counterbalanced increasing efficacy.

The apparent effect of calcium that we observed is consistent with epidemiological data and is supported by a large body of experimental data in humans and in animals. Inasmuch as this agent is inexpensive and relatively nontoxic, and because it may confer other benefits (e.g., reduction of the risk of osteoporosis[31]), its risk–benefit balance is likely to be favorable. However, it would be desirable to confirm our results, clarify effects on invasive carcinoma, and understand the risk–benefit balance in more detail.

ACKNOWLEDGMENTS

In addition to the authors, the Polyp Prevention Study Group investigators included Leila A. Mott, David W. Nierenberg, Marguerite M. Stevens, Thérèse Stukel, Tor D. Tosteson (all at the Dartmouth Medical School), Douglas Howell (Maine Medical Center), James Church (Cleveland Clinic Foundation), and Joseph Truszkowski (University of Iowa). Study coordinators were Hennie Hasson and Janine Bauman (Cleveland Clinic), Kim Wood (Dartmouth-Hitchcock Medical Center), Beth Cheyne, Robin Thompson, and Dorothy Finke (University of Iowa), Joyce Blomquist and Sarah Waldemar (University of Minnesota), Colleen McAuliffe and Barbara Schliebe (University of North Carolina), and Patricia Harmon (University of Southern California).

Safety and Data Monitoring Committee members for the trial were Sam Greenhouse (George Washington University), James Grizzle (Fred Hutchinson Cancer Research Center), Richard Hunt (McMaster University), Gordon Luk (Wayne State University), Francis M. Giardiello (Johns Hopkins University), and Walter C. Willett (Harvard University).

This study was supported in part by NIH Grants CA37287 and CA23108. Study agents were provided by Lederle (now Whitehall-Robins, Pearl River, NY).

REFERENCES

1. NEWMARK, H.L., M.J. WARGOVICH & W.R. BRUCE. 1984. Colon cancer and dietary fat, phosphate, and calcium: A hypothesis. J. Natl. Cancer Inst. **72:** 1323–1325.
2. PENCE, B.C. 1993. Role of calcium in colon cancer prevention: Experimental and clinical studies. Mutat. Res. **290:** 87–95.
3. PENCE, B.C. & F. BUDDINGH. 1988. Inhibition of dietary fat-promoted colon carcinogenesis in rats by supplemental calcium of vitamin D_3. Carcinogenesis **9:** 187–190.
4. BLERGSMA-KADIJK, J.A., P. VAN'T VEER, E. KAMPMAN & J. BUREMA. 1996. Calcium does not protect against colorectal neoplasia. Epidemiology **7:** 590–597.
5. MARTINEZ, M.E. & S.C. WILLETT. 1998. Calcium, vitamin D, and colorectal cancer: A review of the epidemiologic evidence. Cancer Epidemiol. Biomarkers Prev. **7:** 163–168.
6. BLOCK, G., A.M. HARTMAN, C.M. DRESSER, M.D. CARROLL, J. GANNON & L. GARDNER. 1986. A data based approach to diet questionnaire design and testing. Am. J. Epidemiol. **124:** 453–469.
7. SNEDECOR, G.W. & W.G. COCHRAN. 1980. Statistical Methods (7th ed.). Iowa State University Press. Ames, Iowa.
8. MCCULLAGH, P. & J.A. NELDER. 1989. Generalized Linear Models (2nd ed.). Chapman & Hall. New York.
9. WILLETT, W. 1990. Nutritional Epidemiology. Oxford University Press.
10. BOSTICK, R.M., J.D. POTTER, T.A. SELLERS, D.R. MCKENZIE, L.H. KUSHI & A.R. FOLSOM. 1993. Relation of calcium, vitamin D, and dairy food intake to incidence of colon cancer among older women: The Iowa women's health study. Am. J. Epidemiol. **137:** 1302–1317.
11. BOUTRON, M.C., J. FAISTIVRE, P. MARTEAU, C. COUILLAULT, P. SENESSE & V. QUIPOURT. 1996. Calcium, phosphorus, vitamin D, dairy products and colorectal carcinogenesis—A French case control study. Br. J. Cancer **74:** 141–151.
12. KAMPMAN, E., R.A. BOLDBOHM, P.A. VAN DEN BRANDT & P. VAN'T VEER. 1994. Fermented dairy products, calcium, and colorectal cancer in the Netherlands cohort study. Cancer Res. **54:** 3186–3190.
13. LITTLE, J., R.F.A. LOGAN, P.G. HAWTIN, J.D. HARDCASTLE & I.D. TURNER. 1993. Colorectal adenomas and diet: A case-control study of subjects participating in the Nottingham faecal occult blood screening programme. Br. J. Cancer **67:** 177–184.
14. KAMPMAN, E., E. GIOVANNUCCI, P. VAN'T VEER et al. 1994. Calcium, vitamin D, dairy foods, and the occurrence of colorectal adenomas among men and women in two prospective studies. Am. J. Epidemiol. **139:** 16–29.
15. TSENG, M., S.C. MURRAY, L.L. KUPPER & R.S. SANDLER. 1996. Micronutrients and the risk of colorectal adenomas. Am. J. Epidemiol. **144:** 1005–1014.
16. NEUGUT, A.I., K. HORVATH, R.L. WHELAN et al. 1996. The effect of calcium and vitamin supplements on the incidence and recurrence of colorectal adenomatous polyps. Cancer **78:** 723–728.
17. VAN DER MEER, R., J.A. LAPRÉ, M.J.A.P. GOVERS & J.H. KLEIBEUKER. 1997. Mechanisms of the intestinal effects of dietary fats and milk products on colon carcinogenesis. Cancer Lett. **114:** 75–83.
18. CATS, A., J.H. KLEIBEUKER, R. VAN DER MEER et al. 1995. Randomized, double-blinded, placebo-controlled intervention study with supplemental calcium in families with hereditary nonpolyposis colorectal cancer. J. Natl. Cancer Inst. **87:** 598–603.
19. LUPTON, J.R., G. STEINBACH, W.C. CHANG et al. 1996. Calcium supplementation modifies the relative amounts of bile acids in bile and affects key aspects of human colon physiology. J. Nutr. **126:** 1421–1428.
20. ALBERTS, D.S., C. RITENBAUGH, J.A. STORY et al. 1996. Randomized double-blinded, placebo-controlled study of effect of wheat bran fiber and calcium on fecal bile

acids in patients with resected adenomatous colon polyps. J. Natl. Cancer Inst. **88:** 81–92.

21. LAPRÉ, J.A., H.T. DEVRIES, D.S.M.L. TERMONT, J.H. KLEIBEUKER, E.G.E. DEVRIES & R. VAN DER MEER. 1993. Mechanism of the protective effect of supplemental dietary calcium on cytolytic activity of fecal water. Cancer Res. **53:** 248–253.

22. STERN, H.S., R.C. GREGOIRE, H. KASTAN, J. STADLER & R.W. BRUCE. 1990. Long-term effects of dietary calcium on risk markers for colon cancer in patients with familial polyposis. Surgery **108:** 528–533.

23. GREGOIRE, R.C., H.S. STERN, K.S. YEUNG *et al.* 1989. Effect of calcium supplementation on mucosal cell proliferation in high risk patients for colon cancer. Gut **30:** 376–382.

24. ALDER, J.F., G. MCKEOWN-EYSSEN & E. BRIGHT-SEE. 1993. Randomized trial of the effect of calcium supplementation on fecal risk factors for colorectal cancer. Am. J. Epidemiol. **138:** 804–814.

25. LIPKIN, M. & M.S. NEWMARK. 1985. Effect of added dietary calcium on colonic epithelial-cell proliferation in subjects at high risk for familial colonic cancer. N. Engl. J. Med. **313:** 1381–1384.

26. WARGOVICH, M.J., G. ISBELL, M. SHABOT *et al.* 1992. Calcium supplementation decreases rectal epithelial cell proliferation in subjects with sporadic adenoma. Gastroenterology **103:** 92–97.

27. BARON, J., T. TOSTESON, M.J. WARGOVICH *et al.* 1995. Calcium supplementation and rectal mucosal proliferation: A randomized controlled trial. J. Natl. Cancer Inst. **87:** 1303–1307.

28. BOSTICK, R.M., L. FOSDICK, J.R. WOOD *et al.* 1995. Calcium and colorectal epithelial cell proliferation in sporadic adenoma patients: A randomized, double-blinded, placebo-controlled clinical trial. J. Natl. Cancer Inst. **87:** 1307–1315.

29. ARMITAGE, N.C., P.S.ROONEY, K-A. GIFFORD, P.A. CLARKE & J.D. HARDCASTLE. 1995. The effect of calcium supplements on rectal mucosal proliferation. Br. J. Cancer **71:** 186–190.

30. PEIPINS, L.A. & R.S. SANDLER. 1994. Epidemiology of colorectal adenomas. Epidemiol. Rev. **16:** 273–297.

31. DAWSON-HUGHES, B., S.S. HARRIS, E.A. KRALL & G.E. DALLAL. 1997. Effect of calcium and vitamin D supplementation on bone density in men and women 65 years of age or older. N. Engl. J. Med. **337:** 670–676.

Breast Cancer Prevention by Antiestrogens

MICHAEL P. OSBORNE[a]

Strang Cornell Breast Center, New York, New York 10021, USA

ABSTRACT: A new era has been entered with the first demonstration that an antiestrogen can prevent breast cancer. In a landmark study tamoxifen was shown to reduce the incidence of breast cancer by ~50%. The reduction was observed in pre- and postmenopausal women at increased risk of breast cancer. Invasive cancers were reduced, the reduction being in the estrogen receptor–positive cancers. No preventive effect was observed for estrogen receptor–negative tumors. *In situ* cancers were also significantly reduced. A collateral benefit was a significant reduction in fractures due to osteoporosis. Adverse effects included a very small increase in the incidence of endometrial cancer, cataracts, and stroke. The benefits appear to outweigh the risks for those at high risk. Preliminary studies of a new selective estrogen receptor modulator (SERM 2), raloxifene, developed for the prevention of osteoporosis, have shown that the breast cancer rate was reduced by more than 50% without any concomitant increase in endometrial cancer. The search for a SERM 3, and beyond, may lead to the development of drugs that have the beneficial effects of estrogen while preventing breast cancer and osteoporosis.

The end of the twentieth century has been marked by the demonstration that an antiestrogen can delay, and perhaps prevent, the onset of breast cancer in women at risk for the disease. Until now the only options available to women at increased risk for breast cancer have been close surveillance[1] or prophylactic bilateral mastectomy[2,3]

Based on the development of tamoxifen by Walpole over 30 years ago, as an anti-fertility drug, and the discovery of the estrogen-receptor by Elwood Jenson, the initial pioneering work by Craig Jordan[4,5] showed that this drug could prevent mammary carcinoma in rats. It was also observed that carcinogen-initiated rat mammary epithelial cells were rendered into a resting (G0) phase by tamoxifen.[6] Initial concerns were that an unselective antiestrogen might increase osteoporosis and heart disease. Successful clinical studies of tamoxifen for the treatment of stage IV metastatic breast cancer led to its introduction as an adjuvant endocrine therapy for earliest stage patients with estrogen receptor–positive tumors. It was noted in many trials and their meta-analysis that not only were recurrences reduced and overall survival enhanced but that contralateral breast cancer was reduced by nearly 50 percent.[7] During the course of these trials it was noted that tamoxifen was a selective antiestrogen. Contrary to initial expectations tamoxifen did not increase coronary ar-

[a]Address for communication: Strang Cornell Breast Center, 428 East 72d Street, Suite 600, New York, NY 10021. Voice: 212-794-4900 ext. 148; fax: 212-396-1244.
e-mail: osborne@strang.org

tery disease but exerted an estrogenic effect on the uterus, resulting in endometrial hyperplasia and an increase in the very low rate of endometrial cancer.

Sufficient preclinical and clinical data were available by the late 1980s to justify large randomized clinical trials to determine the worth of tamoxifen in preventing breast cancer in women at increased risk. Three groups embarked on these prevention trials: the United Kingdom's Royal Marsden Hospital group led by Trevor Powles, in 1986; the European Institute of Oncology in Italy led by Umberto Veronesi, in 1992; and the United States North American Surgical Adjuvant Breast and Bowel Project (NSABP) led by Bernard Fisher in 1992 proposed preventive trials. All three groups published their results in 1998.

UNITED STATES NSABP TAMOXIFEN PREVENTION TRIAL

The NSABP initiated the Breast Cancer Prevention Trial (BCPT) P-1, recruiting 13,388 women randomly assigned to placebo or tamoxifen 20 mg/day for 5 years.[8] The participants were women at increased risk because of the following factors: 60 years of age or older, 35–59 years of age with a five-year predicted risk for breast cancer of at least 1.66%, and lobular carcinoma *in situ* (lobular neoplasia). The five-year predicted risk was calculated from an algorithm based on a logistic regression model using a combination of risk factors: age, number of first-degree relatives with breast cancer, nulliparity or age at first live birth, number of breast biopsies, pathologic diagnosis of atypical hyperplasia, and age at menarche. The trial was stopped early and unblinded because the Independent Endpoint Review, Safety Monitoring and Advisory Committee determined that there was sufficient evidence that the tamoxifen significantly reduced the incidence of invasive breast cancer.

Breast Cancer Preventive Effects

The major finding of the trial was that the risk of invasive breast cancer was reduced by 49% ($p < 0.00001$), with a cumulative incidence, at 69 months of follow-up, of 43.4 versus 22.0 breast cancer cases per 1000 women in the placebo and tamoxifen groups, respectively. The risk of noninvasive breast cancer was reduced by 50% ($p < 0.002$), with a cumulative incidence of 15.9 versus 7.7 breast cancer cases per 1000 women in the placebo and tamoxifen groups, respectively. It was noted that the occurrence of estrogen receptor (ER) –positive tumors was reduced by 69%, but there was no difference in the occurrence of estrogen receptor–negative tumors.

Collateral Benefit

The antiosteoporosis effects of tamoxifen were manifest by a 19% reduction in hip, radius, and spine fractures. There was no difference in the average annual rate of ischemic heart disease between placebo and tamoxifen groups.

Adverse Effects

An increase in the endometrial cancer rate from 0.91 per 1000 women per year in the placebo group to 2.30 per 1000 women per year in the tamoxifen group was observed. This represents an increase in the relative risk (RR) of 2.53 and a 95% confidence interval (CI) of 1.35–4.97. The increased risk was mostly observed in women 50 years of age or older, and all the endometrial cancers in the tamoxifen group were early FIGO stage I.

Other adverse effects in the tamoxifen group included pulmonary embolism (RR = 3.01; 95% CI = 1.15–9.27); deep vein thrombosis (RR = 1.60; 95% CI = 0.91–2.86); stroke, in women 50 years of age or older (RR = 1.75; 95% CI = 0.98–3.20); and development of cataracts (marginally increased) (RR = 1.14; 95% CI = 1.01–1.29). Hot flashes increased from 28.7% in the placebo group to 45.7% in the tamoxifen group, and vaginal discharge increased from 13.0% in the placebo group to 29.0% in the tamoxifen group.

Death Rate

The ultimate end point of death in the trial occurred in 71 in the placebo group and 57 in the tamoxifen group (RR = 0.81; 95% CI = 0.56–1.16). In reviewing the causes of death, the absolute reduction in cancer deaths was 0.28% (42 in the placebo group and 23 in the tamoxifen group), with a relative risk reduction of 45 percent. This was counterbalanced by an increase of 0.10% in cardiac and vascular deaths (15 in the placebo group and 22 in the tamoxifen group), with a relative risk increase of 47.5 percent. The absolute chance of being alive on tamoxifen over the 69 months of the study was increased by approximately 0.18% or the relative increased chance of being alive was 19 percent. There were no differences in other causes of death.

ITALIAN TAMOXIFEN PREVENTION STUDY

Between 1992 and 1997 5,408 women, who had undergone prior hysterectomy with or without ovariectomy, were recruited and randomly assigned to receive placebo or tamoxifen 20 mg/day for 5 years.[9] At a median follow-up of 46 months, 41 cases of breast cancer occurred, of which 22 were in the placebo arm and 19 in the tamoxifen arm. The trial permitted entry of women on estrogen-replacement therapy (ERT), and 14% of participants took ERT. Of 390 women on ERT in the placebo group, there were eight cases of breast cancer compared with one case in 362 women on ERT in the tamoxifen group ($p = 0.216$).

In a subset analysis of women who were on their assigned treatment for more than one year, there were 19 cases of breast cancer in the placebo group and 11 in the tamoxifen group ($p = 0.02$). The investigators predicted that in this group there was an estimated probability of 0.87 (SE 0.02) of reporting a significant difference (at 5%) between the two arms after a further 5 years of follow-up, given the observed difference of 33 percent. There were no differences in the status of ER between those developing breast cancer either in the placebo or tamoxifen arms.

The power of this study is low ($\propto = 0.05$; power = 0.34). Simulation showed that the probability of obtaining a significant hazard rate is only 22%, to prove the initial hypothesis of a 33% reduction in breast cancer by tamoxifen.

THE ROYAL MARSDEN HOSPITAL TAMOXIFEN
CHEMOPREVENTION TRIAL

Between 1986 and 1996, 2,494 women with a family history of breast cancer were recruited and randomly assigned to placebo versus tamoxifen 20 mg/day for 8 years.[10] At a median follow-up of 54.6 months, the overall frequency of breast cancer was the same for women on placebo or tamoxifen. Thirty-six women developed breast cancer on placebo and 34 on tamoxifen. In this trial 1,030 women (41%) were on ERT, and there was no difference in breast cancer occurrence if they were in placebo or tamoxifen arms.

Critique

The NSABP trial has enormous power to detect small differences in outcomes. The trial was well conducted, with thorough audits during its progress. The level of enhanced risk in the study population was significant (on average five times the normal population). The study has 52,401 women years of follow-up, with a drop-out rate of 19.7% in the placebo group and 23.7% in the tamoxifen group, and only 8% were lost to follow-up. Although there is a clear reduction in both invasive and noninvasive cancers the effect was confined to the ER-positive group, which tended to have a slightly better prognosis than patients with ER-negative tumors. One question is whether those patients developing ER-positive tumors while on tamoxifen are resistant and whether they will derive any benefit from tamoxifen as an adjuvant therapy. The early breaking of the blindedness of the study, thereby giving the participants the opportunity to take tamoxifen, may not permit determination of the key end point of death due to breast cancer.

The Italian trial clearly has a low level of risk in the participants, which may be reduced below normal levels in those having an ovariectomy at a younger age. The drop-out rate was 26.3% and significantly less at 11.7% for women over 60 years. The power of this trial to detect a significant preventive effect of tamoxifen was low.

The United Kingdom trial has 26% of the women years of follow-up compared to the NSABP. There is possibly a high breast cancer risk level due to the frequency of family histories, consistent with a BRCA 1 or 2 mutation. The authors estimated that about 36% of all participants and 60% of those who developed breast cancer have a greater than 80% chance of having an alteration in a breast cancer gene. The U.K. study also experienced a drop-out rate of 35% overall and 40% in the tamoxifen arm; 26% were on ERT during the trial.

FUTURE DIRECTIONS

Continuing follow-up of the United States and the United Kingdom studies may yield further information concerning the preventive effects of tamoxifen. The International Breast Cancer Intervention Study (IBIS) plans to enroll 7,000 women in a tamoxifen prevention trial, which may help to yield a definitive answer.

Selective estrogen receptor modulators (SERMS) are either undergoing clinical testing or are in preclinical studies for the prevention of osteoporosis and potential breast cancer preventive effects.[11] During the course of European trials of raloxifene, a SERM II for osteoporosis prevention, it was noted that the breast cancer rate was significantly lower than those on placebo.[12,13] Raloxifene will be tested against tamoxifen in 22,000 women at 200 institutions by the NSABP (Study of Tamoxifen and Raloxifene, STAR) or P-02 study, which started in 1999. SERM IIIs, such as droloxifene and idoxifene, are under development. Understanding the complexities of the estrogen receptor has recently moved forward, and this will provide the basis for new drug discovery.

CONCLUSIONS

The critical question is, Why do the European studies fail to confirm the U.S. study? Clearly the answers are complex and uncertain.[14] Differences in power, age, risk, compliance, and the use of ERT in the European studies may be relevant. The efficacy of tamoxifen in BRCA 1 or 2 carriers is an important issue; recent data have shown a DNA repair defect in those with BRCA 1 gene alterations.[15] The known genotoxicity of tamoxifen is of concern; however, the NSABP study did show a significant reduction in breast cancer risk in those with first degree relatives with breast cancer, including those likely to have a hereditary predisposition gene. The issue will be clarified when the BRCA 1 or 2 status of these individuals is determined, as DNA samples were stored for all participants.

Should tamoxifen be used outside of a clinical trial? The FDA has approved its use to delay breast cancer, but the word *prevention* has been the subject of polemics. For the individual woman, every day that breast cancer is delayed is a day that it has been prevented. *Risk reduction* is technically a more accurate phrase but lacks meaning to the woman. Elimination of breast cancer is an ideal that is probably unattainable; the current goal is to reduce the incidence, and ultimately the mortality, of this disease.

REFERENCES

1. OSBORNE, M.P. & J.P. CROWE. 1987. The identificaiton of enhanced risk patients and their management in a special surveillance breast clinic. *In* Breast Cancer: Diagnosis and Treatment. I.M. Ariel & J.B. Cleary, Eds.: 75–86. McGraw Hill. New York.
2. SIMMONS, R.M. & M.P. OSBORNE. 1999. Prophylactic mastectomy. Breast J. **3:** 372–379.
3. HARTMAN, L.C., D.J. SCHAID, J.E. WOODS *et al.* 1999. Efficacy of bilateral prophylactic mastectomy in women with a family history of breast cancer. N. Engl. J. Med. **340:** 77–84.
4. JORDAN, V.C. 1976. Effect of tamoxifen (ICI 46, 474) on initiation and growth of DMBA-induced rat mammary carcinomata. Eur. J. Cancer **12:** 419–424.
5. JORDAN, V.C., M.K. LABABIDI & M.K LANGAN-FAHEY. 1991. Suppression of mouse mammary tumorgenesis by long-term tamoxifen therapy. J. Natl. Cancer Inst. **83:** 492–496.
6. OSBORNE, M.P., J.F. RUPERTO, J.P. CROWE *et al.* 1992. The effect of tamoxifen on preneoplastic cell proliferationin *N*-nitroso-*N*-methylurea-induced mammmary carcinogenesis. Cancer Res. **52:** 1477–1480.
7. EARLY BREAST CANCER TRIALISTS COLLABORATIVE GROUP. 1998. Tamoxifen for early breast cancer: An overview of the randomized trial. Lancet **351:** 1451–1467.

8. FISHER, B., J.P CONSTANTINO, D.L. WICKERHAM et al. 1998. Tamoxifen for prevention of breast cancer: Report of the National Surgical Adjuvant Breast and Bowel Project P–1 study. J. Natl. Cancer Inst. **90:** 1371–1388.
9. VERONESI, U., P. MAISONNEUVE, A. COSTA et al. 1998. Prevention of breast cancer with tamoxifen: Prelimminary findings from the Italian randomized trial among hysterectomized women. Lancet **352:** 93–97.
10. POWLES, T., R. ELES, S. ASHLEY et al. 1998. Interim analysis of the incidence of breast cancer in the Royal Marsden Hospital tamoxifen randomized prevention trial. Lancet **352:** 98–101.
11. MITLAK, B.M. & F.J. COHEN. 1997. In search of optimal long-term female hormone replacement: The potential of selective estrogen receptor modulators. Horm. Res. **48:** 155–163.
12. CUMMINGS, S.R., S. ECKERT, K.A. KRUEGER et al. 1999. The effect of raloxifene on risk of breast cancer in menopausal women. Results from the MORE randomized trial. J. Am. Med. Assoc. **281:** 2189–2197.
13. JORDAN, V.C., J.E. GLUSMAN, S. ECKERT et al. 1998. Incident primary breast cancers are reduced by raloxifene: Integrated data from multicenter, double blind, randomized trials in ~12,000 post-menopausal women [abstract]. Proc. Am. Soc. Clin. Oncol. **17:** 122a.
14. PRITCHARD, K.I. 1998. Is tamoxifen effective in prevention of breast cancer? Lancet **352:** 80–81.
15. SCULLY, R., J. CHEN, A. PLUG et al. 1997. Association of BRCA 1 with Rad 51 in mitotic and meiotic cells. Cell **88:** 265–275.

European Trials on Dietary Supplementation for Cancer Prevention

GUIDO BIASCO[a,c] AND GIAN MARIA PAGANELLI[b,d]

[a]Istituto di Ematologia ed Oncologia Medica "Ludovico e Ariosto Seràgnoli," University of Bologna, 40138 Bologna, Italy

[b]Divisione di Pneumologia, Azienda Ospedaliera di Bologna, 40138 Bologna, Italy

ABSTRACT: European institutions aimed at cancer research and control are spending sizable resources to develop preclinical and clinical chemoprevention trials. Pilot studies showed positive effect on colorectal cell proliferation from supplementation with calcium; vitamins A, C, and E; Ω-3 fatty acids; and folic acid. A significant reduction in adenoma recurrence after polypectomy was found in patients randomly assigned to take vitamin A, C, and E supplementation or, to a lesser extent, lactulose. Although first reports showed a disquieting higher incidence of lung cancer in male smokers who took β-carotene supplementation, the European Organization of Research and Treatment of Cancer (EORTC) planned a chemoprevention study on the prevention of second primary tumors in patients with curatively treated head and neck or lung cancer (EUROSCAN). Retinol palmitate or N-acetylcysteine or both are given for two years. The European Cancer Prevention Organization (ECP) is carrying out a clinical trial in patients with previous adenomas of the large bowel, to test the efficacy of calcium or fiber supplementation on adenoma recurrence. ECP in collaboration with EURONUT has also started a multinational intervention study of the effect of H. pylori eradication and/or dietary supplementation with vitamin C on intestinal metaplasia.

INTRODUCTION

In recent years, the proposal of using natural or synthetic agents in order to reverse or inhibit cancer development can be considered one of the most important advances in cancer prevention. Among potential chemopreventive agents, dietary constituents are often preferred because they are regarded as naturally occurring and safe. In particular, studies on the molecular biology of the neoplastic process focused on the importance of micronutrients as candidates for chemoprevention of specific tumors.

Therefore, European institutions conducting cancer research and control spent sizable resources to develop preclinical and clinical chemoprevention trials.[1] Be-

[c]Address for communication: Istituto di Ematologia ed Oncologia Medica "Ludovico e Ariosto Seràgnoli," University of Bologna, Divisione di Pneumologia, Azienda Ospedaliera di Bologna, Policlinico S. Orsola-Malpighi, Via Massarenti 9, 40138 Bologna, Italy. Voice: 39-51-6363111 ext. 4078; fax: 39-51-398973.
e-mail: gbiasco@med.unibo.it
[d]Divisione di Pneumologia, Azienda Ospedaliera di Bologna, Policlinico S. Orsola-Malpighi, Via Palagi 9, 40138 Bologna, Italy. Voice: 39-51-6362465; fax: 39-51-6362557.
e-mail: pneumo@orsola-malpighi.med.unibo.it

cause the definitive end point of cancer chemoprevention is cancer incidence, these trials need thousands of patients monitored for several years in order to detect a significant efficacy of treatment. Pioneer studies were aimed to assay the effect of potential chemopreventive substances on intermediate end points that are associated with cancer risk, among which are cell proliferation abnormalities.

CELL PROLIFERATION AS AN INTERMEDIATE BIOMARKER IN CHEMOPREVENTION STUDIES OF COLORECTAL CANCER

The first report of a normalization of rectal cell proliferation as an intermediate chemopreventive effect was done by Martin Lipkin and Harold Newmark in 1985, using a 1.5–2 g/day dietary calcium supplementation. These results were confirmed by other trials, some of which were carried out in Europe.[2]

In 1992, a pilot study carried out at the University of Bologna suggested that antioxidant vitamins are able to reduce the expansion of the proliferative compartment of the rectal mucosa, which is frequently found in conditions at increased risk of colorectal cancer. In this trial, vitamins A, C, and E were given daily for 6 months at doses of 30,000 IU, 1000 mg, and 70 mg, respectively, to patients with previous adenomas of the large bowel after colonoscopic polypectomy.[3]

Similarly, another preclinical study was carried out in Italy on the basis of the epidemiological evidence of an inverse correlation between the consumption of seafood and colorectal cancer incidence. In this study, the supplementation of fish oil rich in Ω-3 fatty acids reduced the expansion of the proliferative compartment of the rectal mucosa of subjects at increased risk of colorectal cancer.[4] We also mention a study that showed that short-chain fatty acids, such as butyric acid, are able to reduce inflammation and mucosal hyperproliferation in patients affected by ulcerative colitis.[5]

It has been suggested that increased colon cancer risk in ulcerative colitis is correlated to a reduced bioavailability of folate, presumably because of an impaired absorption induced by a common medication, sulfapyridine. Recently, we studied the effect of folate supplementation on rectal cell proliferation of patients with longstanding ulcerative colitis, which are at increased risk of colorectal cancer. In this pilot trial, the administration of folic acid (as calcium folate 15 mg/day for 3 months) was able to normalize cell kinetic abnormalities, whereas no significant change was observed in the placebo group.[6]

These preliminary results gave impulse to the development of phase II clinical trials aimed at evaluating the effect of dietary consituents and/or micronutrients on later end points related to cancer development, that is, epithelial dysplasia, or the recurrence of cancer or second primary malignancies of the gastrointestinal tract and respiratory system.

BETA-CAROTENE AND LUNG CANCER: WHAT'S GOING WRONG?

Epidemiological evidence indicates that the consumption of diets rich in carotenoids; selenium; and vitamins A, C, and E are associated with reduced lung cancer risk. On the basis of these findings, large chemoprevention trials were planned in the

1980s and early1990s. In 1994 the results of a Finnish study (sponsored by the National Public Health Institute of Finland with the United States National Cancer Institute) were published on the effect of α-tocopherol and β-carotene on male smokers. The report was quite disquieting: a minimal reduction in lung cancer incidence was demonstrated in men who received vitamin E, but, by contrast, an 18% higher incidence of lung cancer and an 8% higher total mortality were found among the subjects who took 20 mg/daily of β-carotene. Subjects who took both vitamin E and β-carotene showed an increase in lung cancer similar to those with β-carotene alone, suggesting the absence of any significant interaction between those supplements.[7]

These results were further confirmed by the United States CARET trial, which was therefore abruptly stopped.[8] However, additional analyses of these studies pointed out that we cannot exclude the possibility that the increase of lung cancer incidence observed in the β-carotene supplementation arms was due to active smoking throughout the period of intervention in a large proportion of subjects. As a matter of fact, the percentage of current smokers at the beginning and at the end of the study were 100–80% in the ATBC study and 80–48% in the CARET study. Because it is possible to hypothesize an increase of metabolic activation of carcinogens from tobacco smoke by high-dose β-carotene or a promoter effect at a later carcinogenetic step, some authors suggested that it is mandatory to concentrate future chemoprevention programs on former smokers before endorsing a causative role by β-carotene.[9]

CHEMOPREVENTION OF HEAD, NECK, AND LUNG CANCERS

In 1988 the European Organization of Research and Treatment of Cancer (EORTC) began a chemoprevention study on the prevention of second primary tumors in patients with head and neck or lung cancer (EUROSCAN). This was a double-blind controlled study with a 2×2 factorial design, started in June 1988, which recruited patients curatively treated with oral, laryngeal, or lung cancer. Retinol palmitate, 300,000 IU/daily, was given for one year and 150,000 IU/daily for another year, or N-acetylcysteine (NAC), 600 mg/daily, for two years, or both drugs. The end points of this study are the rate of recurrence and occurrence of second primary tumors. More than 60 centers from 14 European countries participated in the study. At present, no data are available in the literature, although the end of the intervention period was expected to be around the end of 1996.[10] However, the investigators are optimists, on the basis of experimental and clinical data regarding the two agents. As a matter of fact, high-dose retinol palmitate was used in an adjuvant trial of surgically resected stage I lung cancer. After a median follow-up of 46 months, a reduction in the percentage of recurrence, or occurrence of new primary tumors, was found in patients treated with retinol palmitate, 300,000 IU/day, for one year, as compared to the control group.[11]

CHEMOPREVENTION OF METACHRONOUS ADENOMAS
OF THE LARGE BOWEL

Concerning the effect of antioxidant vitamins in large-bowel carcinogenesis, Roncucci *et al.* showed a significant reduction in adenoma recurrence in 209 patients who were followed for at least 12–18 months after polypectomy. Patients were randomly chosen to take either vitamins A (30,000 IU daily), C (1000 mg/daily), and E (70 mg) or lactulose (20 mg/daily). A decrease in adenoma recurrence rate was found in both arms but was remarkably higher in vitamin-treated patients; however, a low compliance rate was observed.[12]

A European multicentric intervention study on chemoprevention of colorectal cancer is currently in progress, conducted by the European Cancer Prevention Organization (ECP). This is a double-blind, placebo-controlled clinical trial with a parallel design, which recruited patients aged 35–75 with adenomas of the large bowel previously removed by colonoscopy and a clean colon at entry. The main aim of the study is to test the efficacy of oral calcium supplementation (2 g/day as calcium gluconolactate and carbonate) or oral dietary supplementation with fiber (as 3.8 g/day isphagula husk) on adenoma recurrence. Secondary end points are the effect of treatment on rectal cell proliferation and on concentration of bile acids and sterols in stools. All randomized patients are followed up every 6 months for 3 years. At the beginning and at the end of the study, a colonoscopy is performed and rectal biopsies are taken for cell proliferation analysis (PCNA immunostaining and, when possible, bromodeoxyuridine uptake). Blood samples are obtained for biochemical analyses, including DNA analysis; stool samples are collected for quantitative analysis of bile acids and related compounds; and a dietary questionnaire is administered. Additional blood samples are drawn annually to assess the tolerability of the treatments (e.g., calcaemia, and liver and kidney function). Up to now, about 700 subjects have been included from Belgium, Denmark, France, Germany, Ireland, Israel, Italy, Portugal, Spain and the United Kingdom; there were only nine cases of important side effects, which consisted of major diarrhea or severe abdominal pain that disappeared after discontinuation of intervention.[13]

PERSPECTIVES OF CHEMOPREVENTION OF GASTRIC CANCER: THE ECP-IM STUDY

In 1985 the European Cancer Prevention Organization (ECP) in collaboration with EURONUT set up a case-control study to study the relationship between diet and intestinal metaplasia as a precursor of epithelial dysplasia and gastric cancer. For every intestinal metaplasia case there were two controls matched for age, gender, and residence. Endoscopy and biopsies were performed as well as diet and lifestyle assessment; serum, urine, and gastric juice samples were also collected. From the first phase of the study, it was concluded that when compared to controls, cases with intestinal metaplasia had a low intake of fresh fruit and vegetables, a very low intake of vitamin C, and a high prevalence of *H. pylori* antibodies.[14] In light of these results, ECP has started a large multinational intervention study of the effect of *H. pylori* eradication and/or dietary supplementation with vitamin C on the gastric mucosal histopathology in patients with intestinal metaplasia.[15] Patients will be randomly assigned as follows: *H. pylori*–negative patients will be administered 1 g vitamin C daily for 3 years *vs* placebo; *H. pylori*–positive patients will be given a 2-week eradication regimen (omeprazole, 20 mg twice daily, and clarithromycin, 500 mg, three times daily), then either vitamin C or placebo. The hypotheses to be tested are that *H. pylori* eradication causes a statistically significant change in the pattern of intestinal metaplasia, ascorbic acid supplementation causes a statistically significant change in the pattern of intestinal metaplasia, and there is an interaction between the two regimens (*H. pylori* eradication and vitamin C supplementation).

In conclusion, the large clinical chemoprevention trials are actually being completed in Europe, and in the next few years we are expecting to obtain more information on the efficacy of chemoprevention with dietary constituents and on the feasibility of such programs on large population groups at increased risk of cancer development.

REFERENCES

1. BUIATTI, E., D. BALZI & A. BARCHIELLI. 1994. Intervention trials of cancer prevention: Results and new research programmes. IARC Technical Report 18, Lyon.
2. O'SULLIVAN, K.R., P.M. MATHIAS, S. BEATTIE & C. O'MORAIN. 1993. Effect of oral calcium supplementation on colonic crypt cell proliferation in patients with adenomatous polyps of the large bowel. Eur. J. Gastroenterol. Hepatol. **5:** 85–89.
3. PAGANELLI, G.M. G. BIASCO, G. BRANDI *et al.* 1992. Effect of vitamin A, C, and E supplementation on rectal cell proliferation in patients with colorectal adenomas. J. Natl. Cancer Inst. **84:** 47–51.
4. ANTI, M., G. MARRA, F. ARMELAO *et al.* 1992. Effect of Ω-3 fatty acids on rectal mucosal cell proliferation in subjects at risk for colon cancer. Gastroenterology **103:** 883–891.
5. SCHEPPACH, W., H. SOMMER, T. KIRCHNER *et al.* 1992. Effect of butyrate enemas on the colonic mucosa in distal ulcerative colitis. Gastroenterology **103:** 51–56.
6. BIASCO, G., U. ZANNONI, G.M. PAGANELLI *et al.* 1997. Folic acid supplementation and cell kinetics of rectal mucosa in patients with ulcerative colitis. Cancer Epidemiol. Biomarkers Prev. **6:** 469–471.
7. THE ALPHA-TOCOPHEROL, BETA-CAROTENE CANCER PREVENTION STUDY GROUP. 1994. The effect of vitamin E and beta carotene on the incidence of lung cancer and other cancers in male smokers. N. Engl. J. Med. **330:** 1029–1035.
8. OMENN, G.S., G.E. GOODMAN, M.D. THORNQUIST *et al.* 1996. Effects of a combination of beta carotene and vitamin A on lung cancer and cardiovascular disease. N. Engl. J. Med. **334:** 1150–1155.
9. PASTORINO, U. 1997. β-carotene and the risk of lung cancer. J. Natl. Cancer Inst. **89:** 456–458.
10. DE VRIES, N., U. PASTORINO & N. VAN ZANDWIJK. 1994. Chemoprevention of second primary tumors in head and neck cancer in Europe: EUROSCAN. Eur. J. Cancer B (Oral Oncol.) **6:** 367–368.
11. PASTORINO, U., M. INFANTE, M. MAIOLI *et al.* 1993. Adjuvant treatment of stage I lung cancer with high-dose vitamin A. J. Clin. Oncol. **11:** 1216–1222.
12. RONCUCCI, L., P.D. DI DONATO, L. CARATI *et al.* 1993. Antioxidant vitamins or lactulose for the prevention of the recurrence of colorectal adenomas. Dis. Colon Rectum **36:** 227–234.
13. FAIVRE, J., C. COUILLAULT, O. KRONBORG *et al.* 1997. Chemoprevention of metachronous adenomas of the large bowel: Design and interim results of a randomized trial of calcium and fibre. Eur. J. Cancer Prev. **6:** 132–138.
14. HILL, M.J. ON BEHALF OF THE ECP-EURONUT-IM STUDY GROUP. 1997. ECP-EURONUT study of diet and intestinal metaplasia. Eur. J. Cancer Prev. **6:** 201–204.
15. REED, P.I. 1994. The ECP-IM Intervention Study. Eur. J. Cancer Prev. 3 (Suppl.2): 99–104.

Update from Asia

Asian Studies on Cancer Chemoprevention

TAIK-KOO YUN[a]

Laboratory of Experimental Pathology, Korea Cancer Center Hospital,
215-4 Gongneung Dong, Nowon Ku, Seoul, Korea

ABSTRACT: In Asia, nontoxic dietary products are considered desirable primary prevention vehicles for conquering cancer. As early as 1978, investigators in Korea carried out extensive long-term anticarcinogenicity experiments using the mouse lung tumor model and observed an anticarcinogenic effect of *Panax ginseng* C.A. Meyer extract in 1980. The results showed that natural products can provide hope for human cancer prevention. A newly established nine-week medium-term model using mouse lung tumors (Yun's model) could confirm the anticarcinogenicity of ginseng that varies according to its type and age. Subsequently, the ginseng was shown by epidemiological studies to be a nonorgan-specific cancer preventive agent associated with a dose–response relationship. The anticarcinogenic effects of vegetarian foods common at every dining table in Korea and some synthetics were also studied using Yun's nine-week model. In brief, ascorbic acid, soybean lecithin, capsaicin, biochanin A, *Ganoderma lucidum*, caffeine, and a novel synthetic 2-(allylthio)pyrazine decrease the incidence of mouse lung tumors, whereas fresh ginseng (4 years old), carrot, spinach, *Sesamum indicum*, β-carotene, and 13-*cis* retinoic acid do not. This result regarding beta-carotene is consistent with the ineffective findings of the ATBC trial, the CARET trial, and the Physicians' Health Study. In 1983, a cancer chemoprevention study group was first established in Japan. Subsequently, (-)-epigallocatechin gallate, cryptoporic acid E, and sarcophytol A from natural products, and synthetic acyclic retinoid and canventol were shown to be anticarcinogenic or chemopreventive in human subjects. Despite the frequent consumption of tea wordwide as a beverage and current experimental evidence of anticarcinogenesis, including controversial results of epidemiological studies, more systematic clinical trials for confirmation of preventive activity of tea against cancer are needed. Placebo-controlled intervention trials of dietary fiber are under study in Japan. In the past decade, new triterpenoids were isolated from various natural sources, and its biological activities were investigated in Asia. In the late 1970s a comprehensive chemoprevention program was established at the Institute of Materia Medica, Chinese Academy of Medical Sciences. Since then, many retinoid compounds have been synthesized and screened in the search for chemopreventive cancer agents. The National Cancer Institute (USA) and China are jointly engaged in the two-nutrition intervention in Linxian, China. The results of joint study of the general population and of dysplasia in China should stimulate further research to clarify the potential benefits of micronutrient supplements. We need to clarify if there is a connection between the lower rates of cancer mortality in Korea and the frequent consumption of anticarcinogenic vegetables or traditional foods,

[a]Address for communication: Director, Korea Complementary & Alternative Medicine Institute, Se Dai Building, Suite 1605, 11-3 Hoe Hyun Dong 3 Ka, Chung Ku, 100-053, Seoul, Korea. Voice: 82-2-335-1020; fax: 82-2-335-1020.
e-mail: tkyun@nuri.net

including ginseng and *Ganoderma lucidum*. The constituents of the nontoxic stable dietary products promise to be the future hope for conquering cancers in the coming years.

INTRODUCTION

During the past 2000 years traditional Chinese medicine (TCM) has been disseminated to many countries in Asia. In TCM, health foods are foods that have the ability to maintain and improve health, to prevent and treat disease, and to facilitate rehabilitation. In other words, in TCM, food and medicine are of equal importance in preventing and treating disease;[1] that is traditional Asian philosophy. Despite comprehensive advances in early diagnosis of, and chemotherapy for, cancer, many malignancies remain difficult to cure. Because primary cancer prevention, particularly chemoprevention, could become an increasingly useful strategy in the fight against cancer, it is worthwhile to look at the preclinical, epidemiological, and clincal research into cancer chemoprevention against the background of the traditional cultures of the Orient, particularly Korea, Japan, and China.

CANCER CHEMOPREVENTION RESEARCH IN KOREA

Fifty years have passed since the first chemotherapeutics, alkylating agents, were developed.[2] The total number of new cancers in 1985 was estimated to be 7.62 million worldwide,[3] but many cancers still remain difficult to cure.[4] In Korea, the failure to improve the five-year "observed" survival from one in three in the 1960s to one in two in the 1970s[5] stimulated awareness of the importance of primary prevention. Since then, researchers have been trying to discover nontoxic cancer chemopreventive agents among natural food products, which is part of the traditional Asian philosophy.

GINSENG

The ginseng plant is a deciduous perennial that belongs to the Araliaceae family. Ginseng species include *Panax ginseng* C. A. Meyer, which is cultivated in Korea, Japan, China and Russia; *Panax quinquefolius* L. (American ginseng); *Panax japonicus* C. A. Meyer (Japanese ginseng); *Panax notoginseng* (Burk) F. H. Chen (Sanchiginseng); *Panax trifolius* L. (Dwarf ginseng); *Panax vietnamensis* Ha et Grushv; and *Panax pseudoginseng*. In Korea, *Panax ginseng* C. A. Meyer is collected after 2 to 6 years of cultivation, and it is classified in three ways depending on how it is processed: (a) fresh ginseng (less than 4 years old and can be consumed fresh); (b) white ginseng (4–6 years old and then dried after peeling); and (c) red ginseng, (harvested when 6 years old and then steamed and dried) (FIG. 1). Each type of ginseng can then be used to make various products: for example, fresh sliced ginseng, juice, extract (tincture or boiled extract), powder, tea, tablets, and capsules.

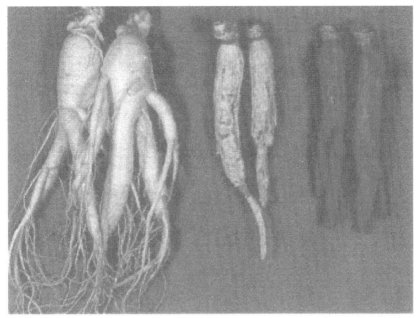

FIGURE 1. *Panax ginseng* C.A. Meyer in Korea is classified as fresh ginseng (left), which is less than 4 years old and can be consumed in the fresh state; white ginseng (center), which is 4–6 years old and dried after peeling; and red ginseng (right), harvested when 6 years old and then steamed and dried.

Preclinical Studies

It is hypothesized that the life-prolongation effect of ginseng described by Shennong[6] during the Liang Dynasty, China, may have been due to the preventive activity of ginseng against the development of cancers. Korean investigators, particularly Yun *et al.* therefore carried out extensive long-term anticarcinogenicity experiments in 1978 to investigate whether ginseng inhibited carcinogenesis induced by 9,10-dimethyl-1,2-benzanthracene (DMBA), urethane, aflatoxin B_1, N-2-fluorenylacetamide (FAA), and tobacco smoke condensates in newborn mice.[7,8] Red ginseng extract was administered orally to the weaned mice. In the group sacrificed at 28 weeks after the treatment (urethane combined with ginseng), there was a 22% decrease ($p<0.05$) in the incidence of lung adenoma. In the group sacrificed at 56 weeks after birth (aflatoxin B_1 combined with ginseng), there was a significant decrease in the incidence of hepatoma (75%) ($p<0.05$). These findings indicated that prolonged administration of red ginseng extract inhibited the incidence of tumors induced by urethane and aflatoxin B_1 (TABLE 1) and showed that natural products are a hope for human cancer prevention.

Establishment of Nine-week Medium-term Anticarcinogenicity Model

In 1983, Yun *et al.* first established a nine-week, medium-term anticarcinogenicity model based on the incidence of mouse pulmonary adenoma induced by ben-

TABLE 1. Effect of red ginseng extract on pulmonary adenoma induced by various chemical carcinogens in long-term *in vivo* experiment[a]

Carcinogens	Sacrifice (wks)	Incidence of Lung Adenoma	Diffuse Infiltration	Incidence of Hepatoma
DMBA[b]	48	21% decrease		63% decrease
Urethane	28		22% decrease**	
Aflatoxin B$_1$	56	29% decrease		75% decrease**

[a]Within 24 hours after birth, various carcinoigens (DMBA, urethane, and aflatoxin B$_1$)were injected subcutaneously in subscapular region of newborn ICR mice. The mice were given a solid-pellet diet, as prescribed by the NIH-7 open formula (1977), and tap water mixed with red ginseng extracts was administered through the drinking water (1 mg/mL), ad libitum; maximum duration, 57 weeks. (Yun *et al.* 1980. Proc. 3rd Int. Ginseng Symp. 87–113.)
[b]DMBA: 9,10-Dimethyl-1,2-benzanthracene.
** $p < 0.05$.

zo(a)pyrene (termed Yun's model).[9] They tried the model using ascorbic acid, β-carotene, and red ginseng extract to verify the utility; there was no anticarcinogenic effect in β-carotene. This result was withheld for five years and then published[10,11] when the Physician's Health Study showed negative results from β-carotene.[12] These results were consistent with ineffective findings of the ATBC trial, which randomly selected 29,133 male smorkers.[13] The CARET trial used more than 18,000 persons with a high risk of lung cancer,[14,15] and the Physicians' Health Study enrolled 22,071 American physicians.[16] Meanwhile, Yun *et al.* tried AOM (colon) and OH-BBN (bladder) models using red ginseng extract, when the Chemoprevention Branch, Division of Cancer Chemoprevention and Control, National Cancer Institute (NCI) made a recommendation in 1992[17,18] without any positive results. It was also negative for 13-*cis* retinoic acid, using Yun's model in 1995.[19,20]

Recently, loci responsible for mouse lung tumor susceptibility have been mapped to chromosomes 6, 9, 17, and 19, whereas those linked to lung tumor resistance have been mapped to chromosome 4, 11, 12, and 18. Known candidate susceptibility or resistance genes include the K-*ras* proto-oncogene on chromosome 6 and the p16 tumor supressor gene on chromosome 4. With evidence of considerable overlap between the genetic alterations that underline human and mouse tumorigenesis, the mouse lung tumor model has been expanded to include preclinical screening of chemopreventive agents against human lung cancer.[21] This mouse lung tumor model is applied among researchers, including those at the Chemoprevention Branch of the NCI. Furthermore, this model system also confirmed the negative anticarcinogenicity effect of 9-*cis* retinoic acid, 4-HPR, and oltipratz that were known to be promising cancer preventive agents in NCI recommended models.[22]

Anticarcinogenicity of Type and Age of Ginseng

Yun *et al.* further investigated whether fresh ginseng and white ginseng have similar anticarcinogenic effects and also whether these effects were related to the type and age of the ginseng used in Yun's model. In this study, fresh ginseng of 1.5, 3, 4, 5, and 6 years of age was used. Significant anticarcinogenic effects were observed in powders and extracts of the 6-year-old dried fresh ginseng, the 5- and 6-year-old

TABLE 2. Anticarcinogenic effects of *Panax ginseng* C.A. Meyer depending on type and age using Yun's 9-week medium-term anticarcinogenicity test model

	Incidence of Lung Adenoma					
	Fresh Ginseng		White Ginseng		Red Ginseng	
Age of Ginseng (years[a])	Powder	Extract	Powder	Extract	Powder	Extract
Benzo(a)pyrene (BP)[b]	41.3	63.9	45.0	41.3	48.6	47.5
BP + 1.5	31.2	48.3	—	—	37.9	40.7
BP + 3	30.0	52.5	41.3	32.0	41.7	35.0
BP + 4	31.3	51.8	38.0	46.0	3 1.7[c]	30.1[c]
BP + 5	30.3	47.5	31.6[c]	44.0	28.3[d]	30.0[c]
BP + 6	27.8[c]	44.1[c]	25.3[c]	26.5[c]	25.41[e]	26.3[c]

[a]Year represents age of ginseng at harvest. Ginseng was given in drinking water at a concentration of 1 mg/mL of red ginseng extract equivalent.

[b]BP, Benzo(a)pyrene. 0.5 mg of BP was injected subcutaneously into mice less than 24 hours old. Significant differences from group that received BP alone are indicated by [c]$p < 0.05$, [d]$p < 0.02$, and [e]$p < 0.01$.[23,24]

ginsengs, and the 4-, 5-, and 6-year-old red ginsengs (TABLE 2). It was concluded that the anticarcinogenicity of ginseng varies according to its type and age.[23-25]

It has been shown that Sanchi ginseng inhibits (1) the early antigen activation of the Epstein-Barr virus in Raji cells, induced by TPA and *N*-butyric acid, (2) pulmonary tumorigenesis induced in mice by 4-nitroquinoline-*N*-oxide and glycerol,[26] and (3) liver cancer induced by diethylnitrosamine in rats.[27] It has also been reported more recently that a tissue culture biomass tincture obtained from cultured cells of *Panax ginseng* C. A. Meyer has a marked inhibitory effect on rat mammary adenocarcinoma induced by *N*-methyl-*N*-nitrosourea administration.[28] In summary, administration of ginseng inhibited the incidence of tumors induced by carcinogens in various rodent tissues, including lung, liver, and mammary glands.

Epidemiological Studies: Case-control Study with 905 Pairs

The effect of ginseng consumption on the risk of cancer was investigated by interviewing 905 pairs of cases and controls matched by age, sex, and date of admission to the Korea Cancer Center Hospital in Seoul.[29] Of the 905 cases, 562 (62%) had a history of ginseng intake, compared to 674 of the controls (75%), a statistically significant difference ($p < 0.01$). The odds ratio (OR) of cancer in relation to ginseng intake was 0.56 [95% confidence interval (CI), 0.45–0.69]. Ginseng extract and powder were shown to be more effective than fresh sliced ginseng, the juice, or tea in reducing the OR (TABLE 3). ORs for decreasing levels of ginseng intake were 1.00, 0.58, 0.43, and 0.25 for males and 1.00, 0.81, 0.56, and 0.52 for females. A trend test showed a significant decrease in the number of cancer cases among those who reported an increased frequency of ginseng intake for males ($p < 10^{-5}$) as well as for females ($p < 0.05$). The reliability of recall for ginseng use was assessed by interviewing one-tenth of the randomly selected subjects twice using the same questionnaire. The overall agreement in reported ginseng use between the two interviews was 0.85, and the Kappa value was 0.71 ($p < 0.01$). These results strongly support the hypothesis that ginseng has cancer preventive effects, as suggested by the previ-

TABLE 3. Odds ratios and 95% confidence intervals for cancers by ginseng intake

	905 pairs		1987 pairs	
Type of ginseng	Odds ratio[a]	95% CI	Odds ratio[a]	95% CI
No intake of ginseng	1.00	Reference	1.00	Reference
Intake of ginseng	0.56	0.46–0.69	0.50	0.44–0.58
Fresh ginseng				
Slice	0.74	0.53–1.04	0.79	0.63–1.01
Juice	0.77	0.46–1.30	0.71	0.49–1.03
Extract	0.14	0.07–0.26	0.37	0.29–0.46
White ginseng				
Powder	0.44	0.26–0.75	0.30	0.22–0.41
Extract	0.64	0.50–0.82	0.57	0.48–0.68
Tea	0.93	0.53–1.61	0.69	0.45–1.07
Red ginseng				
Extract	0.45	0.05–3.32	0.20	0.08–0.50
Combination	0.27	0.13–0.53	0.16	0.10–0.25

[a]Adjusted for age, sex, marital status, education, smoking, and alcohol consumption.[29,31]

ous animal experiments.[29] The Lancet stated in an editorial that ginseng consumption reduces the risks for all cancer types. The article included an example of the "nonorgan specific approach" to cancer chemoprevention.[30]

Case-control Study on 1987 Pairs

In order to explore further (a) the types of ginseng products that have the most prominent cancer preventive effect, (b) the reproducibility of the dose-response relationship, (c) the duration of ginseng consumption that has a significant preventive effect, (d) the types of cancer that can be prevented by ginseng, and (e) the effect of ginseng on cancers associated with smoking, Yun *et al.* extended the number of subjects for a case-control study to 1987 pairs.[31] In this study, as with the other study, ginseng users had a lower risk (OR, 0.50) for cancer compared with nonusers. With respect to the type of ginseng, the ORs for cancer were 0.37 for fresh ginseng extract users, 0.57 for white ginseng extract users, 0.30 for white ginseng extract users, 0.30 for white ginseng powder users, and 0.20 for red ginseng users (TABLE 3). Those who took fresh ginseng slices, fresh ginseng juice, and white ginseng tea, however, showed no decreasing risk. Overall, the risk decreased as the frequency and duration of ginseng intake increased, thus showing a dose–response relationship (TABLE 4). With respect to the site of cancer, the odds ratios were 0.47 for cancer of the lip, oral cavity, and pharynx; 0.20 for esophageal cancer; 0.36 for stomach cancer; 0.42 for colorectal cancer; 0.48 for liver cancer; 0.22 for pancreatic cancer; 0.18 for laryngeal cancer; 0.55 for lung cancer; 0.15 for ovarian cancer; and 0.48 for other cancers (TABLE 5). In cancers of the female breast, uterine cervix, urinary bladder, and thyroid gland, however, there was no association with ginseng intake. In cancer of the lung, lip, oral cavity and pharynx, and liver, smokers who took ginseng showed decreased

TABLE 4. Distribution of ginseng intake frequency for cases and controls by sex: Odds ratios of cancer and 95% confidence interval(CI) in case-control study on 1987 pairs

Ginseng Intake	Male				Female			
	Cases	Controls	OR[a]	95% CI	Cases	Controls	OR[a]	95%CI
Frequency of ginseng intake								
None	409	234	1.00	Reference	512	371	1.00	Reference
1–3 times/year	246	231	0.62	0.49-0.79	171	209	0.60	0.47–0.76
4–11 times/year	197	223	0.48	0.37–0.62	127	171	0.54	0.42–0.71
1 time/month or more	220	384	0.31	0.25–0.39	105	164	0.47	0.39–0.62
Total lifetime consumption of ginseng								
None	409	452	1.00	Reference	512	371	1.00	Reference
1–50	452	501	0.51	0.42–0.63	322	402	0.58	0.48-0.71
51–100	75	100	0.41	0.29–0.58	28	39	0.56	0.34–0.93
101–300	80	131	0.32	0.23–0.44	29	54	0.39	0.25–0.61
301–500	20	29	0.33	0.18–0.62	8	21	0.29	0.14–0.63
500 +	36	77	0.25	0.16–0.38	16	28	0.42	0.23–0.79

[a]Adjusted for age, marital status, education, smoking, and alcohol consumption.[31]

TABLE 5. Odds ratios for various cancers according to ginseng intakers in case-control study on 1987 pairs

Site of Cancer	Cases Never Taken/Taken	Control Never Taken/Taken	OR[a]	95% CI
Lip, oral cavity, and pharynx	67/92	40/119	0.47	0.29 ± 0.76
Esophagus	40/47	14/73	0.20	0.09 ± 0.38
Stomach	142/158	76/224	0.36	0.09 ± 0.52
Colon and rectum	55/63	32/86	0.42	0.24 ± 0.74
Liver	108/156	67/197	0.48	0.33 ± 0.70
Pancreas	12/11	5/18	0.22	0.05 ± 0.95
Larynx	21/19	8/32	0.18	0.06 ± 0.54
Lung	120/156	81/195	0.55	0.38 ± 0.79
Female breast	82/92	70/109	0.63	0.40 ± 1.05
Cervix uteri	156/146	312/170	0.72	0.52 ± 1.01
Ovary	17/5	8/14	0.15	0.04 ± 0.60
Urinary bladder	23/40	16/47	0.64	0.28 ± 1.47
Thyroid gland	16/24	14/26	0.96	0.38 ± 2.44
Other	53/61	35/79	0.48	0.27 ± 0.85

[a]Adjusted for age, sex, marital status, education, smoking, and alcohol consumption.[31]

TABLE 6. Adjusted relative risks (RRs) for selected cancers by ginseng intake in cohort study

Ginseng Intake	No. of Subjects	Cancers (n)								
		Stomach (42)[c]			Lung (24)			Liver (14)		
		No.	RR[a]	95% CI[b]	No.	RR	95% CI	No.	RR	95% CI
No intake	1283	23	1.00	—	14	1.00	—	4	1.00	
Ginseng intake	3167	19	0.33	0.18–0.57	10	0.30	0.14–0.65	10	0.86	0.25–2.94
Fresh ginseng										
Slices & juice	236	2	0.57	0.17–1.94	1	0.67	0.15–3.43	2	1.97	0.34–2.95
Extract	296	1	0.33	0.12–0.88	1	0.28	0.04–2.17	—	—	—
White ginseng										
Powder	147	1	0.24	0.03–1.84	—	—	—	—	—	—
Extract	68	2	1.34	0.30–5.97	—	—	—	—	—	—
Tea	442	6	0.64	0.26–1.61	4	0.80	0.26–2.44	2	1.72	0.15–4.87
Boiled chicken with young ginseng root	381	5	0.43	0.12–1.43	1	0.35	0.08–1.95	1	0.85	0.15–4.87

[a]RR adjusted for age, sex, education, smoking, and alcohol consumption.
[b]CI, Confidence interval.
[c]Values in parentheses indicate number of cancer cases.

OR compared with smokers with no ginseng intake. These findings support the view that ginseng use decreases the risk for most cancer compared to nonuse.

Prospective Study for Population[32]

Because they obtained promising findings at the beginning of our case-control study, and because there were no studies on the preventive effects of ginseng on cancer, Yun *et al.* performed a more reliable cohort study in 1987.[18] This study was conducted in a ginseng cultivation area, Kangwha-eup, from August 1987 to December 1992. They studied 4,634 (2,362 men, 2,272 women) adults over 40 years old who completed a questionnaire on ginseng intake. Among 355 (7.7%) total deaths, cancer accounted for 79 (22.8%). Subjects with cancer totalled 137 (3.0%), with 58 (1.3%) alive at the end of the study period and 79 (1.7%) deaths. Of 4,634 persons eligible for analysis, 70.5% (3,267) were ginseng users. Ginseng users had a decreased risk (RR = 0.40, 95% CI: 0.28–0.56) compared with nonusers. With regard to the type of ginseng, the RRs were 0.31 (95% CI: 0.13–0.74) for fresh ginseng extract users and 0.34 (95% CI: 0.20–0.53) for users of multiple combinations. There were no cancer deaths among the 24 red ginseng users. There was a decreased risk with a rise in the frequency of ginseng intake, showing a dose-response relationship. Newly diagnosed cancer cases were identified: 42 stomach, 24 lung, 14 liver, and 57 at other sites (TABLE 6). The RRs for ginseng users were 0.33 (95% CI: 0.18–0.57) in gastric cancer and 0.30 (95% CI: 0.14–0.65) in lung cancer. Among ginseng preparations, fresh ginseng extract users were significantly associated with a decreased risk of gastric cancer (RR = 0.33, 95% CI: 0.12–0.88). These results strongly suggest that

TABLE 7. Comparison of relative risks for cancer by type of ginseng intake among medium-term experiment, case-control studies, and cohort studies[29,31,32]

Kind of Ginseng	Yun's Medium-term Anticarcinogenicity	Case-control Studies		Cohort Study Morbidity & Mortality
		905 pairs	1987 pairs	4634 participants/ 5 years
Ginseng intake	—	0.56^a	0.50^a	0.40^a
Fresh ginseng				
Fresh slices	6-year-old only	Negative	Negative	Negative
Extract	6-year-old only	0.14	0.37	0.31
White ginseng				
Powder	5- and 6-year-old	0.64	0.57	Negative
Extract	5- and 6-year-old	0.44	0.30	Negative
Red ginseng				
Extract	4-, 5-, and 6-year-old	0.45	0.20	24 participants
Powder	4-, 5-, and 6-year-old			Non-cancer death
Combination	—	0.27	0.16	0.34

^{a}RR adjusted for age, sex, education, smoking, and alcohol consumption.

Panax ginseng C.A. Meyer has nontoxic and nonorgan-specific preventive effects against cancer.[33]

Using Yun's nine-week medium-term test model, Yun *et al.* observed a statistically significant anticarcinogenic effect of ginseng only in the group treated with 6-year-old dried fresh ginseng powder and extract, 5- and 6-year-old white ginseng, and 4-, 5-, and 6-year-old red ginseng powder or extract. The findings are consistent with a negative finding in fresh slice intakers in both case-control studies and cohort analysis. There were no cancer deaths among the 24 red ginseng consumers, and red ginseng showed prominent anticarcinogenicity in medium-term experiments (TABLE 7).

To examine the dose–response relationship between ginseng consumption and cancer, all types and forms of ginseng products were combined and the frequency of ginseng intake was divided into four levels: more than 1–3 times per year, 4–11 times per year, once a month, and more than once a month. A trend test showed a significant decrease of cancer cases with an increasing frequency of intake for both males and females in each case-control and cohort study (TABLE 8).

Ongoing Clinical Trials

Two trials conducted by the Korea Complementary and Alternative Medicine Institute, Seoul, and the Cancer Institute of Zhejiang Medical University, Hangzhou, Zhejiang Province, China are investigating the effect of Korean red ginseng extract (once a week for three years) administration on cancer incidence, including colorectal cancer and stomach cancer. Each research group has been performing a double-blind, placebo-controlled trial since July 1997 with red ginseng extract capsules to observe their preventive effects on cancers, including rectal or gastric cancer. To date, 560 patients have been selected from 2,815 polypectomized patients in Hain-

TABLE 8. Comparison of dose response relation, by frequency of ginseng intake between two case-control studies and three cohort studies

Frequency of Ginseng Intake	Relative risks for cancer			
	Case-control Studies (Patients)			Cohort Studies (Population Bases) Morbidity & Mortality
	905 pairs		1987 pairs	5 years
Sources	Male	Female	Both sexes	Both sexes
No intake	1.00	1.00	1.00	1.00
1–3 times/year	0.58	0.81	0.60	0.46
4–11 times/year	0.43	0.56	0.51	0.35
1 time/month <	0.25	0.52	0.36	0.34

[a]RR adjusted for age, sex, education, smoking, and alcohol consumption.

ing, Zhejiang Province and another 560 patients diagnosed with chronic atrophic gastritis in the Second Zhejiang Medical University Hospital that were screened by the Cancer Institute of Zhejiang Medical University, Hangzhou, China, to determine whether intervention can reduce the cancer incidence end points.

Active Components of Ginseng

It is still unknown what components of ginseng work in reducing cancer risks. Ginseng saponin comprises triterpenoidal glycosides of the dammar type with glucose, arabinose, xylose or rhamnose; the ginsenosides-Rx were recognized as active components in 1965.[34] Thirty-four kinds of ginsenosides have been isolated so far from fresh, white, or red ginseng: twenty-two kinds of ginsenosides are protopanaxadiol, eleven are protopanaxatriol, and only ginsenoside, Ro, is oleanane. The unique components of red ginseng are known as 20(R)-ginsenosides Rh1 and Rh2, 20(S)-ginsenoside Rh2, 20(R)-ginsenoside Rg2, 20(S)-ginsenoside Rg3, and notoginsenoside R4. Malonyl-ginsenoside-Rb1, -Rb2, -Rc, and Rd, found only in white ginseng, are transformed into ginsenosides Rb1, Rb2, Rc, and Rd; and ginsenoside -Rs1 or Rs2, saponin derivatives of red ginseng created by decarboxylation. Other than saponin, the following chemical constituents of ginseng have also been isolated: phenolic compounds, polyacetylene, ginsenoyne, sesquiterpenes, methoxypyrazine, alkypyrazine derivatives, sesquiterpene alcohol, panasinsanols, β-caboline, and neutral or acidic polysaccharides. Other vitamins, inorganic substances, free monosaccharides, and organic acids are also contained in ginseng.[35]

In both medium-term anticarcinogenicity experiments and epidemiological study it was confirmed that red ginseng and heat-processed ginseng, rather than fresh ginseng, showed enhanced anticarcinogenicity and a prominent reduction of relative risks of cancer. If one takes into account the kinds and content of saponin, red ginseng still has its characteristics. Active research is in progress to trace the active cancer-preventive components in ginseng, particularly in red ginseng for its minor ginsenosides Rh1, Rh2, Rg2, Rg3, and Rg5 using Yun's model (FIG. 2).

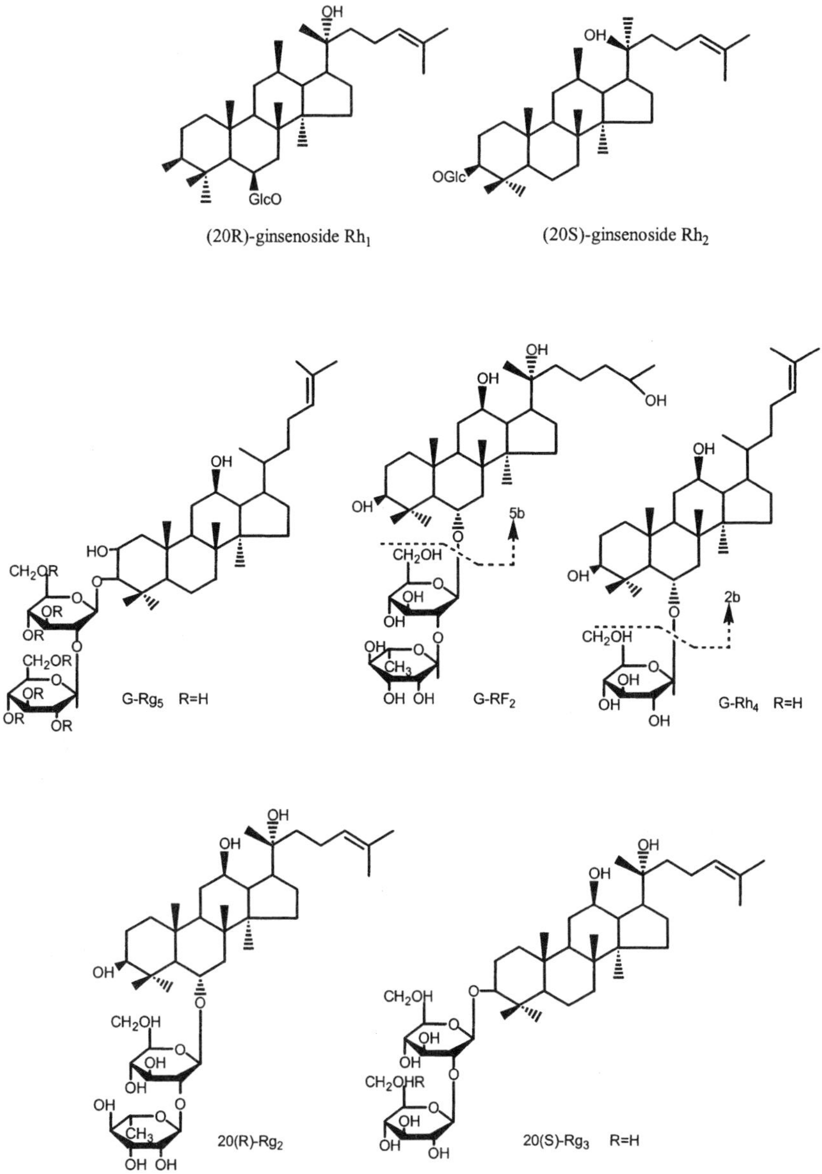

FIGURE 2. Minor ginsenosides in red ginseng.

Summary

Ginseng showed multiorgan anticarcinogenicity in rodent preclinical studies in Korea, Japan, China, and Russia. Epidemiological studies, including two case-control studies and a cohort study from Korea, revealed ginseng, especially red ginseng,

TABLE 9. Anticarcinogenicicty of various foods and synthetics, tested by Yun's 9-week mouse lung tumor model

Anticarcinogenictity	
Negative	Positive
Carrot[9]	Ascorbic acid[9]
β-Carotene[10]	Soybean lecithin[10]
Spinach[10]	Cultivated *G. lucidum* fruiting body[10]
13-*cis* retinoic acid[19]	Red ginseng extract (6 years)[10,47]
Sesamum indicum[10]	Caffeine[10]
French red wine[a]	Capsaicin[67]
Refined rice wine[a]	Biochanin A[93]
Authentic honey[a]	2-(Allylthio)pyrazine[a]

[a]Unpublished.

to have non-organ-specific cancer-preventive effects. One might hope and expect to have positive results from clinical trials in China and hope for worldwide cooporation in the development of wide-range clinical trials to confirm these preclinical and epidemiological studies.

KOREANS' VEGETARIAN FOODS AND THEIR CONSTITUENTS

Koreans are traditionally vegetarian. Therefore, using Yun's anticarcinogenicity test model, vegetarian foods and their constituents, that is, ascorbic acid, soybean lecithin, spinach, *Sesamum indicum*, capsaicin, biochanin A, the fruiting body and mycelia of *Ganoderma lucidum*, carrots, and caffeine, are tested, to assess the nine-week medium-term anticarcinogenicity test model newly established for ginseng. Among these, ascorbic acid, soybean lecithin, *Ganoderma lucidum*, caffeine, capsaicin, and biochanin A showed statistically significant decreased incidence of lung adenoma (TABLE 9). These results suggested that Yun's test model could be used to screen and detect cancer chemopreventive agents among vegetarian foods. Other than these tested foods, several important vegetarian foods and natural products are discussed below.[22–24]

CHLOROPHYLLIN

Preclinical Study

Early work by Lai *et al.*[36] and Kimm *et al.*[37,38] has shown that vegetable extracts containing chlorophylls are antimutagenic in bacterial-based assay systems. Chlorophyllin (CHL), an aqueous soluble chemical derived from chlorophyll, has been intensively studied as an inhibitor of various mutagens.[39] Anticarcinogenic activity of chlorophyllin has been demonstrated. In a study to assess the chemopreventive activity of CHL, mice were gavaged with CHL, or the vehicle alone, prior to the topical application of carcinogenic epoxides, such as benzo[a]pyrene-7,8-dihydrodiol-9,10-

epoxide (BPDE), vinyl carbamate epoxide (VCO), and 2'-(4-nitrophenoxy)oxirane (NPO). The induction of skin tumors in both groups after promotion with 12-O-tetradecanoylphorbol-13-acetate (TPA) was compared in terms of incidence and multiplicity of papillomas.[40] Although almost all mice that received BPDE alone developed skin tumors at 24 weeks after promotion, the incidence of papillomas in the CHL-pretreated group was 70 percent. CHL pretreatment also decreased the multiplicity of skin tumors by 42 percent. The results of this study lend further support to the possibility that CHL can act as an interceptor molecule capable of directly interacting with the active part of the ultimate electrophilic metabolites of the chemical carcinogens, thereby suppressing their genotoxic and oncogenic activities. On the other hand, CHL was tested for its chemopreventive activity against tumorigenesis induced by benzo[a]pyrene and its ultimate electrophilic and carcinogenic metabolite, BPDE.[31] Administration of CHL by gavage to mice prior to a topical application of BP or BPDE resulted in a significant reduction in both incidence and multiplicity of skin tumors initiated by these cacinogens. These results show that CHL is a potential chemopreventive agent.

Summary

Antimutagenicity and anticarcinogenicity of CHL has been observed. Inasmuch as epidemiological and clinical data are not yet available, clinical trials are needed to confirm the chemopreventive potential of chlorophyllin.

GANODERMA LUCIDUM

Ganoderma lucidum (Fr.) Karst, a popular edible mushroom with a reputation rivaling that of ginseng (*Panax ginseng*), has been widely used as a miraculous or auspicious herb for promotion of health and longevity in Korea, Japan, China, and other Asian countries. To date, over one hundred species of oxygenated triterpenes have been isolated from this fungus, many of which have been identified only in this species.[42] There a few reports on biological activities that consist of histamine release-inhibitory action,[43] immunomodulatory activity,[44] antitumor cytokines acting on inhibition of leukemic-cell growth,[45] and differentiation inducing activity,[46] but the chemopreventive activity of *Ganoderma lucidum* remains largely unexplored.

Preclinical Studies

Because the fruiting body of *Ganoderma lucidum* (GL) is reported to have an anticarcinogenic effect *in vivo*, using Yun's model,[9–11,47] we examined whether the mycelia of GL, which contain similar constituents, would have a similar efficacy. Benzo(a)pyrene was injected in the subscapular region of NIH(GP) newborn mice within 24 hours after birth at a dose of 0.5 mg per mouse. Mycelia of GL were extracted sequentially with water, alkali solvent, and ethanol. The total fraction, high-molecular fraction and low-molecular fraction, were respectively administered by drinking water at a dose of 2 or 10 mg/mL for six weeks after weaning. After nine weeks, lung tumors were fixed and counted. The total fraction of GL showed significant inhibition of lung adenoma incidence, and this activity seems to be concentrated in its high-molecular fraction. These results suggest that the mycelia of GL have the same anticarcinogenic effects as the fruiting body of GL in a nine-week medium-term pulmonary tumor model and that the active components might be concentrated it its high molecular fraction.[48]

Summary

Ganoderma lucidum might be a useful candidate for a chemopreventive agent, and further study is necessary for the identification of an active component for chemoprevention.

SOYBEAN PRODUCTS

Soybean seeds have been consumed by humans for thousands of years because they are rich in protein and their oil is of good nutritional quality. Most east Asians consume soybean seeds regularly from childhood via a variety of soybean products.

Preclinical Studies

The antimutagenic effects of Korean fermented soy paste, doenjang, were studied on various carcinogens by using the *Salmonella typhimurium* strains of the TA98 and TA100 Ames test. Doenjang exhibited strong mutagenic activity against aflatoxin B1 and *N*-methyl-*N'*-nitro-*N*-nitrosoguanidine (MNNG). Linoleic acid in doenjang seemed to be one of the active antimutagenic compounds.[49] The Japanese fermented soybean product, miso, also showed significant antimutagenesis,[50] and reduction of mammary cancer incidence and multiplicity was induced by *N*-nitroso-*N*-methylurea (MNU).[51] In an experiment with soybean milk protein that involved two-stage carcinogenesis on mouse skin, the number of tumors was significantly lowered.[50] Japanese-style fermented sauce (shoyu) showed anticarcinogeniticty on benzo(a)pyrene-induced mouse forestomach neoplasm.[51]

Soybean Constituents

Soybean lecithin showed anticarcinogenic effects in mice through the use of Yun's test model early in 1987.[9–12] There has been intensive research on the cancer chemoprevention effects of soybean constituents.[54] Soybean extracts were screened for anticarcinogenic substances by testing their ability to induce quinone reductase [NAD(P)H: (quinone acceptor) oxidoreductase, EC 1.6.99.2], one of the phase II detoxication enzymes, in murine hepatoma cells. Genistein strongly induced quinone reductase whereas daidzein did not.[55] Genistein also inhibited both constitutive and EGF-stimulated invasion in ER-negative human breast carcinoma cell lines.[56] Soybean saponins had a dose-dependent growth inhibtory effect on human carcinoma cells (HCT-15).[57] Soy daidzein exhibited a stimulatory effect on nonspecific immunity, by increasing the phagocytic response of peritoneal macrophages and thymus weight, in a dose-dependent manner. Augmentation of spleen immunoglobulin M-producing cells against sheep red blood cells demonstrated activation of humoral immunity.[58]

Epidemiological Studies

The incidence of breast and colon cancer in Asian people is considerably lower than in those living in Western countries,[59] where soybean products are seldom eaten. Furthermore, a large-scale census-based cohort study in Japan by Hirayama showed significant lower sex- and age-standardized mortality rates in daily consumers than nondaily consumers of soybean paste soup (miso) for stomach cancer.[60,61] Recently in a Hawaiian study it was shown that those who ate tofu or other soybean products had a reduced incidence of uterine corpus carcinoma.[62] These associations suggest that soybeans may play a role in reducing the risk for breast, colon, stomach, and uterine body cancer.

Summary

Although there are few epidemiological studies and no clinical data yet, there is experimental and epidemioligical evidence that the following soybean-derived products suppress carcinogenesis *in vivo*: soybeans; miso or doenjang (Korean soybean paste); isoflavones, including genistein; the primary protease inhibitors (Kunitz trypsin inhibitor,[54] Bowman-Birk inhibitor; BBI, and chymotrypsin inhibitor);[63] inositol hexaphosphate(phytic acid, IP_6);[64] β-sitosterol;[65] and saponins.[57] It is believed that supplementation of human diets with certain soybean products could suppress carcinogenesis and markedly reduce human cancer mortality rates. Dietitians need to become more aware of the phytochemical content of vegetarian foods and the effects of phytochemicals on health and disease.

CAPSAICIN

Capsaicin (*N*-vanillyl-8-methyl-6-nonenamide) (FIG. 3) is a homovanillic acid derivative and the principal pungent and irritating constituent of capsicum fruits (*Capsicun annum* L., Solanaceae). The Korean people are large consumers of capsicum fruit. It has been heavily used as a food additive for approximately 400 years, and the average daily per capita consumption of capsaicin may reach 50 milligrams.[66] The content of capsaicin in capsicum is about 0.02% in fresh fruit and 0.5–1.0% in dried ripe fruit.

Preclinical Studies

To test the modifying effect of capsaicin on benzo(a)pyrene-induced tumors, we used Yun's nine-week medium-term anticarcinogenicity test model, using a benzo(a)pyrene. This test was previously applied on ginseng effects and appears to be

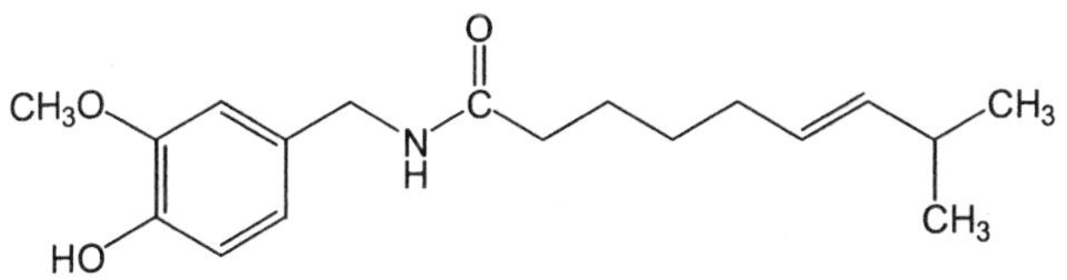

FIGURE 3. Capsaicin (trans-8-methyl-*N*-vanilly-6-nonenamide).

an appropriate experimental model for capsaicin. In this experiment, capsaicin caused a significant inhibitory effect on the frequency of pulmonary adenoma-bearing mice.[67] On the contrary, it has been suspected that spicy foods play some role in human carcinogenesis. Ingestion of large amounts of capsaicin has been reported to cause histopathological and biochemical changes, including erosion of gastric mucosa and hepatic necrosis.[68] There are conflicting data, however, on the modulating effect of capsaicin; in some studies significant tumor-initiating or -promoting effects were observed,[69–73] whereas in others this finding was not confirmed.[74–76] Some studies demonstrated the marked mutagenic activity of the compound in the presence or absence of an external metabolic activation system,[71,77–81] whereas others failed to provide evidence for its genotoxic potential.[82–86] Recent clinical trials revealed that topical cream containing 0.025% capsaicin significantly ameliorated the pain in patients with arthritis.[87] Considering the popular consumption of capsaicin as a food additive and its current therapeutic application, correct assessment of any harmful effects of this compound is important from the public health standpoint.

However, capsaicin competitively inhibited ethylmorphine-N-demethylase activity *in vitro* in rat hepatic microsomes.[88] Capsaicin appears to possess inhibitory activity for cytochrome P-450, a characteristic of other naturally occurring compounds of particular interest for their potential ability to augment the body's defense mechanism against selected environmental carcinogens and mutagens. Furthermore, it is known that capsaicin suppresses vinyl carbamate- and N-nitrosodimethylamine-induced mutagenesis or tumorigenesis, in part, through inhibition of the cytochrome P-450 IIE1 isoform responsible for activation of these carcinogens.[89] A single topical application of capsaicin (10 μmol), followed by twice-weekly applications of TPA onto shaven backs of mice, resulted in no significant increases in incidence and multiplicity of skin tumors compared with the solvent-pretreated control animals.[90]

Epidemiological Studies

Only a single positive correlation between chili pepper consumption and gastric cancer has appeared in the literature. According to a case-control study conducted in Mexico, chili pepper consumers were at about sixfold greater risk for gastric cancer than nonconsumers.[91] By contrast, an Italian case-control study revealed that chili consumption was protective against stomach cancer.[92] It should be noted that the etiology of human gastric cancer is complicated by such multifactorial risk factors as salty, smoked, or pickled foods, cigarette smoking, insufficient daily intake of fruits and vegetables, and *Helicobacter pylori* infection.[82]

Summary

In view of its pronounced antimutagenic and anticarcinogenic activities, capsaicin may represent another important dietary phytochemical with potential chemopreventive activity. However, this compound causes adverse effects in experimental animals, especially at high doses. It is no coincidence that cancer mortality rates in Korean are only 110 per 100,000 persons (Annual Reports from Bureau of Statistics for the past 10 years), which is about half the rate of other countries, taking into account the above-mentioned adverse results. Considering the frequent consumption of capsaicin as a food additive, correct assessment of any harmful effects of capsaicin is important from the public health standpoint.

BIOCHANIN A

Biochanin A, an isoflavone existing in red clover, cabbage, and alfalfa, has an inhibitory effect of benzo(a)pyrene metabolism.

Preclinical Studies

In Yun's nine-week medium-term anticarcinogenicity test model, biochanin A administration significantly reduced the incidence of pulmonary tumors in benzo(a)pyrene-treated mice and the mean number of tumors compared to the benzo(a)pyrene control group.[93] Biochanin A has an inhibitory effect of benzo(a)pyrene metabolism.[94] A 95% ethyl alcohol extract of the red clover *Trifolium pratense* L. Leguminosae significantly inhibited benzo(a)pyrene metabolism and decreased its DNA binding by 30 to 40 percent.[95] In an 18-week study, a biochanin A–supplemented diet significantly reduced the incidence of *N*-nitroso-*N*-nitroso-*N*-methylurea-induced mammary tumors in rats.[96]

Summary

There is no controversial data on anticarcinogenicity of biochanin A. Because the Korean and vegetarian intake of isoflavonoid or flavonoid is potentially very high through daily consumption of dishes like "Kimchi" made of Chinese cabbage and chili peppers, biochanin A is very relevant to public health and should be further studied in preclinical and clinical trials.

A NOVEL SYNTHETIC SULFIDE COMPOUND: 2-(ALLYLTHIO)PYRAZINE

2-(Allylthio)pyrazine (2AP) (FIG. 4), a pyrazine derivative with an allylsulfur moiety, was recently synthesized as a cancer chemopreventive in Korea.[97] 2-AP was effective in inhibiting cytochrome P450 2E1,[98] enhancing cellular glutathione (GSH), preventing the hepatic toxicity caused by acetaminophen or carbon tetrachloride in animals, and significantly reducing the mortality rate induced by toxicants.[99] 2-AP also enhanced the activities of glutathione S-transferase (GST) and the expression of microsomal epoxide hydrolase (mEH) involved in the detoxification of carcinogens.[97] Multiplicities of skin tumors in female ICR mice treated with vinyl carbamate or vinyl

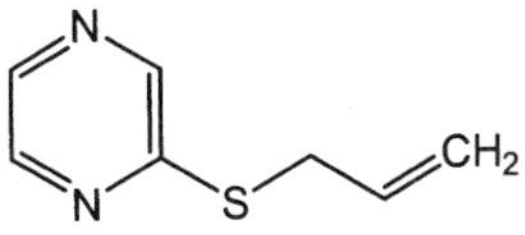

FIGURE 4. 2-(Allylthio)pyrazine(2-AP).

carbamate oxide were inhibited by pretreatment with 2-AP.[100] 2-AP also exhibited protective effects against AFB_1-induced hepatocarcinogenesis in rats with a marked decrease in the level of AFB_1-DNA adduct.[101]

Summary

A novel synthetic pyrazine derivative of 2-(allylthio)pyrazine showed chemopreventive effect in skin and liver tumors in rodents, and the chemopreventitve effects of 2-AP might result from inactivation of the carcinogen through induction of phase II detoxification enzymes that would facilitate the clearance of activated metabolites through conjugation reaction. Further studies on metabolic, systematic toxicological and mechanistic aspects, including clinical trials on 2-AP, would facilitate development of this agent as a clinically useful cancer chemopreventive.

CHEMOPREVENTIVE AGENTS DEVELOPED IN JAPAN

Japanese research groups first established short-term screening tests on the inhibitions of various biochemical and biological activities induced by tumor promoters for the purpose of finding cancer chemopreventive agents.[102] Japanese scientists developed the cancer chemopreventive agents acyclic retinoid (E5166), sarcophytol A, canventol, and tea polyphenols.

ACYCLIC RETINOID, SARCOPHYTOL A, AND CANVENTOL

Preclinical Study

Muto et al. identified acyclic retinoid (a new synthetic derivative of the polyprenoic acid: 3,7,11,15-tetramethyl-2,4,6,10,14-hexadecapentaenoic acid or E5166) (FIG. 5), which competitively inhibited specific binding of all-*trans*-retinoic acid [11,12-^{3}H] to cellular retinoic acid-binding protein (CRABP) as well as CRBP(F).[103] Anticarcinogenicity were observed in rat hepatoma induced by 3'-methyl-*N*-,*N*-dimethly-4-aminoazobenzene and a spontaneous hepatoma in mice.[104] Cryptoporic acids A–G are drimane-type sesquiterpenoid ethers of isocitric acid isolated from the fungus *Cryptoporus volvatus*.[105] Treatment with cryptoporic acids D and E (FIG. 6) showed anticarcinogenic effects in a two-stage carcinogenesis experiment, MNU and 1,2-dimethylhydrazine induced tumors in rats and mice.[106,107] Sarcophytol A treatment inhibited tumors on mouse skin.[108] Further studies showed that sarcophytol A in the diet was effective in inhibiting development of chemical

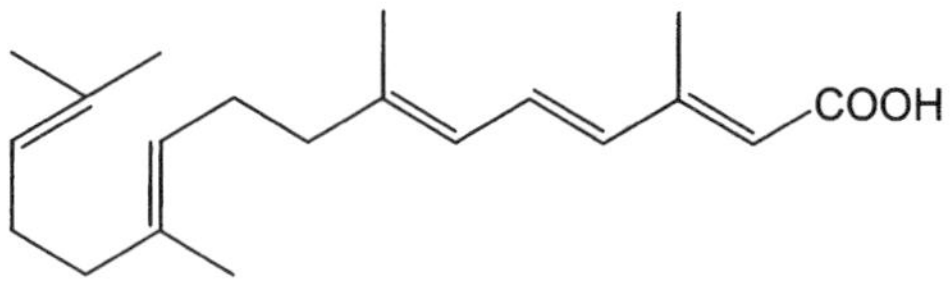

FIGURE 5. Polyprenoic acid, acyclic retinoid, E5166.

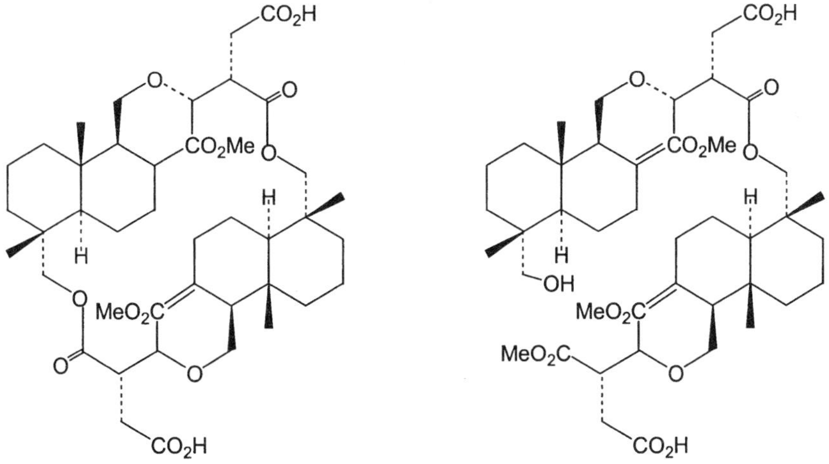

Cryptoporic acid D

Cryptoporic acid E

FIGURE 6. Cryptoporic acid D and E.

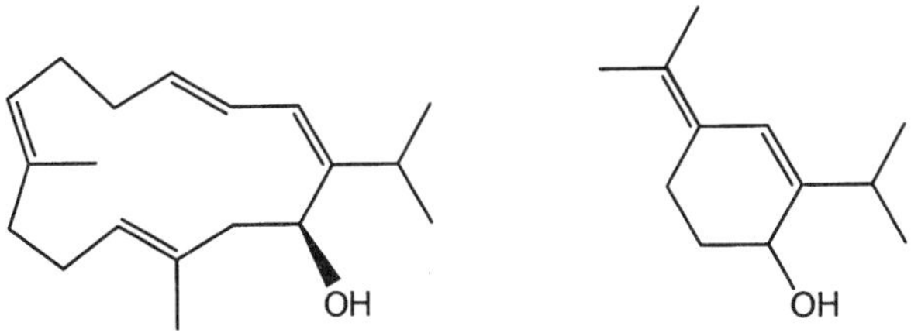

Sarcophytol A

Canventol

FIGURE 7. Sarcophytol A and canventol.

carcinogenesis in various organs, such as colon[109] and pancreas.[110] The new compound, canventol, inhibited tumor promotion of okadaic acid on mouse skin.[111] Sarcophytol A and canventol (FIG. 7) inhibited TNF-α release from Balb/3T3 cells treated with okadaic acid.

Clinical Study

Acyclic retinoid was the first compound designed as a preventive agent for liver cancer in Japan. The randomized placebo-controlled double-blind trial (phase II) enrolled a total of 89 postoperative patients who did not have residual hepatoma at entry. Acyclic retinoid was given orally for 48 weeks. The group treated with acyclic retinoid had a 15% recurrence rate of hepatoma, and the placebo group had a 39% recurrence rate.[112] Based on these results provided by the Japanese scientists, cryptoporic acid E has now been forwarded to the Chemoprevention Program for Preclinical Chemopreventive Agents, supported by the Chemoprevention Branch, NCI.[113] In this experiment, sarcophytol A inhibited TNF-α release about 10 times more effectively than caventol, although caventol is a more potent inhibitor of tumor promotion on mouse skin. Sarcophytol A appears to be an inhibitor of TNF-α release, whereas canventol is bifunctional, inhibiting both TNF-α release and protein isoprenylation. Consequently, canventol potently inhibited tumor promotion. At present, the Chemoprevention Branch is testing the potential of canventol as a preclinical chemopreventive agent.

Clinical Studies Ongoing

Besides the previously described chemopreventive agents being studied in Japan, at least two interventional trials are in progress. One is the Interventional Trial for Colorectal Cancer Prevention in Osaka research group, which established a protocol for an interventional randomized controlled trial (RCT) for prevention of colorectal cancer by attaching special importance to feasibility. The subjects were patients with multiple colorectal tumors. Two regimens were formulated for prevention of colorectal cancer. One was dietary guidance alone (regimen I), and the other was dietary guidance plus eating wheat bran biscuits (regimen II). The main end points of the trial were examinations for occurrence of new colorectal tumors after two and four years. The total number of patients was 200, that is,100 for each group.[114] During the effective 35 months from initial subject recruitment, 63 (94%) of the 67 patients recuited for regimen 1, and 64 (90%) of the 71 patients recruited for regimen II agreed to participate in the trial by 1996.

Summary

Acyclic retinoid, sarcophytol A, and canventol that are developed in Japan show consistent effect. It is hoped that these could turn out to be potent cancer chemopreventive agents through phase II and III clinical studies. It is also hoped that the clinical trial of the fiber biscuit of colon cancer and the red ginseng trial of liver diseases show good results.

TEA POLYPHENOLS

Tea is one of the most popular beverages consumed worldwide. The inhibitory action of tea (*Camellia sinensis*) and tea components has been demonstrated in several animal models in many laboratories.[113,115,116] The relationship between tea consumption and human cancer incidence is an important health concern.

Preclinical Study

In 1987, Fujiki's group first reported that (−)-epigallocatechin gallate (EGCG) (FIG. 8) treatment inhibited tumor promotion of teleocidin on mouse skin. The preparation of EGCG used in this experiment contained 85% EGCG, 10% (−)-epicatechin, and 5% (−)-epicatechin gallate. Initiation was achieved by a single application of 50 μg DMBA, and tumor promotion was conducted by repeated application of

TABLE 10. Anticarcinogenic effects of EGCG[a] and green tea extract in various organs

Organs	Species	Carcinogens/Tumor	Reduction In Tumor Incidence (%)	Reduction In Average Number of Tumors per Animal	Reported Year
Skin	Mouse CD-1	DMBA[b]/teleocidin	53.0 → 13.0	2.1 → 0.1	1987
		DMBA/okadaic acid	73.3 → 0	4.2 → 0	1991
Glandular stomach	Wistar Rat	MNNG[c]	62.0 → 31.0	0.88 → 0.43	1995
Duodenum	C57BL/6 Mouse	ENNG[d]	63.0 → 20.0	1.2 → 0.3	1989
			63.0 → 20.0	0.8 → 0.3	1989
Colon	Rat	AOM[e]	77.3 → 38.1	1.2 → 0.3	1991
	Rat	MNU[f]	67.0 → 33.0	1.2 → 0.5[a]	1993
Liver	C3H/HeN Mouse	Spontaneous	83.3 → 52.2	1.8 → 0.9	1993
Pancreas	Hamster	BOP[g]	54.0 → 33.0	1.0 → 0.5[A]	1990

[a]EGCG: (−)-Epigallocatechin gallate. [b]DMBA, 7,12-Dimethylbenz(a)anthraxcene. [c]MNNG, N-Methyl-N′-nitro-nitrosoguanidine. [d]ENNG, Ethyl-nitro-N-nitrosoguanidine. [e]AOM, Azoxymethane. [f]MNU, Methylnitrosourea. [g]BOP: Nitrosobis-(2-oxopropyl)amine.

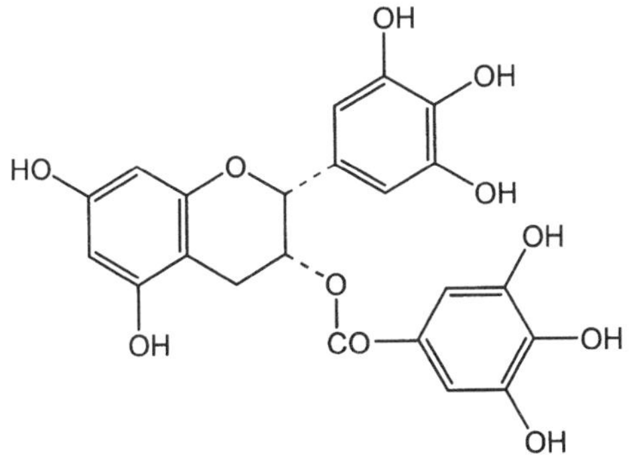

FIGURE 8. (−)-Epigallocatechin gallate.

2.5 μg teleocidin twice a week. EGCG treatment reduced the percentage of tumor-bearing mice from 53% to 13% and the average number of tumors per mouse from 2.1 to 0.1, in week 25.[117] Since then, many laboratories have provided evidence that EGCG and green tea extract in drinking water inhibited carcinogenesis in rat glandular stomach, mouse duodenum, rat colon, hamster pancreas, mouse liver, and mouse lung (TABLE 10).[118–121] Consequently, EGCG and green tea extract are widely believed to be promising agents for cancer preventive activity.

This inhibitory activity is believed to be mainly due to the antioxidative and possible antiproliferative effects of polyphenolic compounds in green and black tea. These polyphenolics may also inhibit carcinogenesis by blocking the endogenous

TABLE 11. Epidemiology studies relationship between tea drinking and human cancer[a]

Organ	Association of Tea Drinking to Cancer	Number of Types of Studies	Reported Years
Bladder and urinary tract	No relationship	I ecological study	1986
		2 cohort studies	1986, 1988
		16 case-control studies	1974, 1975, 1978, 1980, 1983, 1985, 1986×2, 1987, 1988×2, 1989, 1991, 1992×3
Breast	Positive	1 ecological study	1970
	No relationship	5 case-control studies	1985×3, 1986, 1987
	Negative	1 ecological study	1992
Colon and rectum	Positive	1 ecological study	1970
		1 cohort study	1986
		1 case-control study	1992
	No relationship	1 cohort study	
		5 case-control studies	1966, 1979, 1983,1985×2
	Negative	3 case-control studies	1984, 1990, 1991
Esophagus	Positive (with high temperature tea)	3 ecological studies	1975,1977, 1986
		5 case-control studies	1965, 1968, 1974, 1979, 1991
	No relationship (with normal temperature tea)	1 ecological study	1970
		4 case-control studies	1965, 1968, 1974, 1979
		2 case-control studies	1987, 1992
Kidney	Positive	1 cohort study	1988
		1 case-control study	1984
	No relationship	1 ecological study	1970
		5 case-control studies	1976, 1986×2,1988, 1992
Liver	No relationship	1 ecological study	1970
		1 cohort study	1986
		1 case-control study	1992
	Negative	1ecological study	1992
Lung	Positive	1 ecological study	1970
		1 cohort study	1988
		1 case-control study	1990
	Negative	1 ecological study	1992
Nasopharynx	No relationship	3 case-control studies	1974, 1976, 1978
Pancreas	Positive	1 case-control study	1984
	No relationship	3 cohort studies	1986, 1988×2
		7 case-control studies	1981, 1985, 1986, 1987, 1990, 1991, 1992
	Negative	1 cohort study	1983
		1 case-control study	1990
Stomach	Positive	1 cohort study	1988
		1 case-control study	1990
	No relationship	7 case-control studies	1966, 1967×2, 1985×2, 1990, 1992
	Negative	2 ecological studies	1970, 1992
		2 case-control studies	1988, 1991
Uterus	Negative	2 ecological studies	1970, 1992

[a]Data from Yang, C.S. & Z.Y. Wang. 1996. J. Natl. Cancer Inst. **85**: 138–149.

TABLE 12. Relative risk of cancer incidence by green tea consumption[a,124]

	Consumption of Green Tea (cups/day)		
	≤ 3	4–9	≥ 10
Males	1.0	1.03 (0.65–1.63)[b]	0.68 (0.39–1.21)
Smokers	1.0	1.11 (0.39–3.10)	0.76 (0.27–2.19)
Nonsmokers	1.0	1.20 (0.68–2.09)	0.53 (0.23–1.23)
Females	1.0	0.184 (0.59–1.22)	0.57 (0.33–0.98)

[a]Adjusted for cigarette smoking, alcohol consumption, and intake of green/yellow vegetables, rice, fish, fruit, soybean products, and dairy products using age as the fundamental time.
[b]Number in parentheses, 95% CI.

formation of N-nitroso compounds, suppressing the activation of carcinogens, and trapping genotoxic agents.[122]

Epidemiological Studies

Many laboratories as well as epidemiological studies, defining an association between tea consumption and cancer risk and prevention, have been reported. A general overview of the pertinent epidemiologic studies on tea consumption and cancer prevention of different sites is also provided. Both positive and inverse associations of teas have been reported for cancers, including those of esophagus, oropharynx, lung, stomach, pancreas, colon, rectum, uterine corpus, breast, kidney, and bladder.[112,113] The above-mentioned epidemiological studies show inconsistent results. There are two recently published results from Japan and the United States (TABLE 11).

The association between nonherbal tea consumption and cancer incidence in a prospective cohort study of 35,369 postmenopausal Iowa women was reported in 1996. After controlling for confounding factors, the authors found that regular tea consumption was related to a slightly, but not satisfactorily significant, reduced incidence of all cancers combined. Inverse association with increasing frequency of tea drinking was seen for cancers of the digestive tract and urinary tract. No appreciable association of tea drinking was found with melanoma, non-Hodgkin's lymphoma, or cancers of the pancreas, lung, breast, uterine corpus, or ovary. This study concluded that tea may protect against some cancers in postmenopausal women.[123] A negative association between green tea consumption and cancer incidence was observed in Japan, especially among females drinking more than 10 cups a day. Relative risk of cancer incidence was lower among females and males in groups with the highest consumption, although the preventive effects did not achieve statistical significance among males, even when stratified by smoking and adjusted for alcohol and dietary variables (TABLE 12).[124]

Clinical Studies

Chemopreventive effects of green tea and coffee among cigarette smokers were examined in clincally healthy male subjects. The frequencies of sister-chromatid exchange (SCE) in mitogen-stimulated peripheral lymphocytes from each experimental group showed SCE rates were significantly elevated in smokers when compared with nonsmokers.[125] A study aimed to examined an effect of tea polyphenol on serum pepsinogen level among patients in Japan. This interim analysis suggested that additional polyphenol intake among Japanese does not improve the stomach atrophy, which is considered as a high-risk condition of stomach cancer. It was concluded that even if polyphenol is a protective agent, it may work against other processes or stages of stomach carcinogenesis.[126]

Summary

Many laboratory studies have demonstrated *in vitro* and *in vivo* inhibitory effects of tea preparations and tea polyphenols against tumor formation and growth. In contrast to preclinical experimental studies, epidemiologic studies on the relationship between tea consumption and cancer risk have been inconsistent. Such inconsistent associations may be explained partially by differences in tea-drinking habits and types of tea consumed in various study populations or by failure to control for potential. There are no clinical trials for tea polyphenol or catechin in Asian countries yet. Inasmuch as research findings in laboratory animals clearly point to a role of tea components in cancer chemoprevention, the well-defined naturally occurring components found in tea should be evaluated in human clinical trials on cancers of specific organ site or population.

TRITERPENOIDS

Increasing numbers of new triterpenoids are being isolated and their structures established with the advent of powerful analytical methods.[127] There have been widespread reports in recent years on their antitumor-promoting effect and chemopreventive effects against neoplasms.

Preclinical Study

Several oleanane-type triterpenoids, which are chemically derived from oleanolic acid and hederagenin, were tested *in vitro* and *in vivo* against the tumor promotor 12-*0*-tetradecanoylphorbol-13-acetate (TPA). The *in vitro* experiment was monitored by TPA-induced stimultation of ^{32}P incorporation into phospholipids. The *in vivo* test on skin tumor formation in mice was initiated with 7,12-dimethyl-benz(a)anthracene (DMBA) and promoted with TPA. 18β-olean-12-ene-3β,28-diol (erythrodiol), 18β-olean-12-ene-3β,23,28-triol, 18α-olean-12-ene-3β-28-diol, and 18α-olean-12-ene-3β-23,28-triol showed remarkable suppressive effects. In particular, 18α-oleanane derivatives having a –CH$_2$OH group at C-17 were found to be 100-fold more effective than glycyrrhetic acid, a commonly used suppressor both *in vitro* and *in vivo*.[128] Olean-11,13(18)-diene-3β,30-diol and its derivatives were found to inhibit tumor-promoting agents such as TPA. These compounds have greater inhibiting activities on tumors than glycyrrhetinic acid and have fewer side effects. Thus, the increases in phospholipid synthesis in various tumors induced by TPA were inhibited *in vitro* by the title compound and five of its analogues.[129] Oral administration of 18β-olean-12-ene-3β,23,28-triol tri-*0*-hemiphthalate sodium and olean 11,13(18)-dien-3β-ol-30-oic acid 3-*0*-β-D-glucuronopyranosyl-(12)-β-D-glucuronopyranoside sodium(II) suppressed carcinogenesis in mouse skin induced by DMBA and TPA. This is the first report of effective oral administration of triterpenoid compounds suppressing skin tumor pro-motion in mice.[130] Carcinogenesis inhibitors containing Me-3α-methoxy-23-oxo-9β-lanost-7-en-27-oate, 25,26,27-trisnor-23R-hydroxy-3α-methoxy-9β-lanost-7-en-24-oic acid, 3,23-dioxo-9β-lanost-7-en-27-oic acid, olean-12-ene-3β,15α-diol, and/or (3S,7S)-dihydroxy-7(8→9)abeo-9S-D:C-Friedo-B:A-neogammacer an-8-one as ac-tive ingredients have been reported.[121] Betulinic acid (5 μmol) markedly inhibited the tumor-promoting effect of 2.50 μg TPA initiated with 50 μg 7,12-dimethylbenz(a)an-thracene.[132] The cyclozartanoid triterpene 3-oxo-24-cycloartin-21-oic acid, isolated from leaves of *Lansium domesticum* (Meliaceae) and some of its derivatives, showed significant inhibitory activity of skin-tumor promotion on the basis of Epstein-Barr vi-rus associated early antigen (EBV-EA) examination.[133] Abiesenoic acid methyl ester, a triterpenoid compound prepared from abieslactone, suppressed tumor promotor–in-duced phenomena *in vitro* and *in vivo*. The methyl ester inhibited TPA-stimulated ^{32}Pi incorporation into phospholipids of cultured cells and the promoting action of TPA on skin tumor formation in mice initiated with 7,12-dimethylbenz(a)anthracene.[134]

Among 23 triterpenoid hydrocarbons isolated from ferns, 8 triterpenoids, hop-17(21)-ene, neohop-13(18)-ene, neohop-12-ene, taraxerane, multiflor-9(11)-ene, multiflor-8-ene, glutin-5(10)-ene, and taraxastane exhibited remarkable inhibitory effects on EBV activation induced by the tumor promotor, TPA. Further, hop-17(21)-ene and neohop-13(18)-ene exhibited remarkable antitumor-promoting effects on mouse skin tumor promotion in an *in vivo* two-stage carcinogenesis test using DMBA as an initiator and TPA as a promotor.[135]

Summary

Many triterpenoids have been isolated and several oleanane-type triterpenoids an triterpenoid hydrocarbons have shown remarkable antitumor-promoting effects. These compounds have potential as cancer chemopreventive agents, and further sys-tematic studies are warrented for developing their potential.

CHEMOPREVENTION RESEARCH IN CHINA

In the late 1970s a comprehensive chemoprevention program was established at the Institute of Materia Medica, Chinese Academy of Medical Sciences. Since then, more than 200 retinoid compounds have been synthesized and screened in the search for chemopreventive agents of cancer.[136]

Preclinical Studies

N-4-(carboxyphenyl) retinamide showed a significant inhibitory effect on car-cinogenesis of cancers in the buccal pouch of hamsters induced by DMBA and in the forestomach of mice induced by nitrosarcosine ethyl ester.[137] Recently allicin iso-lated from garlic and elemene from the Chinese medicinal herb, *Rhizoma zedoatiae,* were reported. The inhibitory effect of elemene on proliferation of HL-60 cells was associated with cell-cycle arrest from the S to the G_2M phase transition and with in-duction of apoptosis. The inibitory effect of allicin on proliferation of tumor cells was associated with the cell-cycle blockage of the S/G_2M boundary phase and induction of apoptosis.[138]

Clinical Studies

Clinical studies have demonstrated that *N*-4-(carboxyphenyl) retinamide is effective against oral leukoplakia, vulvar leukoplakia, and dysplasia of the uterine cervix and stomach. Field studies among a population at high risk for esophageal cancer in Linxian County, Henan Province, revealed that *N*-4-(ethoxycarbophenyl) retinamide decreased the incidence of esophageal cancer.[136]

Summary

In China, we can see that chemoprevention studies have been extensively used for both synthetic retinoids and natural products.

NCI–CHINA JOINT RESEARCH

In a high-risk population in Linxian, China, two trials conducted by the Cancer Institute of the Chinese Academy of Medical Sciences and the NCI investigated the effect of a daily multiple vitamin and mineral supplement on incidence and mortality rates for esophageal/gastric cardia cancers and on the prevalence of histological dysplasia. The general population trial included more than 30,000 individuals who received one of four combinations of vitamins/minerals daily for approximately five years. Results showed a 9% reduction in deaths from all causes and a 13% reduction in cancer mortality for persons receiving a β-carotene/vitamin E/selenium combination, largely because of a 21% decrease in stomach cancer mortality.[139]

The dysplasia trial included 3,318 individuals with evidence of severe esophageal dysplasia who received either a placebo or a daily supplement containing 14 vitamins and 12 minerals for six years. In the dysplasia trial, subjects receiving supplements showed reductions in mortality due to all causes (8%), esophageal cancer (16%), and stomach cancer (18%) compared with the placebo group. Endoscopic surveys, conducted after 30 and 72 months of intervention, found reduction in risk of 16% and 14%, respectively, for esophageal or gastric cancer or dysplasia (combined).[140] Persons receiving supplements were 1.2 times as likely to have no dysplasia after 30 and 72 months of intervention, compared with persons receiving a placebo. The third joint trial started in 1995. It consisted of treating *Helicobacter pylori* in 3411 people with gastric dysplasia or precancereous gastric lesions from Linque County in China by applying amoxicillin and omeprazole or by giving capsules containing vitamins C and E, and selenium. The last group was given steam-distilled garlic oil and Kyolic aged garlic extract. The chemoprevention between these groups will be compared in 1999 by means of gastroscopy and biopsy.[141] The fourth trial, which began in 1995, studying 234 people in China's Quidong County, were divided into those who were given oltipraz and placebo; this was a phase IIa clinical trial, which measures the level of aflatoxin-albumin adducts in sera. Because there were no differences between the oltipraz and placebo groups, the study was extended to a phase IIb clinical trial.[142–145]

Summary

The results of clincal trials in the general population and dysplasia patients should stimulate further research to clarify the potential benefits of micronutrient supplements. On the other hand, clinical trials on oltipraz are expected to be extended for phase IIb trials.

CONCLUSIONS

Cancer chemopreventive studies in Korea, Japan, and China were reviewed in which traditional Asian herbs or such beverages as ginseng and green tea have been studied experimentally and epidemiologically. Ginseng seems to have non-organ-specific cancer preventive properties epidemiologically, and green tea seems to have multiorgan preventive effects. Further clinical studies on ginseng and green tea are warranted to determine their efficacy in cancers of specific organs and tissues. Vegetarian foods common to every dining table in Korea were also studied experimentally for potential anticarcinogenic or chemopreventive effects. In Japan, besides tea polyphenol, three kinds of cancer chemopreventives were developed. *Ganoderma lucidum* and vegetarian foods (soy products, capsaicin, biochanin A, and chlorophyllin) should be studied further to confirm their anticarcinogenicity and chemopreventive properties by double-blind placebo-controlled clinical trials. The results of joint study in the general population and of dysplasia in China should stimulate further research to clarify the potential benefits of micronutrient supplements. The lower rates of mortality in Korea should be clarified as to whether they are related to frequent consumption of anticarcinogenic vegetables or traditional foods, including ginseng and *Ganoderma lucidum.* The constituents of the nontoxic stable dietary products promise to be the future hope in conquering cancers in the coming century.

ACKNOWLEDGMENTS

I would like to thank the following people for their inspiration and guidance in my early anticancer research: the late Professor Il Sun Yun, former President of Seoul National University (SNU), Emeritus Professor, Department of Pathology, SNU College of Medicine; the late Professor Sung Soo Lee, Professor, Department of Pathology, SNU College of Medicine; the late Dr. Harold L. Stewart, former Chief of the Laboratory of Pathology, National Cancer Institute (NCI), NIH, Bethesda, MD, USA; Professor E. Hyuk Kwon, former President of the Korean Academy of Sciences, Emeritus Professor, Department of Preventive Medicine, SNU; and Professor Ki Yung Lee, Emeritus Professor, Department of Biochemistry, SNU College of Medicine, Seoul, Korea.

I also express my gratitude for valuable advice and fruitful contributions from Professor Je. G. Chi, President of the Korean Academy of Medical Science, Department of Pathology, Seoul National University (SNU) College of Medicine, Seoul; Professor Il Soon Kim, Department of Preventive Medicine, Yonsei Yonsei University Medical College, Seoul; Professor Joung Soon Kim, Department of Epidemiology, School of Public Health, SNU; Professor Young Kyoon Kim, President, Korean

Prostate Health Council, Inc., Professor Emeritus, SNU; Professor Martin Lipkin, Director of Clinical Research, Professor of Medicine, Cornell Medical Center, Strang Cancer Research Laboratory, The Rockefeller University, New York, USA; Dr. Waun Ki Hong, Dr. Jin Soo Lee, Head, Neck and Thoracic Medical Oncology, the University of Texas, M.D. Anderson Cancer Center, Houston, USA; Professor Woo Hyun Chang, Dean of Hallym University Medical School, Chunchon, Korea; Professor Yoon Ok Ahn, Department of Preventive Medicine, SNU College of Medicine; Professor Chong Kook Kim, Laboratory of Physical Pharmacy, College of Pharmacy, SNU; Professor Woon K. Baek, Department of Biochemistry, Ajou University College of Medicine; Professor Jung Koo Youn, Department of Microbiology, Ajou University College of Medicine, Suwon, Korea; Dr. Takahashi Sugimura, former President, National Cancer Center, Tokyo, Japan; Professor Kunio Aoki, former Dean, Nagoya Univeristy, Nagoya, Japan; Professor Osamu Tanaka, former President of Suzugamine Women's College, Hiroshima-ken, Japan; Professor Shoji Shibata, Emeritus Professor, University of Tokyo; Dr. Toru Otani, Dr. Hideki Ishikawa, the Center for Adult Diseases, Osaka, Japan; Dr. Johng S. Rhim, Associate Director, Center for Prostate Disease Research, Uniformed Services University of Health Sciences, Rockville, MD, USA; Dr. Gen-Sun Qian, Department of Chemical Carcinogenesis, Shanghai Cancer Institute, China; Professor Thomas W. Kensler, Department of Environmental Health Sciences, Johns Hopkins School of Hygiene and Public Health, Baltimore, MD, USA; Professor Shu Zheng, President of the Cancer Institute, Dr. Xi Yong Liu, the Cancer Institute, Zhejiang Medical University, Hangzhou, China; Dr. Soo Yong Choi, Dr. Yun Sil Lee, and Dr. Yeon Sook Yun, Korea Cancer Center Hospital, Seoul, Korea.

REFERENCES

1. WANG, W.J. & C.Q. LU. 1992. Nutrition in Traditional Chinese Medicine [in Chinese]. Shanghai Science and Technology Publishing House. Shanghai, China. p. 14.
2. GOODMAN, L.S., M.M. WINTROBE, W. DAMESHEK, M.J. GOODMAN, A. GILMAN & M.T. McLENNAN. 1946. Nitrogen mustard therapy. J. Am. Med. Assoc. **132:** 126–132.
3. MUIR, C.S. & J. NECTOUX. 1996. International patterns of cancer. *In* Cancer Epidemiology and Prevention, 2nd ed. D. Schottenfwld & J. F. Fraumeni, Eds.: 141–167. Oxford University Press. Oxford.
4. BEARDSLEY, T. 1994. Trends in cancer epidemiology: A war not won. Sci. Am. January 130–138.
5. AMERICAN CANCER SOCIETY. 1996. Cancer Facts & Figures-1996. American Cancer Society Inc. Atlanta, GA, USA.
6. JING, T.H. & S.B.A. JING. 1982. Simplified Version of Shennong's Ancient Chinese Medical Book, Liang Dynasty of China, circa 500 A.D., Munkwang Doso. Taipei. p. 40.
7. YUN, T.K., Y.S. YUN & I.W. HAN. 1980. An experimental study on tumor inhibitory effect of red ginseng in mice and rats exposed to various chemical carcinogens. Proc. 3rd Int. Ginseng Symp. Korea Ginseng Research Institute Press. Seoul. pp. 87–112.
8. YUN, T.K., Y.S. YUN & I.H. HAN. 1983. Anticarcinogenetic effect of long-term oral adminstration of red ginseng on newborn mice exposed to various chemical carcinogens. Cancer Detect. Prev. **6:** 515–525.
9. YUN, T.K. S.H. KIM & Y.R. OH. 1987. Medium-term (nine weeks) method for assay of preventive agents against tumor. J. Korean Cancer Assoc. **19:** 1–7.

10. YUN, T.K. & S.H. KIM. 1988. Inhibition of development of benzo(a)pyrene-induced mouse pulmonary adenoma by natural products in medium-term bioassay system. J. Korean Cancer Assoc. **20:** 133–142.

11. YUN, T.K. 1992. Usefulness of medium-term bioassay determining formation of pulmonary adenoma in NIH(GP) mice for finding anticarcinogenic agents from natural products. J. Toxicol. Sci. (Japan) **16:** (Suppl. 1) 53–62.

12. THE STEERING COMMITTEE OF THE PHYSICIANS' HEALTH STUDY RESEARCH GROUP. 1988. Special report: Preliminary report: Findings from the aspirin component of the ongoing physicians' health study. N. Engl. J. Med. **318:** 262–264.

13. THE ALPHA-TOCOPHEROL, BETA CAROTENE CANCER PREVENTION STUDY GROUP. 1994. The effect of vitamin E and beta carotene on the incidence of lung cancer and other cancers in male smorkers. N. Engl. J. Med. **330:** 1029–1035.

14. OMENN, G.S. G.E. GOODMAN, M.D. THORNQUIST et al. 1996. Risk factors for lung cancer and for intervention effects in CARET, the Beta-Carotene and Retinol Efficacy Trial. J. Natl. Cancer Inst. **88:** 1550–1559.

15. OMENN, G.S., G.E. GOODMAN, M.D. THORNQUIST et al. 1996. Effects of a combination of beta carotene and vitamin A on lung cancer and cardiovascular disease. N. Engl. J. Med. **334:** 1150–1155.

16. HENNEKENS, C.H., J.E. BURING, J.E. MANSON, M. STAMPFER, B. ROSNER, N.R. COOK, C. BELANGER, F. LAMOTTE, J.M. GAZIANO, P.M. RIDKER, W. WILLETT & R.PETO. 1996. Lack of effect of long-term disease. N. Engl. J. Med. **334:** 1145–1149.

17. BOONE, C.W., V.E. STEELE & G.J. KELLOFF. 1992. Screening for chemopreventive (anticarcinogenic) compounds in rodents. Mutat. Res. **267:** 251–255.

18. STEELE, V.E., R.C. MOON, R.A. LUBET, C.J. GRUBBS, B.S. REDDY, M. WARGOVICH, D.L. MCCORMICK, M.A. PEREIRA, J.A. CROWELL, D. BAGHERI, C.C. SIGMAN, C.W. BOONE & G. J. KELLOFF. 1994. Preclinical efficacy evaluation of potential chemoprentive agents in animal carcinogenesis models: Methods and results from NCI Chemoprevention Drug Development Program. J. Cell. Biochem. **20:** 32–54.

19. YUN, T.K., S.H. KIM & Y.S. LEE. 1995. Trial of new medium-term model using benzo(a)pyrene induced lung tumor in newborn mice. Anticancer Res. **15:** 839–846.

20. YUN, T-K. 1996. Experimental and epidemiological evidence of the cancer preventive effects of Panax ginseng C.A. Meyer. Nutr. Rev. **54:** S71–S81.

21. HERZOG, C.R., R.A. LUBET & M. YOU. 1997. Genetic alterations in mouse tumors: Implications for cancer chemoprevention. J. Cell. Biochem. Suppl. **28/29:** 49–63.

22. YOU, M. & G. BERGMAN. 1998. Preclinical and clinical models of lung cancer chemoprevention. Hematol. Oncol. Clinics N. Am. **12:** 1037–1053.

23. YUN, T.K & Y.S. LEE. 1994. Anticarcinogenic effect of ginseng powders depending on the types and ages using Yun's anticarcinogenicity test(I). Korean J. Ginseng Sci. **18:** 89–94.

24. YUN, T.K. & Y.S. LEE. 1994. Anticarcinogenic effect of ginseng extracts depending on the types and ages using Yun's anticarcinogenicity test(II). Korean J. Ginseng Sci. **18:** 160–164.

25. YUN, T-K. Y-S. LEE, H-K. KWON & K.J. CHOI. 1996. Saponin contents and anticarcinogenic effects of ginseng depending on types and ages in mice. Acta Pharm. Sin. **17:** 293–298.

26. KONOSHIMA, T., M. TAKASAKI & H. TOKUDA. 1996. Anti-tumor-promoting activities of the roots of notoginseng(1). Nature Med. **50:** 158–162.

27. WU, X.G. & D.H.J. ZHU. 1990. Influence of ginseng upon the development of liver cancer induced by diethylnitrosamine in rats. J. Tongji Med. Univ. China **10:** 141–145.

28. BESPALOV, V.G., V.A. ALEKSANDROV, V.V. DAVYDOV, A. YU. LIMANKO, D.S. MOLOKOVSKII, A.S. PETROV, L.I. SLEPYAN & YA G. TRILIS. 1993. Mammary car-

cinogenesis suppression by ginseng tissue culture biomass tincture. Bull. Exp. Biol. Med. **115:** 63–65.

29. YUN, T.K. & S.Y. CHOI. 1990. A case-control study of ginseng intake and cancer. Int. J. Epidemiol. **19:** 871–876.

30. EDITORIAL. 1992. Cancer screening and prevention: Organ vs. non-organ specific? Lancet **33:** 902–903.

31. YUN, T.K. & S.Y. CHOI. 1995. Preventive effect of ginseng intake against various human cancers: A case-control study on 1987 pairs. Cancer Epidemiol. Biomarkers Prev. **4:** 401–408.

32. YUN, T.K. & S-Y. CHOI. 1998. Non-organ specific cancer prevention of ginseng: A prospective study in Korea. Int. J. Epidemiol. **27:** 359–364.

33. YUN, T-K., S-Y. CHOI & Y-S. LEE. 1998. Nontoxic and nonorgan specific cancer preventive effect of *Panax ginseng* C.A. Meyer. *In* Functional Foods for Disease Prevention II. Medicinal Plants and Other Foods. T. Shibamoto, J. Terao & T. Osawa, Eds.: 162–177. American Chemical Society. Washington, DC.

34. SHIBATA, S., O. TANAKA, K. SOMA, Y. IIDA T. ANDO & H. NAKAMURA. 1965. Studies in saponins and sapogenin of ginseng, the structure of panaxatriol. Tetrahedron Lett. **3:** 207–213.

35. PARK, J.D. 1996. Recent studies on the chemical constituents of Korean ginseng (*Panax ginseng* C.A. Meyer). Korean J. Ginseng Sci. **20:** 389–415.

36. LAI, C.N., M.A. BUTLER & T.S. MATNEY. 1980. Antimutagenic activities of common vegetables and their chlorophill content. Mutat. Res. **77:** 245–250.

37. KIMM, S-W., S-C. PARK & S-J KANG. 1982. Antimutagenic activity of chlorophyll to direct- and indirect-acting mutagnes and its contents in the vegetables. Korean J. Biochem. **14:** 1–8.

38. KIMM, S-W. & S-C. PARK. 1982. Evidences for the existence of antimutagenic factors in edible plants. Korean J. Biochem. **14:** 41–53

39. SARKAR, K., A. SHARM & G. TALUKDER. 1994. Chlorophyll and chlorophyllin as modifiers of genotoxic effects. Mutat. Res. **318:** 239–247.

40. SURH, Y-J., K-K. PARK & M. SHLYANKEVICH. 1995. Inhibitory effects of chlorophyllin on chemically induced mutagenesis and carcinogenesis. Ann. N. Y. Acad. Sci. **768:** 246–249.

41. PARK, K-K. & Y-J. SURH. 1996. Chemopreventive activity of chlorophyllin against mouse skin carcinogenesis by benzo(a)pyrene and benzo(a)pyrne-7,8-dihydrodiol-9,10-epoxide. Cancer Lett. **102:** 143–149.

42. SHIAO, M-S., K. R. LEE, L.J. LIN & C. T. WANG. 1994. Natural products and biological activities of the Chinese medical fungus, *Ganoderma lucidum. In* Food Phytochemicals for Cancer Prevention. II: Teas, Spices, and Herbs. C.T. Ho, T. Osawa, M.T. Huang & R.T. Rosen, Eds.: 342–354. American Chemical Society. Washington, DC.

43. KOHDA, H., W. TOKUMOTO, K. SAKAMOTO, M. FUJII, Y. HIRAI, K. YAMASAKI, Y. KOMODA, H. NAKAMURA, S. ISHIHARA & M. UCHIDA. 1985. The biologically active constituents of *Ganoderma lucidum* (Fr.) Karst. Histamine release-inhibitory triterpenes. Chem. Pharm. Bull. **33:** 1367–1374.

44. MURASUGI, A., S. TANAKA, N. KOMIYAMA, N. IWATA, K. KINO, H. TSUNOO & S. SKUMA. 1991. Molecular cloning of a cDNA and a gene encoding an immunomodulatory protein, Ling Zhi-8, from a fungus, *Ganoderma lucidum.* J. Biol. Chem. **266:** 2486–2493.

45. WANG, S-Y., M-L. HSU, H-C. HSU, C-H. TZENG, S-S. LEE, M-S. SHIAO & C-K. HO, 1997. The anti-tumor effect of *Ganoderma lucidum* is mediated by cytokines released from activated macrophages and T lymphocytes. Int. J. Cancer **70:** 699–705.

46. LIEU, C-W., S-S. LEE & S-Y. WANG. 1992. The effect of *Ganoderma lucidum* on induction of differentiation in leukemic U937 cells. Anticancer Res. **12:** 1211–1216.

47. YUN, T.K. & Y.S. LEE. 1993. Effect of *Ganoderma lucidum* on mouse pulmonary adenoma induced by benzo(a)pyrene. J. Korean Cancer Assoc. **25:** 531–538.

48. YUN, T-K. & Y-S. LEE. 1997. Anticarcinogenicity of *Ganoderma lucidum*. J. Korean Assoc. Cancer Prev. **2:** 108–112.

49. PARK, K-Y., S-H. MOON, H-S. CHEIGH & H-S. BAIK. 1996. Antimutagenic effects of doenjang (Korean soy paste). J. Food Sci. Nutr. **1:** 151–158.

50. ASAHARA, N., X.B. ZANG & Y. OHTA. 1992. Antimutagenicity and mutagen-binding activation of mutagenic pyrolysates by microorganisms isolated from Japanese miso. J. Sci. Food Agric. **58:** 395–401.

51. GOTOH,T., K. YAMADA, A. ITO, H. YIN, T. KATAOKA & K. DOHI. 1998. Chemoprevention of *N*-nitroso-*N*-methylurea-induced rat mammary cancer by miso and tamoxifen, alone and in combination. Jpn. J. Cancer Res. **89:** 487–495.

52. LIMTRAKUL, P., M. SUTTAJIT, R. SEMURA, K. SHIMADA & S. YAMAMOTO. 1993. Suppressive effect of soybean milk protein on experimentally induced skin tumor in mice. Life Sci. **53:** 1591–1596.

53. BENJAMIN, H., STORKSON, A. NAGAHARA & M.W. PARIZA. 1991. Inhibition of benzo(a)pyrene-induced mouse forestomach neoplasia by dietary soy sauce. Cancer Res. **51:** 2940–2942.

54. KENNEDY, A.R. 1995. The evidence for soybean products as cancer preventive agents. J. Nutr. **125:** 733S–743S.

55. KIM, J-S., Y-J. NAM & T-W. KWON. 1996. Induction of quinone reductase activity by genistein, soybean isoflavone. Foods & Biotech. **5:** 70–75.

56. SHAO, Z.M., J. WU, Z.Z. SHEN & S.H. BARSKY. 1998. Genistein inhibits both constitutive and EGF-stimulated invasion in ER-negative human breast carcinoma cell lines. Anticancer Res. **18:** 1435–1439.

57. RAO, A.V. & M.K. SUNG. 1995. Saponins as anticarcinogen. J. Nutr. **125:** 717S–724S.

58. ZHANG, R. Y. LI & F.W. WANG. 1997. Enhancement of immune function in mice fed high doses of soy daidzein. Nutr. Cancer **29:** 24–28.

59. KURIHARA, M., K. AOKI & F. HISAMICHI. 1989. Cancer Mortality Statistics in the World, 1950–1985. UICC Publication. 1–93. The University of Nagoya Press. Nagoya , Japan.

60. HIRAYAMA, T. 1982. Relationship of soybean paste soup intake to gastric cancer risk. Nutr. Cancer **3:** 223–233.

61. HIRAYAMA, T. 1990. Life-style and mortality. *In* Contributions to Epidemiology and Biostatistics. J. Wahrendorf, Ed.: **6:** 1–137. Karger. München, Germany.

62. GOODMAN, M.T., L.R. WILKENS, J.H. HANKIN, L-C. LYU, A.H. WU & L.N. KOLONEL. 1997. Association of soy and fiber consumption with the risk of endometrial cancer. Am. J. Epdidemiol. **146:** 294–306.

63. MESSINA, M. & V. MESSINA. 1991. Increasing use of soyfoods and their potential role in cancer prevention. J. Am. Diet. Assoc. **91:** 836–840.

64. SHAMSUDDIN, A.M., I. VUCENIK & K. E. COLE. 1997. IP$_6$: A novel anti-cancer agent. Life Sci. **61:** 343–354.

65. AWAD, A.B., R.L. VON HOLTZ, J.P. CONE, C.S. FINK & Y-C. CHEN. 1998. β-Sitosterol inhibits growth of HT-29 human colon cancer cells by activating the sphingomyelin cycle. Anticancer Res. **18:** 471– 473.

66. BUCH, S.H. & T.F. BURKS. 1983. Hot new pharmacological tool. Trends Pharmacol. Sci. **4:** 84–87.

67. JANG, J.J., S.H. KIM & T.K. YUN. 1989. Inhibitory effect of capsaicin on mouse lung tumor development. In Vivo **3:** 49–53.

68. Monsereenusorn, Y., S. Kongsamut & P. D. Pezalla. 1982. Capsaicin—A literature survey. CRC Crit. Rev. Toxicol. **10:** 321–339.
69. Hoch-Legetti, C. 1951. Production of liver tumors by dietary means: Effect of feeding chillies [capsiucum frutescens and annum (Linn.)] to rats. Acta Unio Int. Contra Cacrum **7:** 1011–1026.
70. Adamia, I.K. 1971. Effect of red pepper on the induction of hepatoma. Acad. Nauk Gruz. SSR. Soobschride **65:** 237–240.
71. Toth, B., E. Rogan & B. Walker. 1984. Tumorigenicity and mutagenicity studies with capsaicin of hot peppers. Anticancer Res. **4:** 117–120.
72. Agrawal, R.C. & S.V. Bhide. 1987. Biological studies on carcinogenicity of chillies in BALB/c mice. Indian J. Med. Res. **86:** 391–396.
73. Hahn, C.K. 1961. Studies on the influences of long term administration of red-pepper upon rabbits. 2. Histopathological changes of rabbits administered with red-pepper. Recent Med. **4:** 1315–1327.
74. Lee, S.D. 1963. Influences of diets and lipotrophic substances upon the various organs and metabolic changes in rabbits on long term feeding with red pepper. 1. Histopathological changes of the liver and spleen. Korean J. Int. Med. **6:** 383–395.
75. Agrawal, R.C. & S.V. Bhide. 1988. Histopathological studies on toxicity of chilli (capsaicin) in Syrian Golden hamsters. Ind. J. Exp. Biol. **26:** L377–382.
76. Agrawal, R.C., M. Weissler, E. Hecker & S.V. Bhide. 1986. Tumor-promoting effect of chilli extract in BALB/c mice. Int. J. Cancer **38:** 689–695.
77. Azizan, A. & R.D. Blevins. 1995. Mutagenicity and antimutagenicity testing of six chemicals associated with the pungent properties of specific spices as revealed by Ames Salmonella/microsome assay. Arch. Environ. Contam. Toxicol. **28:** 248–258.
78. Lawson, T. & P. Gannett. 1989. The mutagenicity of capsaicin and dihydrocapsaicin in V79 cells. Cancer Lett. **49:** 109–113.
79. Nagabhushan, M. & S.V. Bhide. 1985. Mutagenicity of chilli extract and capsaicin in short-term tests. Environ. Mut. **7:** 881–888.
80. Nagabhushan, M. & S.V. Bhide. 1986. No mutagenicity of curcumin and its antimutagenic action versus chilli and capsaicin. Nut. Cancer **8:** 201–210.
81. Jang, J.J & S.H. Kim. 1988. The promoting effect of capsaicin on the development of diethylnitrosamine-initiated enzyme altered hepatic foci in male Sprague-Dawley rats. J. Korean Cancer Assoc. **20:** 1–7.
82. Buchanan, R.L., S. Goldstein & J.D. Budroe. 1981. Examination of chilli pepper and nutmeg oleoresins using the Salmonella/mammalian microsome mutagenicity assay. J. Food Sci. **47:** 330–333.
83. Gannett, P.M., D.L. Nagel, P.J. Reilly, T. Lawson, J. Sharpe & B. Toth. 1988. The capsaicinoids: Their separation, synthesis, and mutagenicity. J. Org. Chem. **53:** 1064–1071.
84. Kim, S-H., K-Y. Park & M-J. Suh. 1991. Inhibitory effect of aflatoxin B_1 mediated mutagenicity by red pepper powder in the Salmonella assay system. J. Korean Soc. Food Nutr. **20:** 156–161.
85. Muralidhara & K. Narasimhamurthy. 1988. Non-mutagenicity of capsaicin in albino mice. Food Chem. Toxicol. **26:** 955–958.
86. Viniketkumnuen U., C. Sasagwa C. & T. Matsushima. 1991. Mutagenicity study of chilli and its pungent principles, capsaicin and dihydrocapsaicin. Mutat. Res. **215:** 115.
87. Cordell, G.A. & O.E. Araujo. 1993. Capsaicin: Identification, nomenclature, and pharmacotherapy. Ann. Pharmacother. **27:** 330–336.
88. Miller, M.S., K. Brendel, T.F. Burks & J.G. Sipes. 1983. Interaction of capsaicinoids with drug metabolizing systems. Relationship to toxicity. Biochem. Pharmacol. **32:** 547–551.

89. SURH, Y-J., R.C. LEE, K-K. PARK, S.T. MAYNE, A. LIEM & J.A. MILLER. 1995. Chemoprotective effects of capsaicin and diallyl sulfide against mutagenesis or tumorigenesis by vinyl carbamate and N-nitrosodimethylamine. Carcinogenesis **16:** 2467–2472.

90. PARK, K.K & Y-J. SURH. 1997. Effects of capsaicin on chemically-induced two-stage mouse skin carcinogenesis. Cancer Lett. **114:** 183–184.

91. LOPEZ-CARILLO, L., M.H. AVILA & R. DUBROW. 1994. Chilli pepper consumption and gastric cancer in Mexico: A case control study. Am. J. Epidemiol. **139:** 263–271.

92. BUIATTI E., D. PALLI, A. DECARLI et al. 1989. A case-control study of gastric cancer and diet in Italy. Int. J. Cancer **44:** 611–616.

93. BIOCHANIN A., Y-S. LEE, T-H. KIM & J.J. JANG. 1991. Effects of biochanin A on mouse lung tumor and lymphocyte proliferation. J. Korean Cancer Assoc. **23:** 479–484.

94. CASSADY, J.M., T.M. ZHENNIE, Y-H. CHAE, M.A. FERIN, N.E. PORTUONDO & W.M. BAIRD. 1988. Use of mammalian cell culture benzo(a)pyrene metabolism assay for the detection of potential anticarcinogens from natural products: Inhibition of metabolism by biochanin A, an isoflavone from Trifolium pratense L. Cancer Res., **48:** 6257–6261.

95. CASSADY, J.M. 1990. Natural products as a source of potential cancer chemotherapeutic and chemopreventive agents. J. Nat. Prod. **53:** 23–41.

96. GOTOH, T., K. YAMADA, H. YIN, A. ITO, T. KATAOKA & K. DOHI. 1998. Chemoprevention of N-nitroso-N-methylurea-induced rat mammary carcinogenesis by soy foods or biochanin A. Jpn. J. Cancer Res. **89:** 137–142.

97. KIM., N.K, S.G. KIM & M.K. KWAK. 1994. Enhanced expression of rat microsomal epoxide hydrolase gene by orgnosulfur compound. Biochem. Pharmacol. **47:** 541–547.

98. KIM, N.D., M. K. KWAK & S.G. KIM. 1997. Inhibition of cytochrome P450 2E1 expression by 2-(allylthio)pyrazine, a potential chemopreventive agent: Hepatoprotective effects. Biochem. Pharmacol. **53:** 261–269.

99. KIM, N.D., S.G. KIM & M.K. KWAK. 1995. Induction of rat hepatic glutathione S-transferase by allyl sulfide, allylmercaptan, allylmethyl sulfide and 2-(allylthio)pyrazine. The Int. Toxicologists (Abstracts of the 7th Int. Congress of Toxicology. July 2–6, Seattle, WA, USA), Abstract No. 69-P-8.

100. SURH, Y-J., R. C-J. LEE, K-K. PARK, S.T. MAYNE, A. LIEM & J.A. MILLER. 1995. Chemopreventive effects of capsaicin and diallyl sulfide against mutagenesis or tumorigenesis by vinyl carbamate and N-nitroso-dimethylamine. Carcinogenesis **13:** 901–904.

101. HA, T.G. & N.D. KIM. 1998. 2-(Allylthio)pyrazine inhibition of aflatoxin B1-induced hepatotoxicity in rats: Inhibition of cytochrome P450 2B- and 3A2-mediated bioactivation. Res. Commun. Mol. Pathol. Pharmacol. **102:** 69–78.

102. MUTO, Y., M. NINOMIYA & H. FUJIKI. 1990. Present status of research on cancer chemoprevention in Japan. Jpn. J. Clin. Oncol. **20:** 219–224.

103. MUTO, Y., H. MORIWAKI & M. OMORI. 1981. In vitro binding affinity of novel synthetic poly-prenoids (polyprenoic acids) to cellular retinoid-binding proteins. GANN **72:** 974–977.

104. MUTO, Y. & H. MORIWAKI. 1984. Antitumor activity of vitamin A and its derivatives. J. Natl. Cancer Inst. **73:** 1389–1393.

105. ASAKAWA, Y., T. HASHIMOTO, Y. MIZUNO et al. 1992. Cryptoporic acids A–G, drimane-type sesquiterpenoid ethers of isocitric acid from the fungus Cryptoporus volvatus. Phytochemistry **31:** 579–592.

106. MATSUNAGA, S., H. FURUY-SUGURI, S. NISHIWAKI et al. 1991. Differential effects of cryptoporic acids D and E, inhibitors of superoxide anion radical release, on tumor promotion of okadaic acid in mouse skin. Carcinogenesis **12:** 1129–1131.

107. NARISAWA, T., Y. FUKAURA, H. KOTANAGI et al. 1992. Inhibitory effect of cryptoporous volvatus on colon carcinogenesis induced with N-methyl-N-nitrosourea in rats and with 1,2-dimethylhydrazine in mice. Jpn. J. Cancer Res. **83:** 830–834.

108. FUJIKI, H. & S. SUGANUMA, S. YOSHIZAWA et al. 1989. Codon 61 mutations in the c-Harvey–ras gene in mouse skin tumors induced by 7,12-dimethylbenz(a)-anthracene plus okadaic acid class tumor promoters. Mol. Carcinog. **2:** 184–187.

109. NARISAWA, T., M. TAKAHASHI, M. NIWA, Y. FUKAURA & H. FUJIKI. 1989. Inhibition of methylnitrosourea-induced large bowel cancer development in rats by sarcophytol A, a product from a marine soft coral Sarcophyton glaucum. Cancer Res. **49:** 3287–3289.

110. YOKOMATSU, H., K. SATAKE, A. HIURA et al. 1994. Sarcophytol A: A new chemotherapeutic and chemopreventive agent for pancreatic cancer. Pancreas **9:** 526–530.

111. KOMORI, A., M. SUGANUMA, S. OKABE, X. ZOU, M.A. TIUS & H. FUJIKI. 1993. Canventol inhibits tumor promotion in CD-1 mouse skin through inhibition of tumor necrosis factor α release and of protein isoprenylation. Cancer Res. **53:** 3462–3464.

112. FUJIKI, H., A. KOMORI & M. SUGANUMA. 1997. Chemoprevention of cancer. *In* Comprehensive Toxicology. G.T. Bowden & S.M. Fischer, Eds.: 453–471. Pergamon. Cambridge, UK.

113. MUTO, Y., H. MORIWAKI, M. NINOMIYA, S. ADACHI, A. SAITO & H. FUJIKI et al. 1996. Prevention of second primary tumors by an acyclic retinoid, polyprenoic acid, in patients with hepatocellular carcinoma. N. Engl. J. Med. **334:** 1521–1567.

114. ISHIKAWA, H., I. AKEDO, T. SUZUKI, T. OTANI & T. SOBUE. 1997. Interventional trial for colorectal cancer prevention in Osaka: An introduction to its protocol. *In* Food Factors for Cancer Prevention. H. Ohigashi, T. Osawa, J. Terao, S. Watanabe & T. Yoshikawa, Eds.: 665–668. Springer. Tokyo.

115. YANG, C.S. & Z-Y. WANG. 1993. Tea and Cancer: A review. J. Natl. Cancer Inst. **85:** 1038–1049.

116. KATIYAR, S. & H. MUKHTAR. 1996. Tea in chemoprevention of cancer: Epidemiologic and experimental studies (review). Int. J. Oncol. **8:** 221–238.

117. YOSHIZAWA, S., T. HORIUCHI, H. FUJIKI, T. YOSHIDA, T. OKUDA & T. SUGIMURA. 1987. Antitumor promoting activity of (-)epigallocatechin gallate, the main constituent of "tannin" in green tea. Phytother. Res. **1:** 44–47.

118. FUJITA, Y., T. YAMANE, M. TANAKA, K. KUWATAS, J. OKUZUMI, T. TAKAHASHI, H. FUJIKI & T. OKUDA. 1989. Inhibitory effect of (−)-epigallocatechin gallate on carcinogenesis with N-ethyl-N′-nitro-N-nitrosoguanidine in mouse duodenum. Jpn. J. Cancer Res. **80:** 503–505.

119. XU, Y., C.T. HO, S.G. AMIN, C. HAN & F.L. CHUNG. 1992. Inhibition of tobacco-specific nitrosamine-induced lung tumorigenesis in A/J mice by green tea and its major polyphenol as antioxidants. Cancer Res. **52:** 3875–3879.

120. NARISAWA, T. & Y. FUKAURA. 1993. A very low dose of green tea polyphenols in drinking water prevents N-methyl-N-nitrosourea-induced colon carcionogenesis in F 344 rats. Jpn J. Cancer Res. **84:** 1007–1009.

121. YAMANE, T., T. TAKAHASHI, K. KUWATA, K. OYA, M. INAGAKE, Y. KITAO, M. SUGANUMA & H. FUJIKI. 1995. Inhibition of N-methyl-N′-nitro-N-nitrosoguanidine-induced carcinogenesis by (-)-epigallocatechin gallate in the rat glandular stomach. Cancer Res. **55:** 2081–2084.

122. YANG, C.S., G-Y., YANG, M-J. LEE & L. CHEN. 1997. Mechanistic considerations of the inhibition of carcinogenesis by tea. *In* Food Factors for Cancer Prevention. H. Ohigashi, T. Osawa, J. Terao, S. Watanabe & T. Yoshikawa, Eds.: 113–117. Springer. Tokyo.

123. ZHENG, W., T.J. DOYLE, L.H. KUSHI, T.A. SELLERS, C-P. HONG & A.R. FOLSOM. 1996. Tea consumption and cancer incidence in a prospective cohort study of postmenopausal women. Am. J. Epidemiol. **144:** 175–182.

124. IMAI, K., K. SUGA & K. NAKACHI. 1997. Cancer-preventive effects of drinking green tea among a Japanese population. Prev. Med. **26:** 769–775.

125. LEE, I.S.P., Y.H. KIM, M.H. KANG, C. ROBERTS, J.S. SHIM & J.K.ROH. 1996. Chemopreventive effect of green tea (*Camellia sinensis*) against cigarette smoke-induced mutations (SCE) in humans. J. Korean Assoc. Cancer Prev. **1:** 26–38.

126. NOBUYUKI, H., K. TAJIMA, S. TOMINAGA, A. MATSUURA & K. OKUMA. 1998. Tea polyphenol capsule intake and serum pepsinogens. 17th Int. Cancer Congress. Abstract Book, p. 233.

127. MAHATO, S.B. & S. SEN. 1997. Advances in triterpenoid research, 1990–1994. Phytochemistry **44:** 1185–1236.

128. NISHINO, H., A. NISHINO, J. TAKAYASU, T. HASEGAWA, A. IWASHIMA, K. HIRABAYASHI, S. IWATA & S. SHIBATA. 1988. Inhibition of the tumor-promoting action of 12-O-tetradecanoylphorbol-13-acetate by some oleanane-type triterpenoid compounds. Cancer Res. **48:** 5210–5215.

129. SHIBATA, S., H. NISHINO & N. NAGATA. 1987. Steroidal inhibitors of tumor promotors. Jpn. Kokai Tokyo Koho JP 61,243,017 [86,243,017], Chem. Abst. **107:** 67, 109342s.

130. TAKAYASU, J., H. NISHINO, K. HIRABAYASHI, S. IWATA, N. NAGATA & S. SHIBATA. 1989. Antitumor-promoting activity of 18β-olean-12-ene-3β,23,28-triol tri-O-hemiphthalate sodium and olean-11,13(18)-dien-3β-ol-30-oic acid 3-O-β-D-glucuronopyranosyl-(12)-β-D-glucuronopyranoside sodium by oral administration. Kyoto-furitsu Ika Daigaku Zasshi **98:** 13–16. Chem. Abstr. **110:** 24, 225092w.

131. MATSUNAGA, S. & H. NISHINO. 1991. Carcinogenesis promotor inhibitors containing tetracyclic triterpenoids. Jpn. Kokai Tokyo Koho JP 03,271,220 [91,271,220], Chem. Abstr. **116:** 78, 143845d.

132. YUSUKAWA, K., M. TAKIDO, T. MATSUMOTO, M. TAKEUCHI & H. TOKUDA. 1989. Tetrahedron Lett. **30:** 5625.

133. NISHIZAWA, M., M. EMURA, H. YAMADA, M.C. SHIRO, Y. HAYASHI & H. TOKUDA. 1989. Isolation of a new cycloartanoid triterpene from leaves of *Lansium domesticum*. Novel skin-tumor promotion inhibitor. Tetrahedron Lett. **30:** 5615–5618.

134. TAKAYASU, J., R. TANAKA, S. MATSUNAGA & A. IWASHIMA. 1990. Anti-tumor-promoting activity of derivatives of abieslactone, a natural triterpenoid isolated from several Abies genus. Cancer Lett. **53:** 141–144.

135. KONOSHIMA, T., M. TAKASAKI, H. TOKUDA, K. MASUDA, Y. ARAI, K. SHOJIMA & H. AGETA. 1996. Anti-tumor promoting activities of triterpenoids from ferns. I. Biol. Pharm. Bull. **19:** 962–965.

136. HAN, J. 1993. Highlights of the cancer chemoprevention studies in China. Prev. Med. **22:** 712–722.

137. CAI, H.Y., J.S. ZHANG & X.X. CUI. 1981. Inhibitory effects of some new retinoids on carcinogenesis. Acta Pharm. Sin. **16:** 648–653.

138. ZHENG, S., H. YANG, S. ZHANG, X. WANG, L. YU, J. LU & J. LI. 1997. Initial study on naturally par occurring products from traditional Chinese herbs and vegetables for chemoprevention. J. Cell. Biochem. Suppl. **27:** 106–112.

139. BLOT, W.J., J-Y. LI, P.R. TAYLOR, W. GUO, S. DAWSEY, G-Q. WANG, C.S. YANG, S-F. ZHENG, M. GAIL, G-Y. LI, Y.YU, B-Q. LIU, J. TANGREA, Y-H. SUN, F. LIU, J.F. FRAUMENI, JR., Y-H. ZHANG & B. LI. 1993. Nutrition intervention trials in Linxian, China: Supplementation with specific vitamin/mineral combinations, cancer incidence, and disease specific mortality in the general population. J. Natl. Cancer Inst. **85:** 1483–1492.

140. LI, J-Y., P.R. TAYLOR, B. LI, S. DAWSEY, G-Q. WANG, A.G. ERSHOW, W. GUO, S-F. LIU, C.S. YANG, Q. SHEN, W. WANG, S.D. MARK, X-N. ZOU, P. GREENWALD, Y-P. WU & W.J. BLOT. 1993. Nutrition intervention trials in Linxian, China: Multiple

vitamin/mineral supplementation, cancer incidence, and disease-specific mortality among adults with esophageal dysplasia. J. Natl. Cancer Inst. **85:** 1492–1498.

141. TAYLOR, P.R., J.Y. LI & B. LI. 1994. Nutrition intervention trials in Linxian, China: Supplementation with specific vitamin/mineral combinations, cancer incidence, and disease-specific mortality in the general population. J. Natl. Cancer Inst. **86:** 1645–1649.

142. YU, S-Y., Y-J. ZHU, W-G. LI, Q-S. HUANG, Z-H. CHANG, Q-N. ZHANG & C. HOU. 1991. A preliminary report on the intervention trials of primary liver cancer in high-risk populations with nutritional supplementation of selenium in China. Biol. Trace Element Res. **29:** 289–294.

143. GAIL, M.H., W.C. YOU, Y-S. CHANG, L. ZHANG, W.J. BLOT, L.M. BROWN, F.D. GROVES, J.P. HEINRICH, J. HU, M-I. JIN, J-Y. LI, W-D. LIU, J-I. MA, S.D. MARK, C.S. RABKIN, J.F. FRAUUMENI & G-W. XU. 1998. Factorial trial of three interventions to reduce the progression of precancerous gastric lesions in Shandong, China: Design issues and initial data. Controlled Clin. Trials **19:** 352–369.

144. KENSLER, T.W., X. HE, M. OTIENO, P.A. EGNER, L.P. JACOBSON, B. CHEN, J-S. WANG, Y-R. ZHU, B-C. ZHANG, J-B. WANG, Y. WU, Q-N. ZHANG, G-S. QIAN, S-Y. KUANG, X. FANG, Y-F. LI, L-Y. YU, H.J. PROCHASKA, N.E. DAVIDSON, G.B. GORDON, M.B. GORMAN, A. ZARBA, C. ENGER, A. MUNOZ, K. J. JHELZLSOUER & J.D. GROOPMAN. 1998. Oltipraz chemoprevention trial in Qidong, People's Republic of China: Modulation of serum aflatoxin albumin adduct biomarkers. Cancer Epidemiol Biomarker Prev. **7:** 127–134.

145. JACOBSON, L.P., B-C. ZHANG, Y-R. ZHU, J-B. WANG, Y. WU, Q-N. ZHANG, L-Y. YU, G-S. QIAN, S-Y. KUANG, Y-F. LI, X. FANG, A. ZARBA, B. CHEN, C. ENGER, N.E. DAVIDSON, M.B. GORMAN, G.B. GORDON, H.J. PROCHASKA, P.A. EGNER, J.D. GROOPMAN, A. MUNOZ, K.J. HELZLSOUER & T.W. KENSLER. 1997. Oltipraz chemoprevention trial in Qidong, People's Republic of China: Study design and clinical outcomes. Cancer Epidemiol. Biomarkers Prev. **6:** 257–265.

Squalene, Olive Oil, and Cancer Risk

Review and Hypothesis

HAROLD L. NEWMARK[a]

Strang Cancer Research Laboratory at The Rockefeller University,
New York, New York 10021, USA and
Rutgers University, Laboratory for Cancer Research,
Piscataway, New Jersey 08854-8020, USA

ABSTRACT: Epidemiologic studies of breast and pancreatic cancer in several Mediterranean populations have demonstrated that increased dietary intake of olive oil is associated with a small decreased risk, or no increased risk, of cancer, despite a high overall lipid intake. Experimental animal models in high dietary fat and cancer also indicate that olive oil either has no effect, or a protective effect, on the prevention of a variety of chemically induced tumors. As a working hypothesis, it is proposed that the high squalene content of olive oil, as compared to other human foods, is a major factor in the cancer-risk reducing effect of olive oil. Experiments in animal models suggest a tumor-inhibiting role for squalene. A mechanism is proposed for the tumor-inhibitory activity of squalene based on its known strong inhibitory activity of HMG-COA reductase catalytic activity *in vivo*, thus reducing farnesyl pyrophosphate (FPP) availability for "prenylation" of ras oncogene, which relocates this oncogene to cell membranes and is required for the signal-transducing function of ras. Reduction of mutated ras oncogene activation may be useful in breast and colon cancer and may be particularly applicable to pancreatic cancers that are strongly associated with ras oncogenes.

Olive oil has been a significant food item for several thousands of years, mentioned in the Old Testament and ancient Greek mythology among others. In modern times it remains an important source of dietary fat (as vegetable oil) in countries surrounding the Mediterranean Sea, including Southern Europe, North Africa, and the Middle East. Scientific interest in dietary intake of olive oil has increased in recent decades due to early observations that suggested an inverse correlation between olive oil intake and risk of some types of cancer.

EPIDEMIOLOGY

Epidemiological studies suggest a cancer-protective effect of dietary olive oil relative to other types of nonmarine fat sources. In Greece, women with approximately

[a]Address for communication: Rutgers University, Laboratory for Cancer Research, Department of Chemical Biology, College of Pharmacy, 164 Frelinghuysen Road, Piscataway, NJ 08854-8020. Fax: 732-445-0687.

40% of energy intake from fat, mainly as olive oil, have a breast cancer rate of only about one-third that of women in the United States, who have until recently also consumed about 40% of energy from fat.[1–3] A case-control study in Spain showed a reduced risk for breast cancer in women with the highest olive oil consumption.[4] In a large case-control study in Greece, a similar lack of overall association with total fat intake was seen, but breast cancer risk was 25% lower in women consuming olive oil more than once a day.[5] In another case-control study in Spain,[6] women in the highest third of monounsaturated fat intake (largely from olive oil) had reduced risk of breast cancer (relative risk = 0.30; 95% confidence interval, 0.1–0.8). A recent report of a case-control study performed in Italy[7] indicated a decreased risk of breast cancer with increased intake of unsaturated fatty acids from edible oils. In Italy, about 80% of edible oil is olive oil, suggesting a protective effect of olive oil intake. A recent case-control study in Italy reported a significant inverse trend of edible oil (mainly olive oil) intake and risk of pancreatic cancer.[8]

LABORATORY ANIMAL STUDIES

Animal studies on fat and cancer have generally shown that olive oil either has no effect, or a protective effect, on the prevention of a variety of chemically induced tumors. Olive oil did not increase tumor incidence or growth, in contrast to corn and sunflower oil, in some mammary cancer models[9–11] and also in colon cancer models,[12,13] although in an earlier report, olive oil exhibited mammary tumor-promoting properties similar to that of corn oil,[14] in contrast to the later studies.[15]

The protective or, at the least, nonpromoting activity of olive oil previously was ascribed to its high content (about 72%) of the monoenoic unsaturated fatty acid, oleic acid (C18:1, n9). This fatty acid is also found in the fat of beef and poultry, in the range of 22–53%, and in appreciable levels in such other vegetable oils as corn, palm, peanut, soybean, and sunflower oils, in the range of 23–50% (see TABLE 1). Many of the other fats and oils rich in oleic acid are largely associated with increased risk of colon and breast cancer in humans and generally act as promoters of chemically induced tumors in rodents, including beef tallow, lard, corn, and sunflower seed oils. Thus it seems that the monoenoic unsaturated fatty acid (oleic acid) content of olive oil cannot fully account for its protective effect or lack of promotion effect in cancer development.

In further confirmation of the inadequacy of oleic acid content as explanation of reduced cancer risk from olive oil intake, a recent report of a case-control study of adipose tissue stores of individual monounsaturated fatty acids in relation to breast cancer in women also indicated that the oleic acid in olive oil does not account for any protective property of this oil.[18]

The chemical composition of olive oil has been extensively studied, with the associated variabilities due to region of origin, seasonal changes and differences in processing techniques.[19] A consideration was made of components unique to olive oil, qualitatively or quantitatively different from other fats and oils, as a possible explanation for its protective or nonpromoting effects. Squalene, at up to 0.7%, is uniquely high in olive oil as compared to other common human food fats and oils.[20,21] Other vegetable oils and animal fats are considerably lower, in the range of

TABLE 1. Oleic acid content of food fats[16,17]

	% of Fatty Acids
Olive Oil:	
European	75
Tunisian	59
Other Plant Oils:	
Peanut	50
Palm	43
Sunflower seed	33
Corn	28
Soybean	23
Animal Fats:	
Duck	53
Pork (Lard)	44
Beef (Tallow)	42
Chicken	40
Lamb	38
Butterfat	23
Turkey	22

0.002–0.03% squalene content.[20] Food-regulatory agencies often rely on the squalene content to determine the purity of commercial olive oil. Squalene is a hydrocarbon of the triterpene type, containing six isoprene units with a pleasant, bland taste. It is a key intermediate in the biosynthetic pathway to steroids in both plants and animals. Thus, it can be considered as almost ubiquitous in most plant and animal cells, although at enormously different levels.

The chemical structure of squalene is shown in FIGURE 1, A and B, where the former is a simple linear mode of presentation, and the latter is in the form to visualize the next major biosynthetic step, the cyclization of squalene to form lanosterol, the first steroid in the metabolic series of the pathway to cholesterol (animals) or sitosterol and stigmasterol (plants).

SQUALENE AS A TUMOR INHIBITOR

A literature search indicated only a few reports of an inhibiting effect of squalene in rodent cancer models. Van Duuren and Goldschmidt noted that squalene applied topically to mouse skin almost completely inhibited benzo(a)pyrene-induced skin carcinogenicity.[22] D-Limonene only partly inhibited skin tumors in the same experiment. In a later study, Murakoshi et al.[23] reported that topically applied squalene markedly suppressed the promoting effect of 12-O-tetradecanoylphorbol-13-acetate (phorbol ester, TPA) on mouse skin tumors initiated with 7,12-dimethylbenz(a)anthracene. Other studies on the antitumor activity of squalene have been reported in Japan.[24–26]

In our published studies, by ourselves or in collaboration with others, the purpose was to demonstrate whether squalene given orally would have an inhibitory effect on

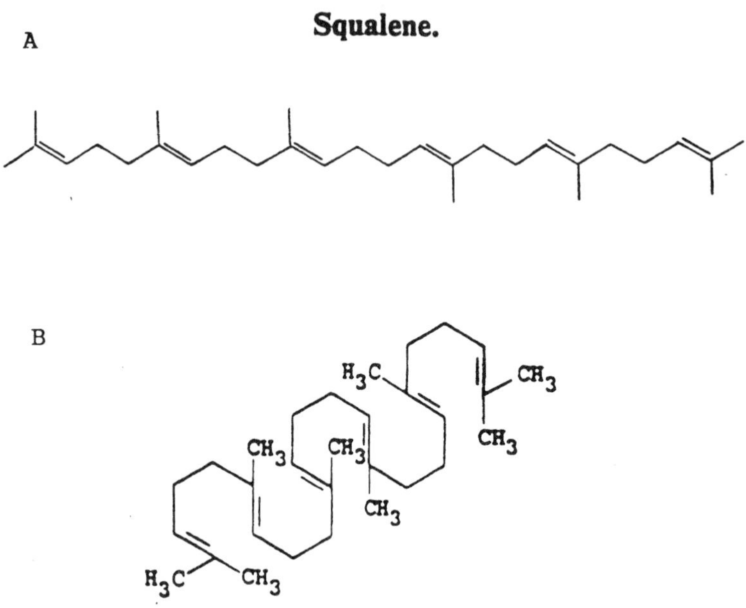

A

Squalene.

B

FIGURE 1.

tumors of internal organs. We demonstrated potent inhibition of aberrant hyperproliferation in a mammary epithelial cell line *in vitro*.[27] Using 1% squalene in the diet of rats treated with the colon chemical carcinogen, azoxymethane, a 45% suppression of induced aberrant crypt foci was seen. This latter study, to our knowledge, is the first experimental demonstration of the inhibitory action of dietary squalene on carcinogenesis.[28] Using either 2% squalene or 19.6% olive oil in the diet of mice inhibited lung tumorigenesis induced by the carcinogen NNK (4-(methylnitrosamino)-1-(3-pyridyl)-1-butanone) found in tobacco smoke.[29]

A hypothetical mechanism for antitumor activity of squalene has been proposed[30] and is further discussed here. In rats given 1% squalene in the diet for five days, serum squalene rose about 20-fold. This was accompanied by a strong inhibition (about 80%) of HMG-CoA reductase activity in hepatic microsomes.[31] This effect has been confirmed in mice by Dr. Theresa Smith, Rutgers University (unpublished observation). It is not clear whether this inhibition stems from squalene itself or one or more of its metabolites, such as steroids,[32] produced endogenously, particularly the methyl steroids first formed (sequentially) on cyclization of squalene *in vivo*, that is, lanosterol, 4,4 dimethyl steroids, and 4 monomethyl steroid, leading to zymosterol (FIG. 2). These methyl steroids are also strongly elevated as a group in rat serum on feeding squalene, but not the desmosterol or cholesterol levels.[31] Inhibition of HMG-CoA reductase activity, the rate-limiting control step in the normal biosynthetic pathway to cholesterol, presumably also reduces the levels of the series of intermediates between HMG-CoA reductase and cholesterol,[32] including mevalonate, geranyl pyrophosphate, and farnesyl pyrophosphate (FPP). FPP is a source for the biosynthesis of ubiquinone, heme a, dolichol, and particularly for the preny-

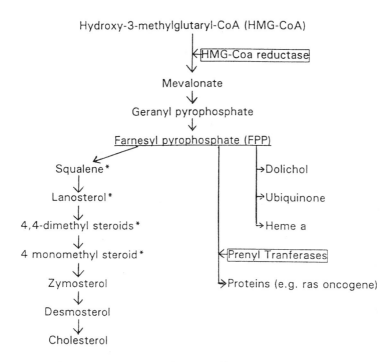

Hydroxy-3-methylglutaryl-CoA (HMG-CoA)
↓ ←HMG-Coa reductase
Mevalonate
↓
Geranyl pyrophosphate
↓
Farnesyl pyrophosphate (FPP)

Squalene*   →Dolichol
↓
Lanosterol*   →Ubiquinone
↓
4,4-dimethyl steroids*   ↳Heme a
↓
4 monomethyl steroid*   ←Prenyl Tranferases
↓
Zymosterol   ↳Proteins (e.g. ras oncogene)
↓
Desmosterol
↓
Cholesterol

*Elevated in serum on feeding 1% squalene

FIGURE 2.

lation (farnesylation) of certain proteins. Protein farnesylation, a posttranslational modification process, mediates the COOH-terminal lipidation of specific cellular signaling proteins, including the Ras oncogene protein p21, guanosine triphosphatases (GTPases), trimeric GTP-binding protein, nuclear lamin B, and yeast mating pheromone α-factor. In each of these cases, farnesylation increases membrane association and cellular activity of these proteins. Thus, farnesylation plays an essential role in signal transduction cascades of yeast and mammalian cells. Several oncogenes, such as *Ras* p21 are proteins produced in the aqueous environment of the cell cytosol but require relocation to the lipophilic cell plasma membrane for activation. This relocation is achieved by attachment of farnesol supplied from FPP via a specialized enzyme system.[33,34] Prevention of prenylation prevents the activation of these proteins as signal-transducing agents in the regulation of cell-transforming activity (FIG. 2).

In small pilot studies with Dr. Kan Yang, we fed 1% squalene in the diet to mice carrying a mutation in the Apc gene that resulted in multiple intestinal neoplasia (MIN). We had hoped to reduce the incidence of intestinal neoplasia and possibly prolong the short life span (about 4–5 months) of these mice. Unfortunately squalene feeding had no effect (unpublished). In retrospect this should not have been surprising, inasmuch as no Ras-activating mutations were detected in tumors from these mice in a recent report.[35] Similar negative results with feeding 1% squalene were obtained with the *Apc1638* mouse, another mouse with a mutated Apc gene that spontaneously develops intestinal neoplasia. This mouse was also recently reported to have no detectable ras mutations in its tumors.[36] These "negative" results from increased dietary squalene in two types of mice that spontaneously develop intestinal neoplasia, but that do not involve detectable ras oncogene mutations, suggest that squalene may indeed act via inhibition of mutated ras function, as in asoxymethane-induced colon carcinogenesis,[28] but not in genetically altered mice without mutated ras.

These seemingly discordant observations on the possible preventive effect of squalene raise the possibility of specificity of its action on the mutant Ras oncogene rather than on the protooncogene. It is also noteworthy that Ras mutations are rare in clinical breast cancer, whereas overexpression of the normal Ras protooncogene is frequently observed in this organsite cancer.[34,37] Furthermore, targeted overexpression of Ras protooncogene is equally effective to that of Ras oncogene in inducing tumorigenic transformation of mammary epithelial cells.[38] Thus, mechanisms responsible for preventive efficacy of squalene may differ depending on the site of the cancer.

Several other dietary isoprenoids are also known to act as inhibitors of the mevalonate pathway and act similarly to reduce cellular availability of FPP, resulting in reduction of tumor growth.[39] In the report of Strandberg,[31] where 1% squalene was fed to rats, there resulted an approximate 20-fold increase in serum squalene, and almost a 30-fold increase in total methyl sterols, including lanosterol, 14 desmethyl lanosterol, and 4 monomethylated sterols. However, sterols further downstream in the biosynthetic pathway (zymosterol, desmosterol, and cholesterol) remained largely unchanged. Thus squalene itself, or one or more of the methyl sterols, or their biochemical intermediates, could be functioning as the key signal to inhibit HMG-CoA reductase, as shown in the Strandberg report.[31]

We and our collaborators are currently testing lanosterol, and other metabolites of squalene *in vitro* and *in vivo*, for potential as tumor inhibitors. Preliminary studies, *in vitro*, on V-Ha Ras-transformed mammary epithelial cells have compared the preventive efficacy of squalene with that of other terpenoid metabolites suggested by Dr. Pamela Crowell. These experiments demonstrate that geraniol, lanosterol, and farnesol are 7.9-, 12.0-, and 12.7-fold more effective as growth inhibitors compared to squalene at equivalent dose levels in the Ras-transformed cell culture model of mammary carcinogenesis.[27] Furthermore, administration of 2% lanosterol in the diet to C-57 mouse recipients bearing transplanted V-Has Ras cells resulted in a 47% decrease in tumor weight, compared to that seen in recipients on a 4% squalene diet. Taken together these preliminary observations suggest that squalene metabolites or unphosphorylated precursor substances for posttranslational modification of Ras p21 may possess a stronger chemopreventive effect than those exhibited by squalene.

There have been several research programs aimed at development of (drug) inhibitors of protein farnesylation as potential cancer chemotherapeutic agents.[40] Some of these agents are targeted to the specific enzymes involved in protein farnesylation, without interfering with the downstream squalene and cholesterol biosynthesis. Dietary squalene presumably inhibits HMG-Coa reductase activity to reduce FPP formation in the cells, without deprivation of any squalene to cholesterol precursors, presumably by enhancing these squalene metabolites.

The squalene inhibition effect on HMG-CoA reductase activity is probably part of the normal feedback regulation control of cholesterol biosynthesis. Increasing dietary intake of squalene (e.g., from increased intake of olive oil) to augment endogenous levels of squalene thus serves to lower FPP levels and therefore to reduce oncogene product activation via prenylation, and thus it can potentially reduce tumor growth without markedly disturbing a normal biochemical pathway. Reduction of tumor growth and development could be expected in tumor types strongly dependent on oncogenes requiring prenylation for activation, such as *ras*. Colon, breast, melanoma, and pancreas develop such tumor types, particularly pancreatic adenocarcinomas, in which up to 90% are associated with activated *ras* oncogene mutation.[33,34] All these tumors represent potential targets for squalene use as a chemopreventive agent, or as an adjunct to drug therapy using inhibitors of prenylase enzymatic activity.

Increased dietary squalene intake could theoretically augment cholesterol and bile acid production, resulting in enhanced atherosclerotic disease. However, a few studies in rabbits and humans indicate that a high intake does not seem to be associated with an increased risk of atherosclerosis. Kritchevsky *et al.*[41] fed 3% squalene in a high-cholesterol diet to rabbits for 14 weeks; the rabbits failed to develop more atheromas than similar cholesterol-fed controls. Our recent colon study also indicates that 1% squalene in the diet had no effect on serum cholesterol in rats.[28] Strandberg *et al.* fed 900 mg of squalene daily to humans for 7–30 days, demonstrating about 60% absorption with a 17-fold increase in serum squalene, but produced no consistent increases in serum cholesterol levels.[42] Chan *et al.* fed 860 mg of squalene daily to elderly patients with hypercholesterolemia for 20 weeks and found a statistically significant 17% decrease of total serum cholesterol.[43] These short-term feeding studies are insufficient, however, to fully answer questions of long-term effects of higher-than-normal dietary squalene intake on metabolism of cholesterol and other steroids, as well as adequacy of biosynthesis of ubiquinones, heme a, and dolichols for normal cell function. However, the combined available data of human epidemiology, human short-term squalene feeding to humans, and laboratory animal feeding studies suggest that increased squalene intake does not pose a problem of hypercholesterolemia.

Squalene in humans is normally supplied by both endogenous biosynthesis and dietary sources. The Rockefeller University group[20] measured squalene in normal human tissues and plasma and found it to be widely distributed, but at great variations in level. Sebum was reported to contain 12% squalene, and adipose tissue contained 0.01–0.04% squalene, with other tissues having lower levels. Plasma squalene levels, normally about 1–2 micromolar in rats and humans, rose strikingly with increased dietary squalene. Generally, there was a direct relationship between plasma levels of squalene and triglycerides, but not with cholesterol. No data are yet available on changes in tissue levels, or tumor levels, of squalene or its metabolites, when dietary intake of squalene is increased, in either animals or humans.

The average dietary intake of squalene in the United States has been estimated to be only about 30 mg/day,[20] with a possible high intake up to 200 mg/day on a 2000-Kcal diet rich in fish and salads dressed with olive oil.[20] In such Mediterranean coun-

TABLE 2.

Country	Estimated Daily Dietary Squalene
Greece	400 mg
Italy	230 mg
USA	30 mg

tries as Greece, where olive oil intake is about 20 kg/year/person (60 g/day), or Italy, where olive oil intake is 12 kg/year/person (35 g/day), average squalene daily intake is more likely to be in the range of 200–400 mg/day[44] based on about 0.6–0.7% squalene content[19,21] of olive oil. This large difference in average dietary intake of squalene between Mediterranean countries and the United States (7- to 13-fold) may be one of the factors related to lower cancer mortality in the Mediterranean basin countries[1–5] (TABLE 2).

Sharks, which have been claimed to be resistant to cancer,[45] have unusually high tissue levels of squalene. Shark liver oil contains 40% or more squalene.[20,21] Dogfish liver oil is very high, reported to be over 90% squalene.[21] It is interesting to speculate whether the high squalene content is related to the reputed cancer resistance in sharks.

SUMMARY

Increased dietary intake of olive oil is associated with a small decreased risk or no increased risk of cancer, despite high lipid intake, in epidemiological studies of colon, breast, and pancreatic cancer in several Mediterranean populations. As a working hypothesis, it is proposed that the high squalene content of olive oil, as compared to other human foods, is a major factor in the cancer risk-reducing effect of olive oil. A few experiments *in vitro* and in animal models suggest a tumor-inhibiting role for squalene. A mechanism is proposed for the tumor-inhibitory activity of squalene, based on its known strong inhibitory activity of HMG-CoA reductase activity, thus reducing FPP availability for prenylation of some oncogenes (e.g., *ras* prenylation as a step in relocation to cell membranes for function as a signal-transducing agent). Further studies are needed to ascertain the potential antineoplastic potential of the squalene metabolites produced during normal biosynthetic pathways to plant and animal sterols. The mechanism proposed above may be only a part of the activity of squalene and/or its metabolites in tumor inhibition.

ACKNOWLEDGMENTS

The author gratefully acknowledges the excellent collaborators who made these studies possible: Dr. Nitin Telang, Dr. Kan Yang (Strang Cancer Research Laboratory, New York, NY), Dr. Bandaru Reddy, Dr. C.V. Rao (American Health Foundation, Valhalla, NY), Dr. Chung S. Yang, Dr. Theresa J. Smith (Rutgers University, Piscataway, NJ), and Dr. Pamela Cromwell (Indiana University/Perdue University, Indianapolis, IN).

REFERENCES

1. GERBER, M. 1991. Olive oil and cancer. *In* The Mediterranean Diet and Cancer Prevention. A. Giacosa & M.J. Hill, Eds. European Cancer Prevention Organization. Cosenza, Italy.

2. TRICHOPOULOU, A., N. TOUPADAKI, A. TZONOU, K. KATSOUYANNI, O. MANOUSOS, E. KADA *et al.* 1993. The macronutrient composition of the Greek diet: Estimates derived from six case-control studies. Eur. J. Clin. Nutr. **47:** 549–558.

3. WILLETT, W.C. 1994. Diet and health: What should we eat? Science **264:** 532–537.

4. MARTIN-MORENO, J.M., W.C. WILLETT, L. GORGOJO, J.R. BANEGAS, F. RODRIGUEZ-ARTALEJO, J.C. FERNANDEZ-RODRIGUEZ *et al.* 1994. Dietary fat, olive oil intake and breast cancer risk. Int. J. Cancer **58:** 774–780.

5. TRICHOPOULOU, A., K. KATSOUYANNI, S. STUVER, L. TZALA, C. GNARDELLIS, E. RIMM *et al.* 1995. Consumption of olive oil and specific food groups in relation to breast cancer risk in Greece. J. Natl. Cancer Inst. **87:** 110–116.

6. LANDA, M.C., N. FARGO & A. TRES. 1994. Diet and the risk of breast cancer in Spain. Eur. J. Cancer Prev. **3:** 313–320.

7. FRANCESCHI, S., A. FAVERO, A. DECARLI, E. NEGRI, C. LAVECCHIA, M. FERRARONI *et al.* 1996. Intake of macronutrients and risk of breast cancer. Lancet **347:** 1351–1356.

8. LA VECCHIA, C. & E. NEGRI. 1997. Fats in seasoning and the relationship to pancreatic cancer. Eur. J. Cancer Prev. **6(4):** 370–373.

9. COHEN, L.S., D.G. THOMPSON, Y. MAUERA, K. CHOI, M.E. BLANK & D.P. ROSE. 1986. Dietary fat and mammary cancer. I. Promotion of effect of different fats on *N*-nitrosomethylurea-induced rat mammary tumorigenesis. J. Natl. Cancer Inst. **77:** 33–42.

10. KATZ, E.B. & E. BOYLAN. 1989. Effect of the quality of the dietary fat in tumor growth and metastasis from a rat mammary adenocarcinoma. Nutr. Cancer **12:** 343–350.

11. LASEKAN, J.B., M.K. CLAYTON, A. GENDRON FITZPATRICK & D.M. NEY. 1990. Dietary olive and safflower oil in promotion of DMBA-induced mammary tumorigenesis in rats. Nutr. Cancer **13:** 153–163.

12. REDDY, B.S. 1992. Dietary fat and colon cancer: Animal model studies. Lipids **27:** 807–813.

13. RAO, C.V. & B.S. REDDY. 1993. Modulating effect of amount and types of dietary fat on ornithine decarboxylase, tyrosine protein kinase and prostaglandins production during colon carcinogenesis in male F344 rats. Carcinognesis (Lond.) **14:** 1327–1333.

14. CARROLL, K.K. & H.T. KHOR. 1971. Effects of level and type of dietary fat on incidence of mammary tumors induced in female Sprague-Dawley rats by 7,12-dimethylbenz(alpha)anthracene. Lipids **6:** 415–420.

15. COHEN, L.A. *In* Diet, Nutrition, and Cancer: A Critical Evaluation. B.S. Reddy & L.A. Cohen, Eds.: **1:** 92. CRC Press. Boca Raton, FL.

16. MCCANCE & WIDDOWSON. 1978. The Composition of Food, 4th ed. Elsevier. 294–299.

17. C. LENTNER, Ed. 1981. Geigy Scientific Tables, vol. 1, p. 264. Medical Education Division. Ciba Geigy Corp. West Caldwell, NJ.

18. SIMONSEN, N., J. FERNANDEZ-CREHUET, J. MARTIN-MORENO, J. STRAIN, B. MARTIN, M. THAMM, A. KARDINAAL, P. VAN'T VEER, F. KOK & L. KOHLMEIER. 1997. Tissue stores of individual monounsaturated fats and breast cancer. FASEB J. **11:** A578.

19. BOSKOU, D., Ed. 1996. Olive Oil: Chemistry and Technology. American Oil Chemists Society Press. Champaign, IL.

20. LIU, C.K., E.H. AHRENS JR., H. SCHREIBMAN & R. CROUSE. 1976. Measurement of squalene in human tissues and plasma: Validation and application. J. Lipid Res. **17:** 38–45.

21. BECKER, R. 1989. Preparation, composition and nutritional implications of amaranth seed oil. Cereal Foods World **34:** 950–953.
22. VAN DUUREN, B.L. & B.M. GOLDSCHMIDT. 1976. Co-carcinogenic and tumor-promoting agents in tobacco carcinogenesis. J. Natl. Cancer Inst. **56:** 1237–1242.
23. MURAKOSHI, M., H. NISHINO, H. TOKUDA, A. IWASHIMA, J. OKUZUMI, H. KITANO et al. 1992. Inhibition by squalene of the tumor-promoting activity of 12-O-tetradecanoylphorbol-13-acetate in mouse-skin carcinogenesis. Int. J. Cancer **52:** 950–952.
24. YAMAGUCHI, T., M. NAKAGAWA, K. HIDAKA, T. YOSHIDA, T. SASAKI, S. AKIYAMA et al. 1985. Potentiation by squalene of antitumor effect of 3-[(4-amino-2-methyl-5-pyrimidinyl)methyl 1]-1-(2-chloroethy)-nitrosourea in a murine tumor system. Jpn. J. Cancer Res. **76:** 1021–1026.
25. IKIKAWA, T., M. UMEJI, T. MANABE, S. YANOMA, K. ORINODA, H. MIZUNUMA et al. 1986. Studies on antitumor activity of squalene and its related compounds (in Japanese). J. Pharm. Soc. Jpn. **106:** 578–582.
26. OHKIMA, T., K. OTAGIRI, S. TANAKA & T. IKEKAWA. 1983. Intensification of host's immunity by squalene in sarcoma 180-bearing ICR mice. J. Pharmacobio-dyn. **6:** 148–151.
27. KATDARE, M., H. SINGHAL, H. NEWMARK, M.P. OSBORNE & N.T. TELANG. 1997. Prevention of mammary preneoplastic transformation by naturally-occurring tumor inhibitors. Cancer Lett. **111:** 141–147.
28. RAO, C.V., H.L. NEWMARK & B.S. REDDY. 1998. Chemopreventive effect of squalene on colon cancer. Carcinogenesis **19:** 287–290.
29. SMITH, T.J., G-Y. YANG, D.N. SERIL, J. LIAO & S. KIM. 1998. Inhibition of 4-(methylnitrosamino)-1-(3-pyridyl)-1-butanone-induced lung tumorigenesis by dietary olive oil and squalene. Carcinogenesis **19:** 703–706.
30. NEWMARK, H.L. 1997. Squalene, olive oil, and cancer risk: A review and hypothesis. Cancer Epidemiol. Biomarkers Prev. **6:** 1101–1103.
31. STRANDBERG, E., R. TILVIS & T.A. MIETTINEN. 1989. Variations of hepatic cholesterol precursors during altered flows of endogenous and exogenous squalene in the rat. Biochem. Biophys. Acta **1001:** 150–156.
32. GOLDSTEIN, J.L. & M.S. BROWN. 1990. Regulation of the mevalonate pathway. Nature (Lond.) **343:** 425–430.
33. KATO, K., A.D. COX, M.M. HISAKA, S.M. GRAHAM, J.E. BUSS & C.J. DER. 1992. Isoprenoid addition to Ras protein is the critical modification for its membrane association and transforming activity. Proc. Natl. Acad. Sci. USA **89:** 6403–6407.
34. BOS, J.L. 1989. Ras oncogenes in human cancer: A review. Cancer Res. **49:** 4682–4689.
35. SHOEMAKER, A.R., C. LUONGO, A.R. MOSER, L.J. MARTON & W.F. DOVE. 1997. Somatic mutational mechanisms involved in intestinal tumor formation in Min mice. Cancer Res. **57:** 1999–2006.
36. SMITS, R., A. KARTHEUSER, S. JAGMOHAN-CHANGUR, C.B. LEBLANC, A. DE VRIES, H. VAN KRANEN, J.H. VAN KRIEKEN, S. WILLIAMSON, W. EDELMANN, R. KUCHERLAPATI, P.M. KHAN & R. FODDE. 1997. Loss of Apc and the entire chromosome 18 but absence of mutations at the Ras and Tp53 genes in intestinal tumors from Apc1638N, a mouse model for Apc-driven carcinogenesis. Carcinogenesis **18(2):** 321–327.
37. ZACHOS, G. & D.A. SPANDIDOS. 1997. Expression of ras proto-oncogenes: Regulation and implications in the development of human tumors. Crit. Rev. Oncol. Hematol. **26:** 65–75.
38. TELANG, N.T., R. NARAYANAN, L. BRADLOW & M.P. OSBORNE. 1991. Coordinated expression of intermediate biomarkers for tumorigenic transformation in RAS-

transfected mouse mammary epithelial cells. Breast Cancer Res. Treat. **18:** 155–163.

39. ELSON, C.E. 1995. Suppression of mevalonate pathway activities by dietary isoprenoids: Protective roles in cancer and cardiovascular disease. J. Nutr. **125:** 1666S–1672S.

40. KELLOFF, G., R.A. LUBET, J.R. FAY, V.E. STEELE, C.W. BOONE, J.A. CROWELL & C.C. SIGMAN. 1997. Farnesyl protein transferase inhibitors as potential cancer chemopreventives. Cancer Epidemiol. Biomarkers Prev. **6:** 267–282.

41. KRITCHEVSKY, D., A.W. MOYER, W.C. TESAR, J.B. LOGAN, R.A. BROWN & G. RICHMOND. 1954. Squalene feeding in experimental atherosclerosis. Circ. Res. **11:** 340–343.

42. STRANDBERG, T.E., R.S. TILVIS & T.A. MIETTINEN. 1990. Metabolic variables of cholesterol during squalene feeding in humans: Comparison with cholestyramine treatment. J. Lipid Res. **31:** 1637–1643.

43. CHAN, P., B. TOMLINSON, C.B. LEE & Y.S. LEE. 1996. Effectiveness and safety of low-dose pravastatin and squalene, alone and in combination, in elderly patients with hypercholesterolemia. J. Clin. Pharmacol. **36:** 422–427.

44. GERBER, M. 1994. Olive oil and cancer. *In* Epidemiology of Diet and Cancer. M.J. Hill, A. Giacosa & C.P.J. Caygill, Eds. Ellis Horwood. New York.

45. MATHEWS, J. 1992. Sharks still intrigue cancer researchers. News report. J. Natl. Cancer Inst. **84:** 1000–1002.

Multifunctional Aspects of the Action of Indole-3-Carbinol as an Antitumor Agent

H. LEON BRADLOW,[a] DANIEL W. SEPKOVIC, NITIN T. TELANG,
AND MICHAEL P. OSBORNE

Strang Cancer Research Laboratory, New York, New York 10021, USA

ABSTRACT: Previous studies from this laboratory have suggested that 2-hydroxyestrone is protective against breast cancer, whereas the other principal metabolite, 16α-hydroxyestrone, and the lesser metabolite quantitatively, 4-hydroxyestrone, are potent carcinogens. Attempts to directly decrease the formation of the 16-hydroxylated metabolite were either unsuccessful or required such high levels of the therapeutic agent as to be impractical. On the other hand the concentration of the protective metabolite, 2-hydroxyestrone, proved to be readily modulated by a variety of agents, both in the direction of increased protection and the opposite direction, increased risk by a variety of agents and activities. We have focussed our attention on indole-3-carbinol, a compound found in cruciferous vegetables, and its further metabolites in the body, diindolylmethane (DIM) and indolylcarbazole (ICZ), because of its relative safty and multifaceted activities. It has been shown that it induces CyP4501A1, increasing 2-hydroxylation of estrogens, leading to the protective 2-OHE1, and also decreases CyP1B1 sharply, inhibiting 4-hydroxylation of estradiol, thereby decreasing the formation of the carcinogenic 4-OHE1. In addition to these indirect effects as a result of altered estrogen metabolism, indole-3-carbinol has been shown to have direct effects on apoptosis and cyclin D, resulting in blockage of the cell cycle. In addition to its antitumor activity in animals, it has also been shown to be effective against HPV-mediated tumors in human patients. All of these responses make the study of its behavior as a therapeutic agent of considerable interest.

In studies dating back to the early 1980s, we have shown that increased 16α-hydroxylation of estradiol relative to 2-hydroxylation was observed in newly diagnosed breast cancer cases[1] and that cancer-inducing viruses, oncogenes, and carcinogens[2–4] all acted to increase this reaction. This reaction was also elevated in cell culture by the addition of chlorinated but not by phosphorus-based pesticides.[5] See FIGURE 1 for the structure of the estrogen metabolites.

The product of this reaction, 16α-hydroxyestrone (16α-OHE1), is a potent inducer of unscheduled DNA synthesis, as well as proliferation and anchorage-independent growth,[6] all markers of increased tumorigenicity. Studies by other investigators[7,8] have also pointed to 4-hydroxyestrogens as potent carcinogens be-

[a]Address for communication: Strang Cancer Prevention Center, The Rockefeller University, Box 231, 1230 York Avenue, New York, NY 10021. Voice: 212-746-5431; fax: 212-746-5413.
e-mail: leon@rockvax. rockefeller.edu

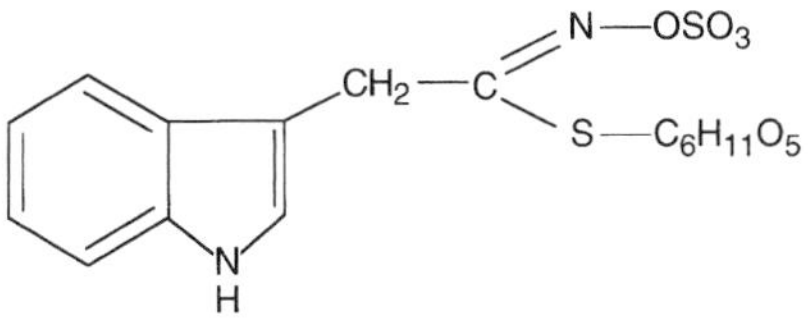

Indole-3-glucosinolate

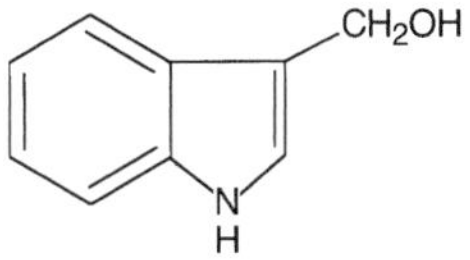

Indole-3-carbinol (I3C)

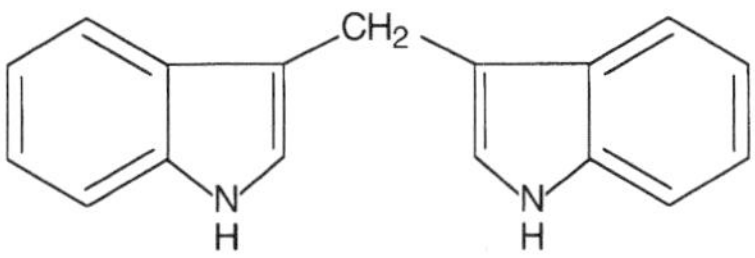

Diindolylmethane

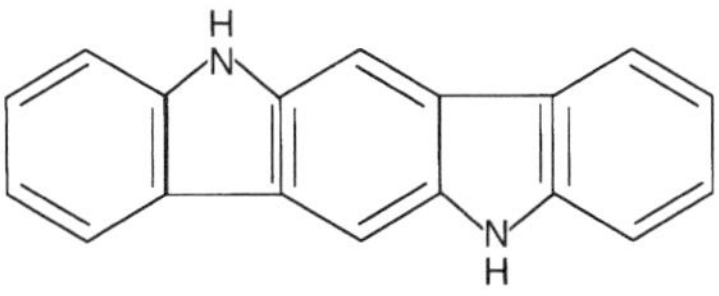

Indole (3, 2, b) carbazole (ICZ)

FIGURE 1. Structure of estrogen metabolites.

cause of their ability to enter into redox cycling leading to free radicals capable of effecting DNA damage. 2-Hydroxyestrone (2-OHE1), on the other hand, was shown to be protective against all of the parameters elevated by 16α-OHE1.[9] Attempts to alter the risk of breast cancer by decreasing the formation of 16α-OHE1 in human subjects were largely unsuccessful except at such high doses of thyroid hormone that undesirable side effects resulted. The results suggested that the extent of 16α-hydroxylation was relatively constitutive and not readily altered.[10]

The extent of 2-hydroxylation, on the other hand, proved to be relatively easy to modulate.[11–14] At least two of these modulators, smoking and dioxin exposure, were clearly not feasible approaches for long-term chemoprevention. Because it had been reported that indole-3-carbinol (I3C) was capable of inducing CyP4501A1, the same enzyme induced by smoking and dioxin, we turned to exploring the application of this compound (found in cruciferous vegetables) to the induction of estradiol 2-hydroxylation.

I3C is present as a glucosinolate complex (FIG. 2) in cruciferous vegetables (broccoli, brussels sprouts, cabbage, cauliflower, and bok choy) along with many other glucosinolates, including one that yields sulforaphane, another antitumor drug as its hydrolysis product. The actual concentration of the various glucosinolates var-

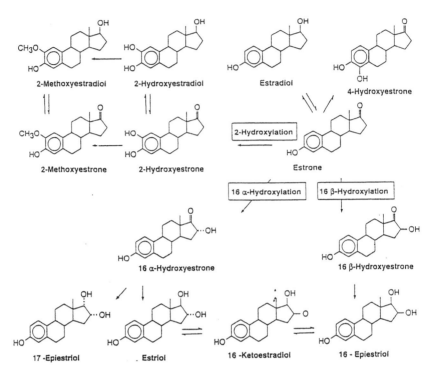

FIGURE 2. Structure of glucobrassicanin, indole-3-carbinol, and its metabolites, diindolylmethane (DIM) and indolylcarbazole (ICZ).

ies widely, depending on the seed strain as well as the soil, climate, and rainfall.[15] Because of this wide range in concentration, which makes it difficult to carry out large-scale feeding studies in a uniform manner using foods as a source of I3C, we have resorted to using the pure compound (given as a capsule) in order to insure uniformity over the course of the study period.

Early studies demonstrated that I3C was effective only when given orally and not when given ip or iv.[16] The reason for this was shown to be the fact that I3C is actually a prodrug that is converted by stomach acid to diindolylmethane (DIM) and indolylcarbazole (ICZ), which are active inducers of CyP4501A1.[17,18] In addition I3C is converted quantitatively at 37°C in tissue culture media to DIM.[19] Stomach acid also converts some of the I3C to a complex mixture of multimers with unknown biological activities. Studies by Niwa *et al.* and Tiwari *et al.*[19,20] showed that of the indole derivatives studied, I3C was the most potent at inducing 2-hydroxylation of estradiol. Cell culture studies also showed that I3C shows a greater inducing ability in Er+ cell lines than in Er– cell lines, where the response was only minimal. This response is similar to our previous observations when dioxin was studied.[14]

More recent studies have expanded our understanding of its role in altering cell-cycle regulation and apoptosis[21,22] and inhibition of 1B1mRNA, and the formation of 4-OHE1,[23] a known carcinogen, as well as noncancer-related effects on enzymes and heart muscle cells.[24,25]

In cell culture studies, the compound was added as a 1% solution in alcohol, whereas in animal studies the compound was incorporated into a standard AIN76A formula. In human studies the compound was administered as a capsule.

Following a single dose by gavage in rats, 2-hydroxylation rose rapidly, peaked at 12 hours, and then declined to baseline by 24 hours. One-week studies in human subjects showed a consistent increase in 2-hydroxylation in both men and women.[26] Chronic studies using a 400 mg/day dose over three months showed a continuous response to I3C, with no adverse biochemical side effects.[27] A similar six-week study, comparing 0, 50, 100, 200, 300, and 400 mg/day showed that no response was observed at the lower doses, although the responses to 300 and 400 mg were comparable.[28] Cell-culture studies showed that I3C can normalize a pattern of estrogen metabolism in cells treated with DMBA. A similar improvement in the metabolic pattern was also induced by the addition of tamoxifen or HPR to cells treated with DMBA.[29]

ANTITUMOR STUDIES

Studies from this laboratory showed that spontaneous mammary tumors could be inhibited by feeding 2000 ppm of I3C in an AIN76A diet base.[30] Both the total number of tumor-bearing animals and the number of tumors per animal were reduced at a time when almost all of the control animals had tumors. A lesser response was observed when 500 ppm of I3C was used. When the animals were maintained on a commercial diet, containing some protective compounds, prior to being placed on the I3C/AIN76A diet, the tumor incidence was decreased and the effect of I3C was less apparent.[31]

Grubbs showed that both DMBA- and NMU-induced mammary tumors were inhibited by feeding I3C, starting after the carcinogen initiation. The effect was most dramatic when DMBA was used as the inducing agent where I3C virtually eliminated tumor formation. A lesser but still substantial response was observed following initiation with NMU.[32]

Following the observation in cell culture that the HPV virus increased 16α-hydroxylation of estradiol and that viral proliferation was inhibited by the addition of 2-OHE1,[33] animal studies were carried out. These showed that feeding I3C to nude mice resulted in the inhibition of the formation of papillomatosis cysts.[34] Subsequent human studies showed that these lesions could be inhibited in children treated with I3C.[35] The overall response rate was ~70% in treated individuals. The therapeutic response correlated with an increase in the 2/16α estrogen metabolite ratio. Studies in the endometrium,[36] lung by several groups,[37–41] tongue,[42] colon,[43] and liver[44, 45] all showed protective effects by feeding I3C in animal models.

In the case of aflatoxin-induced tumors, the situation is more complex. Bailey *et al.*, using the brown trout, reported that although I3C inhibited tumor formation induced by feeding aflatoxin to the fish, when given before or during drug treatment, when I3C was given only after initiation with aflatoxin, it appeared to exhibit promotional activity.[46] When aflatoxin was used as a tumor inducer in the F344 rat, Manson *et al.* found that I3C was able to inhibit tumor formation when given before aflatoxin treatment, as well as when given afterwards during the promotional phase.[47]

When DEN-induced hepatocarcinogenesis was studied in the infant-mouse model by Organesian *et al.*, dietary I3C (1500 ppm) given after initiation for the duration of the study served to inhibit hepatocarcinogenesis. The protective effect was observed both in the number and size of the tumors in these mice.[48] The effect is different from the results reported in rats by Stresser (unpublished in ref. 53), where some degree of promotion was observed. They suggested that the situation in humans depends on whether humans are more like mice than rats.[48] Unpublished observations from our laboratory in the adult F-344 rat primed with DEN, using the protocol described by Williams,[50] also showed an absence of promotional effects.

EFFECT OF I3C ON ENZYMES

Studies by Manson and colleagues showed that I3C could inhibit the induction of ornithine decarboxylase (ODC) in both human breast and colon cell lines. This decrease in enzyme activity correlated in part with a decrease in cell growth in these cell lines. A similar decrease in tyrosine kinase activity in these cell lines was also observed.[51] Whereas the results suggest that these enzymes are involved in the inhibitory effect of I3C, they are clearly not responsible for the total effect of I3C on these cell lines. In male rat liver this group showed that I3C induced CYP450 1A1, 1A2, and 2B1 among phase I enzymes, and GST Ye2, as well as quinone oxidoreductase among phase II enzymes. When I3C or its acid condensation products were added directly to liver cell incubation systems, inhibition of enzyme activity was observed, contrasting with the stimulation of enzyme activity observed when liver preparations from animals fed I3C were studied.

Modulation of multiple CyP450 enzymes by indole-3-carbinol has been described by Baldwin and LeBlanc.[52] They explored induction of 7-ethoxy-resorufin (EROD) activity, estradiol 2-hydroxylase, and seven different testosterone hydroxylases. Of these seven, only testosterone 6α-hydroxylase was stimulated. *In vitro* experiments showed that testosterone-6β-hydroxylase was inhibited by I3C and its acid condensation products. Although I3C and its acid condensation products potently stimulate EROD activity and 2-hydroxylase when fed to animals, no direct effect of I3C or its acid condensation products could be detected when added directly to microsomal systems, although Stresser had previously reported that diindolylmethane (DIM) inhibited EROD activity in trout liver microsomes.[53] The acid condensation product apparently contains too little DIM for this inhibitory activity to be detected in their model. The difference between the activation of 2-hydroxylase and EROD activity suggests that different P450s may be involved in these activities. CYP4501A1 primarily accounts for EROD activity, whereas P4501A2 and P4502C11 primarily account for 2-hydroxylase in rat liver. Testosterone 6α-hydroxylase is primarily attributed to CYP-2A1. CYP-3A family members are the major testosterone 6β-hydroxylases and also affect metabolic activation of benzpyrene. The acid condensation products of I3C inhibit CyP450-3A, resulting in decreased activation of chemical carcinogens, so that part of the activity of I3C is to inhibit the activation of chemical carcinogens. These conclusions are further supported by

Wortelboer who showed that 6β-hydroxylation of testosterone was significantly inhibited by I3C in feeding studies and in direct *in vitro* inhibition.[54]

EFFECTS OF I3C ON CELL CYCLE REGULATORY STEPS

Treatment of cultured MCF-7 cells with I3C reversibly decreased the incorporation of [^{3}H]thymidine into cells without affecting viability or estrogen receptor responsiveness. Cell-cycle analysis showed that the cells were arrested in G1/G0. At the same time it was shown that cyclin-dependent kinase 6 (CDK6) is reduced by I3C in a dose-dependent manner. The levels of P21 and P27 CDK inhibitors were increased by 50 percent. These changes were also observed in MDA-MB-231 breast cancer cell lines, showing that the inhibition of cell growth is independent of estrogen receptor signaling.[22]

Telang and colleagues demonstrated in mammoplasty-derived B-184 cells, initiated with BP or her-2-neu, that I3C inhibited aberrant proliferation in initiated and transformed cells. This was shown to be associated with altered cell-cycle progression, estradiol metabolism, and apoptosis. The initiated cells showed a 55–67% decrease in the Go/(S+M) transition phase of the cell cycle, a 72–90% decrease in apoptosis, a 76–106% increase in anchorage-independent growth, and an 88–90% decrease in the 2/16α-metabolite ratio. Exposure to 50 mM I3C caused a 137–210% increase in the Qo/(S+M) ratio, a 4- to 18-fold increase in 2/16α, a 2-fold increase in cellular apoptosis, and a 54–61% inhibition of growth. The preventive effect is due, in part, to its ability to alter all three of these parameters. No such reponse was seen when 16α-OHE1 was used as the test steroid.[23]

CARDIAC-RELATED EFFECTS OF I3C

The effect of the I3C-induced metabolites, 2-OHE1 and 2-MeOE1, on the oxidizability of low-density lipoproteins was explored by Seeger *et al.*[24] They found that the C-2 metabolites inhibited the oxidation of LDL, which converts it into a toxic product when taken up by macrophages. Ox-LDL also directly increases the formation of endothelin-1. The C-2 metabolites were more potent than E2 or 16α-OHE1. The antioxidative potency of the C-2 metabolites exceeded that of vitamin E.

These compounds also inhibited smooth muscle cell proliferation, with the 2-methoxy compound being twice as potent as E2 with no estrogenic side effects, whereas 16α-OHE1 was devoid of such activity.[25] In the first study using breast cancer cells and looking for synergistic responses, Bjeldanes and colleagues reported that I3C plus tamoxifen resulted in a greater inhibitory response in MCF-7 cells than either compound alone.[55]

CONCLUSIONS

The results described above show a remarkable variety of therapeutic responses to I3C, not only against cancers but also against heart disease. In some animal models a promotional response has been reported when I3C was given after initiation by a carcinogen, but this has not been confirmed in other studies. Long-term studies in human subjects have not shown any harmful responses. Further studies on the benefits of combination therapy are under way and offer promise of benefits at lower doses of I3C and other compounds. Because of its relative stability and the absence of the multimers, the use of DIM, instead of I3C, has attracted some attention but has not displaced I3C thus far.

REFERENCES

1. SCHNEIDER, J., D. KINNE, A. FRACCHIA, V. PIERCE, K.E. ANDERSON, H.L. BRADLOW & J. FISHMAN. 1982. Abnormal oxidative metabolism of estradiol in women with breast cancer. Proc. Natl. Acad. Sci. USA 79(9): 3047–3051.
2. BRADLOW, H.L., R.J. HERSHCOPF, C.P. MARTUCCI & J. FISHMAN. 1985. Estradiol 16α-hydroxylation in the mouse correlates with mammary tumor incidence and presence of murine mammary tumor virus: A possible model for the hormonal etiology of breast cancer in humans. Proc. Natl. Acad. Sci. USA 82: 6295–6299.
3. TELANG, N.T., R. NARAYANEN, H.L. BRADLOW & M.P. OSBORNE. 1991. Coordinated expression of intermediate biomarkers for tumorigenic transformation in Ras-transfected mouse mammary epithelial cells. Breast Cancer Res. Treat. 18: 155–163.
4. TELANG, N.T., H.L. BRADLOW, H. KURIHARA & M.P. OSBORNE. 1989. In vitro biotransformation of estradiol by explant cultures of murine mammary tissues. Breast Cancer Res. Treat. 13: 173–181.
5. BRADLOW, H.L., D. DAVIS, D.W. SEPKOVIC, R. TIWARI & M.P. OSBORNE. 1998. Role of the estrogen receptor in the action of organochlorine pesticides on estrogen metabolism in human breast cancer cell lines. Sci. Total Environ. 202: 9–14.
6. TELANG, N.T., A. SUTO, G.Y. WONG, M.P. OSBORNE & H.L. BRADLOW. 1992. Estrogen metabolite 16α-hydroxyestrone induces genotoxic damage and aberrant cell proliferation in mouse mammary epithelial cells in culture. J. Natl. Cancer Inst. 84: 634–638.
7. LIEHR, J.G. & M.J. RICCI. 1996. 4-Hydroxylation of estrogens as marker of human mammary tumors. Proc. Natl. Acad. Sci. USA 93: 3294–3296.
8. DWIVEDY, I., P. DEVANESAN, P. CREMONESI, E. ROGAN & E. CAVALIERI. 1992. Synthesis and characterization of estrogen 2,3- and 3,4-quinones. Comparison of DNA adducts formed by the quinones versus horseradish peroxidase-activated catechol estrogens. Chem. Res. Toxicol. 5: 828–833.
9. SUTO, A., H.L. BRADLOW, T. KUBOTA, M. KITAJIMA, G.Y. WONG, M.P. OSBORNE & N.T. TELANG. 1993. Alteration in proliferative and endocrine responsiveness of human mammary carcinoma cells by prototypic tumor-suppressing agents. Steroids 58: 215–219.
10. OSBORNE, M.P., R.A. KARMALI, R.J. HERSHCOPF, H.L. BRADLOW, I.A. KOURIDES, W.R. WILLIAMS, P.P. ROSEN & J. FISHMAN. 1988. Omega-3 fatty acids: Modulation of estrogen metabolism and potential for breast cancer prevention. Cancer Invest. 8: 629–631.
11. KAPPAS, A., K.E. ANDERSON, A.H. CONNEY, E.J. PANTUCK, J. FISHMAN & H.L. BRADLOW. 1983. Nutrition-endocrine interactions: Induction of reciprocal changes in the D4-5a-reduction of testosterone and the cytochrome P-450-dependent oxidation of estradiol by dietary macronutrients in man. Proc. Natl. Acad. Sci. USA 80: 7646–7649.
12. ANDERSON, K.E., A. KAPPAS, A.H. CONNEY, H.L. BRADLOW & J. FISHMAN. 1984. The influence of dietary protein and carbohydrate on the principal oxidative biotransformations of estradiol in normal subjects. J. Clin. Endocrinol. Metab. 59: 103–107.
13. MICHNOVICZ, J.J., H. NAGANUMA, R.J. HERSHCOPF, H.L. BRADLOW & J. FISHMAN. 1988. Increased urinary catechol estrogen excretion in female smokers. Steroids 52: 69–83.

14. GIERTHY, J.F., D.W. LINCOLN II, S.J. KAMPCIK, H.W. DICKERMAN, H.L. BRADLOW, T. NIWA & G.E. SWANECK. 1988. Induction of human breast cancer cells by 2,3,7,8-tetrachlorodibenzo-P-dioxin. Biochem. Biophys. Res. Commun. **157:** 50–55.

15. MCDANELL, R., A.E. MCLEAN, A.B. HANLEY, R.K. HEANEY & G.R. FENWICK. 1987. Differential induction of mixed-function oxidase (MFO) activity in rat liver and intestine by diets containing processed cabbage: Correlation with cabbage levels of glucosinolates and glucosinolate hydrolysis products. Food Chem. Toxicol. **25:** 363–368.

16. BRADFIELD, C.A. & L.F. BJELDANES. 1987. Structure-activity relationships of dietary indoles: A proposed mechanism of action as modifiers of xenobiotic metabolism. J. Toxicol. Environ. Health **21:** 311–323.

17. BJELDANES, L.F., J.Y. KIM, K.R. GROSE, J.C. BARTHOLOMEW & C.A. BRADFIELD. 1991. Aromatic hydrocarbon responsiveness-receptor agonists generated from indole-3-carbinol *in vitro* and *in vivo*: Comparisons with 2,3,7,8-tetrachloro-dibenzo-*p*-dioxin. Proc. Natl. Acad. Sci. USA **88:** 9543–9547.

18. JELLINCK, P.H., P.G. FORKERT, D.S. RIDDICK, A.B. OKEY, J.J. MICHNOVICZ & H.L. BRADLOW. 1993. Ah receptor binding properties of indole carbinols and induction of hepatic estradiol hydroxylation. Biochem. Pharmacol. **45:** 1129–1136.

19. NIWA, T., G. SWANECK & H.L. BRADLOW. 1994. Alterations in estradiol metabolism in MCF-7 cells induced by treatment with indole-3-carbinol and related compounds. Steroids **59:** 523–527.

20. TIWARI, R.K., H.L. BRADLOW, N.T. TELANG & M.P. OSBORNE. 1994. Selective responses of human breast cancer cells to indole-3-carbinol, a chemopreventive agent. J. Natl. Cancer Inst. **86:** 126–131.

21. COVER, C.M., S.J. HSIEH, S.H. TRANS, G. HALLDEN, G.S. KIM, L.F. BJELDANES & G.L. FIRESTONE. 1998. Indole-3-carbinol inhibits the expression of cyclin-dependent kinase-6 and induces a G1 cell cycle arrest of human breast cancer cells independent of estrogen receptor signalling. J. Biol. Chem. **273:** 2828–2847.

22. TELANG, N.T., M. KATDARE, H.L. BRADLOW, M.P. OSBORNE & J. FISHMAN. 1997. Inhibition of proliferation and modulation of estradiol metabolism: Novel mechanisms for breast cancer prevention by the phytochemical indole-3-carbinol. Proc. Soc. Exp. Biol. Med. **216:** 246–252.

23. YUAN, F., D.Z. CHEN, K. LIU, D.W. SEPKOVIC, H.L. BRADLOW & K. AUBORN. 1999. Anti-estrogenic activities of indole-3-carbinol in cervical cells: Implication for prevention of cervical cancer. Anticancer Res. **19** (3A): 1673–1680.

24. SEEGER, H., A.O. MUECK & T.H. LIPPERT. 1997. Effect of estradiol metabolites on the susceptibility of low density lipoprotein to oxidation. Life Sci. **61:** 865–868.

25. SEEGER, H., A.O. MUECK & T.H. LIPPERT. 1998. The antiproliferative effect of 17β-estradiol metabolites on human cronary artery smooth muscle cells. Med. Sci. Res. **26:** 481–482.

26. MICHNOVICZ, J.J. & H.L. BRADLOW. 1990. Induction of estradiol metabolism by dietary indole-3-carbinol in humans. J. Natl. Cancer Inst. **50:** 947–950.

27. BRADLOW, H.L., J.J. MICHNOVICZ, G.Y.C. WONG, M.P. HALPER, D. MILLER & M.P. OSBORNE. 1994. Long term responses of women to indole-3-carbinol or a high fiber diet. Cancer Epidemiol. Biomarkers Prev. **3:** 591–595.

28. WONG, G.Y.C., H.L. BRADLOW, D.W. SEPKOVIC, S. MEHL, J. MAILMAN & M.P. OSBORNE. 1998. A dose-ranging study of indole-3-carbinol for breast cancer prevention J. Cell Biol. **28:** 111–116.

29. SUTO, A., H.L. BRADLOW, T. KUBOTA, M. KITAJIMA, G.Y. WONG, M.P. OSBORNE & N.T. TELANG. 1993. Alteration in proliferative and endocrine responsiveness of human mammary carcinoma cells by prototypic tumor-suppressing agents. Steroids **58:** 215–219.

30. BRADLOW, H.L., R.J. HERSHCOPF, C.P. MARTUCCI & J. FISHMAN. 1995. Estradiol 16α-hydroxylation in the mouse correlates with mammary tumor incidence and presence of murine mammary tumor virus: A possible model for the hormonal etiology of breast cancer in humans. Proc. Natl. Acad. Sci. USA **82:** 6295–6299.

31. MALLOY, V.L., H.L. BRADLOW & N. ORENTREICH. 1998. Interaction between a semisynthetic diet and indole-3-carbinol on mammary tumor incidence in Balb-C3H mice. Anticancer Res. **17:** 4333–4338.

32. GRUBBS, C.J., V.E. STEELE, T. CASEBOLT, M.M. JULIANA, I. ETO, L.M. WHITAKER, K.H. DRAGNEV, G.J. KELLOFF & R.L. LUBET. 1995. Chemoprevention of chemically-induced mammary carcinogenesis by indole-3-carbinol. Anticancer Res. **15:** 709–716.

33. NEWFIELD, L., H.L. BRADLOW, D.W. SEPKOVIC & K. AUBORN. 1998. Estrogen metabolism and the malignant potential of human papillomavirus immortalized keratinocytes. Proc. Soc. Exp. Biol. Med. **217:** 322–326.

34. NEWFIELD, L., A. GOLDSMITH, H.L. BRADLOW & K. AUBORN. 1993. Estrogen metabolism and human papillomavirus-induced tumors of the larynx: Chemoprophylaxis with indole-3-carbinol. Anticancer Res. **13:** 337–342.

35. ROSEN, C.A., J.W. THOMPSON, G.E. WOODSON, A.P. HENGESTEG & H.L. BRADLOW. 1998. Preliminary results of the use of indole-3-carbinol for recurrent respiratory apillomatosis. Otolaryngol. Head Neck Surg. **118:** 810–815.

36. KOJIMA, T., T. TANAKA & H. MORI. 1994. Chemprevention of spontaneous endometrial cancer in female Donryu rats by dietary indole-3-carbinol. Cancer Res. **54:** 1446–1449.

37. STONER, G.D., G. ADAM-RODWELL & M.A. MORSE. 1993. Lung tumors in strain A mice: Application for studies in cancer chemprevention. J. Cell. Biochem. Suppl. **17F:** 95–103.

38. CHUNG, F-L., M.A. MORSE, K.I. EKLIND & Y. XU. 1993. Inhibition of tobacco-specific nitrosamine-induced lung tumorigenesis by compounds derived from cruciferous vegetables and green tea. Ann. N.Y. Acad. Sci. **686:** 186–202.

39. MORSE, M.A., S.D. LAGRECA, S.C. AMIN & F.L. CHUNG. 1990. Effects of indole-3-carbinol on lung tumorigenesis and DNA methylation induced by 4-(methylnitrosamino)-1-(3-pyridyl)-1-butanone (NNK) and on the metabolism and disposition of NNK in A/J mice. Cancer Res. **50:** 2613–2617.

40. EL-BAYOUMY, K., P. UPADHYAYA, D.H. DESAI, S. AMIN, D. HOFFMAN & E.L. WYNDER. 1996. Effects of 1,4-phenylenebis(methylene)selenocyanate, phenethyl-iso-thiocyanate, indole-3-carbinol, and D-limonene individually and in combination on the tumorigenicity of the tobacco-specific nitrosamine 4-(methylnitrosamino)-1-(3-pyridyl)-1-butanone in A/J mouse lung. Anticancer Res. **16:** 2709–2712.

41. TAIOLI, E., S. GARBERS, H.L. BRADLOW, S.G. CARMELLA, S. AKERBAR & S.S. HECHT. 1997. Effects of indole-3-carbinol on the metabolism of 4-(methylnitroso-amino)-1-(3-pyridyl)-1-butanone (NNK) in smokers. Cancer Epidemiol. Biomarkers Prev. **6:** 517–522.

42. TANAKA, T., T. KOJIMA, Y. MORISHITA & H. MORI. 1992. inhibitory effects of the natural products indole-3-carbinol and sinigrin during initiation and promotion phases of 4-nitroquinoline 1-oxide-induced rat tongue carcinogenesis. Jpn. J. Cancer Res. **83:** 835–842.

43. GAMET-PAYRASTRE, L., S. LUMEAU, N. GASC, G. CASSAR, P. ROLLIN & J. TULIEZ. 1998. Selective cytostatic and cytotoxic effects of glucosinolate hydrolysis products on human colon cancer cells *in vitro*. Anticancer Drugs **9:** 141–148.

44. TANAKA, T., Y. MORI, Y. MORISHITA, A. HARA, T. OHNO, T. KOJIMA & H. MORI. 1990. Inhibitory effect of sinigrin and indole-3-carbinol on diethylnitroamine-induced hepatocarcinogenesis in male ACI/N rats. Carcinogenesis **11:** 1403–1406.

45. BAILEY, G.S., R.H. DASHWOOD, A.T. FONG, D.E. WILLIAMS, R.A. SCANLAN & J.D. HENDRICKS. 1991. Modulation of mycotoxin and nitrosamine carcinogenesis by indole-3-carbinol: Quantitative analysis of inhibition versus promotion. *In* Relevance to Human Cancer of *N*-Nitroso Compounds. I.K. O'Neill, J. Chen & H. Bartsch, Eds.: 275–280. International Agency for Research on Cancer. Lyon.

46. BAILEY, G.S., J.D. HENDRICKS, D.W. SHELTON, J.E. NIXON & N. PAWLOWSHI. 1987. Enhancement of carcinogenesis by the natural anti-carcinogen indole-3-carbinol. J. Natl. Cancer Inst. **78:** 931–934.

47. MANSON, M.M., E.H. HUDSON, H.W.L. BALL, M.C. BARRETT, H.L. CLARK, D.J. JUDAH, R.D. VERSCHOYLE & G.E. NEAL. 1999. Chemoprevention of aflatoxin B$_1$-induced carcinogenesis by indole-3-carbinol in rat liver—Predicting the outcome using early biomarkers. Carcinogenesis. In press.

48. ORGANESIAN, A., J.D. HENDRICKS & D.E. WILLIAMS. 1997. Long term dietary indole-3-carbinol inhibits diethylnitrosamine-initiated hepatocarcinogenesis in the infant mouse model. Cancer Lett. **118:** 87–94.

49. KIM, D.J., K.K. LEE, B.S. HAN, B. AHN, J.H. BAE & J.J. JANG. 1994. Biphasic modifying effect of indole-3-carbinol on diethylnitrosamine-induced preneoplastic glutathione S-transferase placental form-positive liver cell foci in sprague-Dawley rats. Jpn. J. Cancer Res. **86:** 578–583.

50. WILLIAMS, G.M., M.J. IATROPOULOS, C.X. WANG, N. ALI, A. RIVENSON, L.A. PETERSON, C. SCHULZ & R. GEBHARDT. 1996. Diethylnitrosamine exposure-responses for DNA damage, centrilobular cytotoxicity, cell proliferation and carcinogenesis in rat liver exhibit some non-linearities. Carcinogenesis **17:** 2253–2258.

51. HUDSON, E.A., R.J.L. MUNKS, L. HOOWELLS, H.W.L. BALL, P. PAMAR & M.M. MANSON. 1998. Mechanism of action of indole-3-carbinol as a chemo-preventive agent. Abstr. 1965 AACR meeting.

52. BALDWIN, W.S. & G.A. LEBLANC. 1992. The anti-carcinogenic plant compound indole-3-carbinol differentially modulates P-450 mediated steroid hydroxylase activities in mice. Chem. Biol. Interact. **83:** 155–169.

53. STRESSER, D.M., D.E. WILLIAMS & G.S. BAILEY. 1991. Diindolylmethane (I33′), the linear dimer of indole-3-carbinol (I3C) is a potent inhibitor of P450 1A1 in trout. Toxicologist **11:** 1309.

54. WORTELBOER, H.M., C.A. DE KRUIF, A.A. VAN IERSEL, H.E. FALKE, J. NOORDHOEK & B.J. BLAUBOER. 1992. Acid reaction products of indole-3-carbinol and their effects on cytochrome P450 and phase II enzymes in rat and monkey hepatocytes. Biochem. Pharmacol. **43:** 1439–444.

55. COVER, C.M., S.J. HSIEH, E.J. CRAM, C. HONG, J.E. RIBY, L.F. BJELDANES & G.L. FIRESTONE. 1999. Indole-3-carbinol and tamoxifen cooperate to arrest the cell cycle of MCF-7 human breast cancer cells. Cancer Res. **59:** 1244–1251.

Resveratrol Inhibits Cyclooxygenase-2 Transcription in Human Mammary Epithelial Cells

KOTHA SUBBARAMAIAH,[a,b,c,f] PEDRO MICHALUART,[d] WEN JING CHUNG,[a] TADASHI TANABE,[e] NITIN TELANG,[c] AND ANDREW J. DANNENBERG[a,b,c]

Departments of [a]Medicine and [b]Surgery, the New York Presbyterian Hospital-Cornell, New York, New York 10021, USA

[c]Anne Fisher Nutrition Center at Strang Cancer Prevention Center, New York, New York 10021, USA

[d]Head and Neck Service, Department of Surgery, Memorial Sloan-Kettering Cancer Center, New York, New York 10021, USA

[e]Department of Pharmacology, National Cardiovascular Center Research Institute, Osaka, Japan

ABSTRACT: A large body of evidence suggests that inhibiting cyclooxygenase-2 (COX-2), the inducible form of COX, will be an important strategy for preventing cancer. In this study, we investigated whether resveratrol, a chemopreventive agent found in grapes, could suppress phorbol ester (PMA)-mediated induction of COX-2 in human mammary and oral epithelial cells. Treatment of cells with PMA induced COX-2 mRNA, COX-2 protein, and prostaglandin synthesis. These effects were inhibited by resveratrol. Nuclear runoffs revealed increased rates of COX-2 transcription after treatment with PMA, an effect that was inhibited by resveratrol. Resveratrol inhibited PMA-mediated activation of protein kinase C and the induction of COX-2 promoter activity by c-Jun. Phorbol ester-mediated induction of AP-1 activity was blocked by resveratrol. These data are likely to be important for understanding the anticancer and anti-inflammatory properties of resveratrol.

INTRODUCTION

Cyclooxygenases (COX) catalyze the synthesis of prostaglandins (PGs) from arachidonic acid. There are two isoforms of COX, designated COX-1 and COX-2. COX-1 is expressed constitutively in most tissues and appears to be responsible for housekeeping functions.[1] By contrast, COX-2 is not detectable in most normal tissues but is induced by oncogenes, growth factors, carcinogens, and tumor promoters.[2–4]

Multiple lines of evidence support the idea that COX-2 is important in carcinogenesis. Thus, COX-2 is upregulated in transformed cells[2,5,6] and in malignant tis-

---

[f]Address for communication: New York Presbyterian Hospital-Cornell, Division of Gastroenterology, Room F-201, 1300 York Avenue, New York, NY 10021. Voice: 212-746-4402; fax: 212-746-4885.

e-mail: ksubba@mail.med.cornell.edu

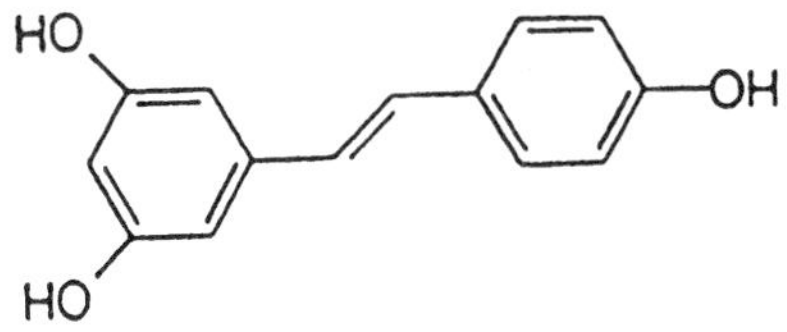

FIGURE 1. Structure of resveratrol. (Subbaramaiah *et al.*[15] With permission from the *Journal of Biological Chemistry.*)

sues.[7–10] A null mutation for *COX-2* in APC$^{\Delta 716}$[11] knockout mice, a murine model of familial adenomatous polyposis, markedly reduces the number and size of intestinal tumors.[11] Furthermore, treatment with a selective inhibitor of COX-2 caused nearly complete suppression of azoxymethane-induced colon cancer.[12] These studies suggest that targeted inhibition of COX-2 is a promising approach to prevent cancer. Although chemopreventive strategies have focused on inhibitors of COX enzyme activity, an equally important strategy may be to identify compounds that suppress amounts of COX-2.[13–15]

Resveratrol, a phytoalexin found in grapes and other foods, has anti-inflammatory and anticancer effects (FIG. 1).[16] It inhibits the development of preneoplastic lesions in carcinogen-treated mouse mammary glands, for example, and it blocks tumorigenesis in a two-stage model of skin cancer that was promoted by treatment with phorbol ester (PMA).[16] The anti-inflammatory properties of resveratrol were demonstrated by suppression of carrageenan-induced pedal edema, an effect attributed to suppression of PG synthesis.[16] In the current work, we have built upon prior observations concerning the effects of resveratrol on PG synthesis by determining if resveratrol modulates the expression of the *COX-2* gene. Our data show that resveratrol suppresses the activation of *COX-2* gene expression by inhibiting the protein kinase C (PKC) signal transduction pathway. These data provide a mechanistic basis for the chemopreventive and anti-inflammatory properties of resveratrol.

MATERIAL AND METHODS

Material

MEM medium, PKC assay kits, and LipofectAMINE were from Life Technologies, Inc. (Grand Island, NY). Keratinocyte basal medium (KBM) and growth medium (KGM) were from Clonetics Corporation (San Diego, CA). PMA, sodium arachidonate, *trans*-resveratrol, epidermal growth factor, hydrocortisone and *O*-nitrophenyl-β-D-galactopyranoside were from Sigma Chemical Co. (St. Louis, MO). Enzyme immunoassay reagents for PGE$_2$ assays were from the Cayman Company (Ann Arbor, MI). [^{32}P]CTP was from DuPont-NEN (Boston, MA). Random-priming kits were from Boehringer Mannheim Biochemicals (Indianapolis, IN). Nitrocellulose membranes were from Schleicher & Schuell (Keene, NH). Reagents for the luciferase assay were from Analytical Luminescence (San Diego, CA). The 18S rRNA cDNA was from Ambion, Inc. (Austin, TX). Rabbit polyclonal antihuman COX-2 antiserum was from Oxford Biomedical Research, Inc. (Oxford, MI). Goat polyclonal antihuman COX-1 antiserum was from Santa Cruz Biotechnology, Inc. (Santa Cruz, CA). Western blotting detection reagents (ECL) were from Amersham (Arlington Heights, Ill.). Plasmid DNA was prepared using a kit from the Promega Corporation (Madison, WI).

Tissue Culture

The 184B5/HER cell line has been described previously.[17] Cells were maintained in MEM-KBM mixed in a ratio of 1:1 (basal medium) containing EGF (10 ng/mL), hydrocortisone (0.5 µg/mL), transferrin (10 µg/mL), gentamicin (5 µg/mL), and insulin (10 µg/mL) (growth medium). Cells were grown to 60% confluence, trypsinized with 0.05% trypsin-2 mM EDTA, and plated for experimental use. MSK Leuk1 was established from a dysplastic leukoplakia lesion adjacent to a squamous cell carcinoma of the tongue in a 46-year-old nonsmoking female.[18] Cells were routinely maintained in KGM and passaged using 0.125% trypsin-2 mM EDTA. In all experiments, 184B5/HER and MSK Leuk1 cells were grown in basal medium for 24 h prior to treatment. Treatment with vehicle (0.2% DMSO), resveratrol, or PMA was always carried out in basal medium.

PGE₂ Production

5×10^4 cells/well were plated in 6-well dishes and grown to 60% confluence in growth medium. The cells were then treated as described below. Levels of PGE_2 released by the cells were measured by enzyme immunoassay. Amounts of PGE_2 produced were normalized to protein concentrations.

Western Blotting

Analysis was done with a rabbit polyclonal anti-COX-2 antiserum or a polyclonal anti-COX-1 antiserum, as described in detail in reference 15.

Northern Blotting

Analysis was done with a radiolabeled human COX-2 cDNA, as described in reference 15.

Nuclear Runoff Assay

2.5×10^5 cells were plated in four T150 dishes for each condition. Cells were grown in growth medium until approximately 60% confluent. Nuclei were isolated and stored in liquid nitrogen. The transcription assay was performed, as described previously.[15]

Plasmids

The *COX-2* promoter construct (−327/+59) has been described previously.[19] The human *COX-2* cDNA was generously provided by Dr. Stephen M. Prescott (University of Utah, Salt Lake City, UT). RSV-c-*jun* was a gift from Dr. Tom Curran (Roche Laboratories, Nutley, NJ). The activator protein 1 (AP-1) reporter plasmid (2 × TRE-luciferase), composed of two copies of the consensus TRE ligated to luciferase, was kindly provided by Dr. Joan Heller Brown (University of California, La Jolla, CA). pSV-βgal was obtained from Promega Corporation (Madison, WI).

Transient Transfection Assays

184B5/HER cells were seeded at a density of 5×10^4 cells/well in 6-well dishes and grown to 50–60% confluence. Transfections and analyses were carried out, as described previously.[15]

Protein Kinase C Assay

The activity of PKC was measured according to directions from Life Technologies, Incorporated. Briefly, cells were plated in 10 cm dishes at 10^6 cells/dish and grown to 60% confluence. Cells were then treated with fresh basal medium containing vehicle (0.2% DMSO), PMA (50 ng/mL), or PMA (50 ng/mL) plus resveratrol (15 μM) for 30 minutes. Total PKC activity was measured in cell lysates. To determine cytosolic and membrane-bound PKC activity, cell lysates were centrifuged at $100,000 \times g$ for 30 minutes. The resulting supernatant contained cytosolic PKC; membrane-bound PKC activity was present in the pellet. Subsequently, DEAE cellulose columns were used to partially purify PKC enzymes. Protein kinase C activity was then measured by incubating partially purified PKC with $[\gamma\text{-}^{32}\text{P}]\text{ATP}$ (3000–6000 Ci/mmol) and the substrate myelin basic protein for 20 min at room temperature. The activity of PKC is expressed as CPM incorporated/μg protein.

Statistics

Comparisons between groups were made by the Student's *t*-test. A difference between groups of $p < 0.05$ was considered significant.

RESULTS

Resveratrol Inhibits the Induction of COX-2 by Phorbol Esters

We investigated whether resveratrol inhibited PMA-mediated induction of PG synthesis by suppressing the induction of COX-2. Cells were cotreated for 4.5 h with PMA and the indicated concentrations of resveratrol. The medium then was replaced, and the synthesis of PGs was measured in the absence of resveratrol over the next 30 minutes. PMA in this setting caused about a twofold increase in synthesis of PGE_2. This effect was suppressed by resveratrol in a dose-dependent manner (FIG. 2). To confirm that these effects of resveratrol were not unique to mammary epithelial cells, we also determined whether resveratrol inhibited PMA-mediated induction of PG synthesis in a premalignant, oral leukoplakia cell line. Treatment of these cells with PMA led to a twofold increase in PG synthesis. This effect was inhibited completely by 20 μM resveratrol (data not shown).

Immunoblotting was performed to determine whether the above effects on production of PGE_2 could be related to differences in levels of COX. FIGURE 3A shows that PMA induced COX-2 in human mammary epithelial cells. Cotreatment with resveratrol caused a dose-dependent decrease in PMA-mediated induction of COX-2; the maximal drug effect was observed at 15–20 μM. Neither PMA nor resveratrol altered amounts of COX-1 (data not shown). The ability of resveratrol to suppress the induction of COX-2 was not limited to mammary cells but was also demonstrable in oral epithelial cells (FIG. 3B).

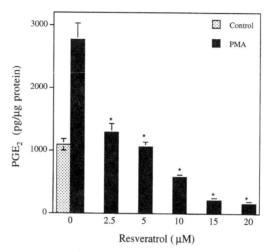

FIGURE 2. Resveratrol inhibits phorbol ester–mediated induction of PGE_2 synthesis. 184B5/HER cells were treated with vehicle (stippled column), PMA (50 ng/mL, black column), or PMA (50 ng/mL) and resveratrol for 4.5 hours. The medium was then replaced with basal medium and 10 μM sodium arachidonate. Thirty minutes later, the medium was collected to measure the amount of production of PGE_2. Synthesis of PGE_2 was determined by enzyme immunoassay. Columns, means; bars, SD; n = 6. *, $p < 0.001$, compared with PMA. (Subbaramaiah et al.[15] With permission from the *Journal of Biological Chemistry*.)

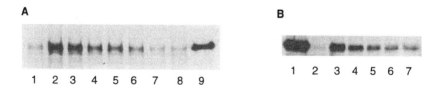

FIGURE 3. Resveratrol inhibits PMA-mediated induction of COX-2 in human mammary and oral epithelial cells. **A:** Lysate protein was from 184B5/HER cells treated with vehicle (lane 1), PMA (50 ng/mL, lane 2), or PMA (50 ng/mL) and resveratrol (2.5, 5, 7.5, 10, 15, 30 μM; lanes 3–8) for 4.5 hours. Lane 9 represents an ovine COX-2 standard. **B:** Lysates were from premalignant oral epithelial (MSK Leuk1) cells treated with vehicle (lane 2), PMA (50 ng/mL, lane 3), or PMA (50 ng/mL) and resveratrol (10, 20, 30, 40 μM; lanes 4–7) for 4.5 hours. Lane 1 represents an ovine COX-2 standard. Cellular lysate protein (25 μg/lane) was loaded onto a 10% SDS-polyacrylamide gel, electrophoresed, and subsequently transferred onto nitrocellulose. Western blots were probed with antibody specific for COX-2. (Subbaramaiah et al.[15] With permission from the *Journal of Biological Chemistry*.)

To further elucidate the mechanism responsible for the changes in amounts of COX-2 protein, we determined steady-state levels of COX-2 mRNA by Northern blotting. Treatment with PMA resulted in a marked increase in levels of COX-2 mRNA, an effect that was suppressed by resveratrol in a concentration-dependent manner (FIG. 4). Differences in levels of mRNA could reflect altered rates of transcription or changes in mRNA stability. Nuclear runoffs were performed to distin-

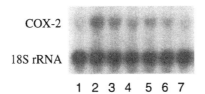

FIGURE 4. Resveratrol inhibits PMA-mediated induction of COX-2 mRNA. 184B5/HER cells were treated with vehicle (lane 1), PMA (50 ng/mL, lane 2), or PMA (50 ng/mL) and resveratrol (2.5, 5, 10, 15, 20 μM; lanes 3–7) for 3 hours. Total cellular RNA was isolated; 10 μg of RNA was added to each lane. The Northern blot was hybridized with probes that recognized mRNAs for COX-2 and 18S rRNA. Results of densitometry in arbitrary units: lane 1, 18; lane 2, 225; lane 3, 135; lane 4, 72; lane 5, 45; lane 6, 42; lane 7, 9. (Subbaramaiah *et al.*[15] With permission from the *Journal of Biological Chemistry*.)

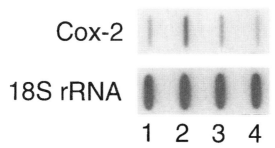

FIGURE 5. Phorbol ester–mediated induction of COX-2 transcription is inhibited by resveratrol. 184B5/HER cells were treated with vehicle (lane 1), PMA (50 ng/mL, lane 2), or PMA (50 ng/mL) and resveratrol (5 μM, lane 3; 10 μM, lane 4) for 3 hours. Nuclear run-offs were performed. The COX-2 and 18S rRNA cDNAs were immobilized onto nitrocellulose membranes and hybridized with labeled nascent RNA transcripts. Results of densitometry in arbitrary units: lane 1, 19; lane 2, 44; lane 3, 29; lane 4, 16. (Subbaramaiah *et al.*[15] With permission from the *Journal of Biological Chemistry*.)

guish between these possibilities. As shown in FIGURE 5, we observed higher rates of synthesis of nascent COX-2 mRNA after treatment with PMA, consistent with the differences observed by Northern blotting. This effect was suppressed by resveratrol.

Determining the Mechanism by Which Resveratrol Inhibits PMA-mediated Induction of COX-2

Tumor promoters like PMA activate PKC and induce AP-1 activity. It was important, therefore, to determine whether resveratrol inhibited PMA-mediated activation of PKC or AP-1. Treatment of cells with PMA stimulated the translocation of PKC activity from cytosol to membrane, an effect that was blocked by resveratrol (FIG. 6). Additionally, transiently overexpressing c-Jun, a component of the AP-1 transcription factor complex, caused about a fourfold increase in *COX-2* promoter activity. This effect was blocked by resveratrol (FIG. 7A). Resveratrol also suppressed the activation of an AP-1 reporter plasmid by PMA (FIG. 7B).

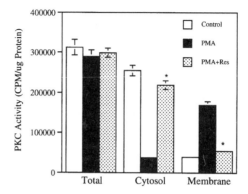

FIGURE 6. Resveratrol inhibits the redistribution of PKC activity mediated by phorbol ester. 184B5/HER cells were treated with vehicle (open column), PMA (50 ng/mL, black column), or PMA (50 ng/mL) and resveratrol (15 μM) (stippled column) for 30 minutes. Total, cytosolic, and membrane PKC activities were determined. Columns, means; bars, SD. n = 6; *, $p < 0.01$ vs. PMA. (Subbaramaiah et al.[15] With permission from the *Journal of Biological Chemistry*.)

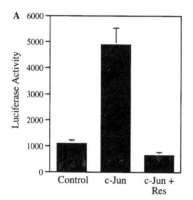 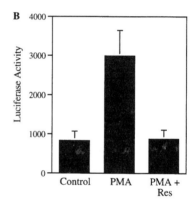

FIGURE 7. Resveratrol inhibits AP-1-mediated induction of COX-2 promoter activity. **A:** 184B5/HER cells were transfected with 0.9 μg of a human *COX-2* promoter construct ligated to luciferase (−327/+59) (control) or 0.9 μg of *COX-2* promoter construct and 0.9 μg of expression vector for c-*jun*. All cells received 0.2 μg of pSVßgal. The total amount of DNA in each reaction was kept constant at 2 μg by using an empty vector. Twenty-four hours later, cells were treated with vehicle or resveratrol (15 μM) for 6 hours. **B:** 184B5/HER cells were cotransfected with 1.8 μg of 2 × TRE-luciferase and 0.2 μg of pSVßgal. Twenty-four hours after transfection, cells were treated with vehicle, PMA (50 ng/mL), or PMA (50 ng/mL) and resveratrol (15 μM) for 6 hours. Luciferase activity represents data that have been normalized with β-galactosidase activity. Six wells were used for each of the conditions. Columns, means; bars, SD. (Subbaramaiah et al.[15] With permission from the *Journal of Biological Chemistry*.)

DISCUSSION

There is considerable evidence that inhibitors of COX-2 are useful for treating inflammation and preventing cancer.[11,12,20] Drugs that interfere with the signaling mechanisms that upregulate COX-2 should also be useful in this regard because they too decrease total COX-2 activity.[13,14] We have shown in the present experiments that resveratrol suppressed PMA-mediated induction of PG synthesis at least, in part, by inhibiting *COX-2* gene expression.[15]

Tumor-promoting phorbol esters induce *COX-2* gene expression by activating the PKC pathway.[21] A downstream target of activated PKC is the AP-1 transcription factor complex. Resveratrol suppressed PMA-mediated activation of *COX-2* transcription by inhibiting the PKC signal transduction pathway at multiple levels. It blocked both PMA-induced translocation of PKC activity from cytosol to membrane (FIG. 6) and the increase in *COX-2* promoter activity mediated by c-Jun (FIG. 7). These inhibitory effects can be explained, in part, by the antioxidant properties of resveratrol inasmuch as other phenolic antioxidants inhibit both PMA-mediated activation of PKC and AP-1.[22,23] These results are significant because PKC activity is upregulated in some cancers and is considered a potential target for anticancer therapy.[24] Additionally, because AP-1 has been implicated in promoting carcinogenesis, these effects are likely to contribute to the antitumor activity of resveratrol.

Xie and Herschman showed that the AP-1 transcription factor complex is important for the activation of the murine *COX-2* promoter via a cyclic AMP response element (CRE).[25] Thus, it is possible that resveratrol blocks PMA-mediated induction of COX-2 by suppressing AP-1-dependent transactivation via the CRE. The anti-AP-1 effect of resveratrol can potentially be explained if resveratrol induced Fra expression like other phenolic antioxidants.[26] Heterodimers of c-Jun and Fra do not activate AP-1-mediated gene expression as effectively as c-Jun homodimers or c-Jun/c-Fos heterodimers.[27] Alternatively, resveratrol could suppress PMA-mediated increases in AP-1 activity by inhibiting the induction or phosphorylation of c-Jun.[28]

We reported previously that retinoids blocked PMA-mediated induction of COX-2 in oral epithelial cells.[13] The same effect of retinoids was observed in the human mammary epithelial cells used in this study. However, whereas resveratrol and retinoids both block PMA-mediated induction of *COX-2* transcription, they appear to do so via different mechanisms. Thus, in contrast to resveratrol, retinoids did not block the PMA-induced redistribution of PKC activity from cytosol to membrane (data not shown). Additionally, resveratrol and retinoids antagonize AP-1 activity via different mechanisms. Retinoids antagonize AP-1 activity via a receptor-dependent mechanism,[29] whereas our data suggest that resveratrol blocks PMA-mediated stimulation of AP-1 activity by inhibiting the PKC signaling cascade. This distinction between resveratrol and retinoids is important for the design of chemopreventive strategies using combinations of drugs that act via different mechanisms. Finally, based on the finding that resveratrol inhibited COX-2, further studies are warranted to determine how effective this compound or its analogues will be in preventing or treating inflammation and cancer.

ACKNOWLEDGMENTS

This work was supported in part by National Institutes of Health Grants CA68136 (A.J. Dannenberg) and P01CA29502 (K. Subbaramaiah and N. Telang). Data in this manuscript were previously reported in Subbaramaiah et al.[15]

REFERENCES

1. FUNK, C.D., L.B. FUNK, M.E. KENNEDY, A.S. PONG & G.A. FITZGERALD. 1991. Human platelet/erythroleukemia cell prostaglandin G/H synthase: cDNA cloning, expression, and gene chromosomal assignment. FASEB J. **5:** 2304–2312.
2. SUBBARAMAIAH, K., N. TELANG, J.T. RAMONETTI, R. ARAKI, B. DEVITO, B.B. WEKSLER & A.J. DANNENBERG. 1996. Transcription of cyclooxygenase-2 is enhanced in transformed mammary epithelial cells. Cancer Res. **56:** 4424–4429.
3. DUBOIS, R.N., J. AWARD, J. MORROW, L.J. ROBERTS & P.R. BISHOP. 1994. Regulation of eicosanoid production and mitogenesis in rat intestinal epithelial cells by transforming growth factor-α and phorbol ester. J. Clin. Invest. **93:** 493–498.
4. KELLEY, D.J., J.R. MESTRE, K. SUBBARAMAIAH, P.G. SACKS, S.P. SCHANTZ, T. TANABE, H. INOUE, J.T. RAMONETTI & A.J. DANNENBERG. 1997. Benzo[a]pyrene upregulates cyclooxygenase-2 gene expression in oral epithelial cells. Carcinogenesis **18:** 795–799.
5. KUTCHERA, W., D.A. JONES, N. MATSUNAMI, J. GRODEN, T.M. MCINTYRE, G.A. ZIMMERMAN, R.L. WHITE & S.M. PRESCOTT. 1996. Prostaglandin H synthase-2 is expressed abnormally in human colon cancer: Evidence for a transcriptional effect. Proc. Natl. Acad. Sci. USA **93:** 4816–4820.
6. SHENG, G.G., J. SHAO, H. SHENG, E.B. HOOTON, P.C. ISAKSON, J.D. MORROW, R.J. COFFEY, R.N. DUBOIS & R.D. BEAUCHAMP. 1997. A selective cyclooxygenase-2 inhibitor suppresses the growth of H-ras-transformed rat intestinal epithelial cells. Gastroenterology **113:** 1883–1891.
7. KARGMAN, S.L., G.P. O'NEIL, P.J. VICKERS, J.F. EVANS, J.A. MANCINI & J.A. JOTHY. 1995. Expression of prostaglandin G/H synthase-1 and -2 protein in human colon cancer. Cancer Res. **55:** 2556–2559.
8. PARETT, M.L., R.E. HARRIS, F.S. JOARDER, M.S. ROSS, K.P. CLAUSEN & F.M. ROBERTSON. 1997. Cyclooxygenase-2 gene expression in human breast cancer. Int. J. Oncol. **10:** 503–507.
9. RISTIMAKI, A., N. HONKANEN, H. JANKALA, P. SIPPONEN & M. HARKONEN. 1997. Expression of cyclooxygenase-2 in human gastric carcinoma. Cancer Res. **57:** 1276–1280.
10. MULLER-DECKER, K., K. SCHOLZ, R. MARKS & G. FURSTENBERGER. 1995. Differential expression of prostaglandin H synthase isozymes during multistage carcinogenesis in mouse epidermis. Mol. Carcinogenesis **12:** 31–41.
11. OSHIMA, M., J.E. DINCHUK, S.L. KARGMAN, H. OSHIMA, B. HANCOCK, E. KWONG, J.M. TRZASKOS, J.F. EVANS & M.M. TAKETO. 1996. Suppression of intestinal polyposis in Apc$^{\Delta716}$ knockout mice by inhibition of cyclooxygenase 2 (Cox-2). Cell **87:** 803–809.
12. KAWAMORI, T., C.V. RAO, K. SEIBERT & B.S. REDDY. 1998. Chemopreventive activity of celecoxib, a specific cyclooxygenase-2 inhibitor, against colon carcinogenesis. Cancer Res. **58:** 409–412.
13. MESTRE, J.R., K. SUBBARAMAIAH, P.G. SACKS, S.P. SCHANTZ, T. TANABE, H. INOUE & A.J. DANNENBERG. 1997. Retinoids suppress phorbol ester-mediated induction of cyclooyxgenase-2. Cancer Res. **57:** 1081–1085.
14. MESTRE, J.R., K. SUBBARAMAIAH, P.G. SACKS, S.P. SCHANTZ, T. TANABE, H. INOUE & A.J. DANNENBERG. 1997. Retinoids suppress epidermal growth factor-induced tran-

scription of cyclooxygenase-2 in human oral squamous carcinoma cells. Cancer Res. **57:** 2890–2895.

15. SUBBARAMAIAH, K., W.J. CHUNG, P. MICHALUART, N. TELANG, T. TANABE, H. INOUE, M. JANG, J.M. PEZZUTO & A.J. DANNENBERG. 1998. Resveratrol inhibits cyclooxygenase-2 transcription and activity in phorbol ester-treated human mammary epithelial cells. J. Biol. Chem. **273:** 21875–21882.

16. JANG, M., L. CAI, G.O. UDEANI, K.V. SLOWING, C.F. THOMAS, C.W.W. BEECHER, H.H.S. FONG, N.R. FARNSWORTH, A.D. KINGHORN, R.G. MEHTA, R.C. MOON & J.M. PEZZUTO. 1997. Cancer chemopreventive activity of resveratrol, a natural product derived from grapes. Science **275:** 218–220.

17. ZHAI, Y.-F., H. BEITTENMILLER, B. WANG, M.N. GOULD, C. OAKLEY, W.J. ESSELMAN & C.W. WELSCH. 1993. Increased expression of specific protein tyrosine phosphatases in human breast epithelial cells neoplastically transformed by the neu oncogene. Cancer Res. **53:** 2272–2278.

18. SACKS, P.G. 1996. Cell, tissue and organ culture as in vitro models to study the biology of squamous cell carcinomas of the head. Cancer Metastasis Rev. **15:** 27–51.

19. INOUE, H., C. YOKOYAMA, S. HARA, Y. TONE & T. TANABE. 1995. Transcriptional regulation of human prostaglandin-endoperoxide synthase-2 gene by lipopolysaccharide and phorbol ester in vascular endothelial cells. J. Biol. Chem. **270:** 24965–24971.

20. MASFERRER, J.L., B.S. ZWEIFEL, P.T. MANNING, S.D. HAUSER, K.M. LEAHY, W.G. SMITH, P.C. ISAKSON & K. SEIBERT. 1994. Selective inhibition of inducible cyclooxygenase-2 in vivo is antiinflammatory and nonulcerogenic. Proc. Natl. Acad. Sci. USA **91:** 3228–3232.

21. SUBBARAMAIAH, K., D. ZAKIM, B.B. WEKSLER & A.J. DANNENBERG. 1997. Inhibition of cyclooxygenase: A novel approach to cancer prevention. Proc. Soc. Exp. Biol. Med. **216:** 201–210.

22. LIU, J-Y., S-J. LIN & J-K. LIN. 1993. Inhibitory effects of curcumin on protein kinase C activity induced by 12-O-tetradecanoyl-phorbol-13-acetate in NIH 3T3 cells. Carcinogenesis **14:** 857–861.

23. HUANG, T-S., S-C. LEE & J-K. LIN. 1991. Suppression of c-Jun/AP-1 activation by an inhibitor of tumor promotion in mouse fibroblast cells. Proc. Natl. Acad. Sci. USA **88:** 5292–5296.

24. GORDGE, P.C., M.J. HULME, R.A. CLEGG & W.R. MILLER. 1996. Elevation of protein kinase A and protein kinase C activities in malignant as compared with normal human breast tissue. Eur. J. Cancer **32A:** 2120–2126.

25. XIE, W. & H.R. HERSCHMAN. 1995. v-src induces prostaglandin synthase-2 gene expression by activation of c-Jun N-terminal kinase and the c-Jun transcription factor. J. Biol. Chem. **270:** 27622–27628.

26. YOSHIOKA, K., T. DENG, M. CAVIGELLI & M. KARIN. 1995. Antitumor promotion by phenolic antioxidants: Inhibition of AP-1 activity through induction of Fra expression. Proc. Natl. Acad. Sci. USA **92:** 4972–4976.

27. SUZUKI, T., H. OKUNO, T. YOSHIDA, T. ENDO, H. NISHINA & H. IBA. 1992. Difference in transcriptional regulatory function between c-Fos and Fra-2. Nucleic Acids Res. **19:** 5537–5542.

28. KARIN, M. 1995. The regulation of AP-1 activity by mitogen-activated protein kinases. J. Biol. Chem. **270:** 16483–16486.

29. PFAHL, M. 1993. Nuclear receptor/AP-1 interaction. Endocr. Rev. **14:** 651–658.

Modification of Dietary Habits (Mediterranean Diet) and Cancer Mortality in a Southern Italian Village from 1960 to 1996

A. DE LORENZO,[a] A. ANDREOLI, R.P. SORGE, L. IACOPINO, S. MONTAGNA, L. PROMENZIO, AND P. SERRANÒ[b]

Human Nutrition Unit, University of Rome "Tor Vergata," 00173 Rome, Italy

[b]*Lega Italiana per la lotta contro i Tumori, Reggio Calabria*

INTRODUCTION

The principal source of information about dietary intake in Italy, in the 1960s, was the survey carried out by the European Atomic Energy Commission. Another source was the Seven Countries Study; therefore the data will only be used to make a rough comparison between Italy and other Mediterranean countries.[1] A more recent study was carried out as a longitudinal study, called the Seven Countries Study.[2–7]

For most types of cancer, genetic factors play only a minor role, as shown by the fact that in populations where the incidence of cancer runs from high to low, depending on the region, cancer incidence has increased in the last few decades. Indeed, environmental factors play a key role: when population studies are performed in developed and underdeveloped countries, the colorectal cancer age-adjusted incidence rate varies by a factor as high as 15-fold.[8–11] According to these studies, the lowest reported cancer rate in a worldwide study should be considered the baseline rate of occurrence, and the increases in rate should be ascribed to such environmental factors as pollution and diet. There is increasing evidence of an association between diet and morbidity or mortality from cancer and coronary heart disease, the two major age-related diseases of Western societies.

The "Mediterranean" effect on mortality is still evident in Italy, where food patterns differ significantly in different geographical areas. In fact there are differences in incidence of cancer between the north and south of Italy (i.e., mortality incidence of gut cancer is 0.363 in northern Italian regions and 0.115 in southern regions; for breast cancer mortality it is 0.264 in the North and 0.089 in the South). Slight differences may be found among Mediterranean countries, according to tradition, local production of food, and even religion: wine is largely consumed in Italy, Spain, and Greece, whereas it is forbidden in Muslim North Africa and Middle East.

The Mediterranean diet is a low-fat, high-carbohydrate, and fiber-rich diet, close to the traditional diet of Mediterranean countries; the diet is rich in cereal products,

[a]Address for communication: Human Nutrition, University Tor Vergata, Via di Tor Vergata, 135. 00173 Rome, Italy. Voice and fax: 39-06-72596415.
e-mail: delorenzo@uniroma2.it

starch, vegetables and fruits, olive oil, and fish.[1,12] Cereals and olive oil were the major sources of energy in the ancient Mediterranean: during the Peloponnesian Wars, the rowers of an Athens trireme had to perform for an extended time in a dramatic situation. Their diet during this performance was mostly bread with olive oil, the best choice in their situation (Thucydides). Bread and olive oil were still common as an afternoon snack in southern Italy 50 years ago.

For people on the Mediterranean diet, according to southern Italian tradition (villages in Campania, Basilicata, and Calabria, 1960),[1] carbohydrates accounted for 60% of calories, fat (95% olive oil) for 28%, and proteins for 12 percent. A large supply of vitamins (A, C, and E) and minerals were obtained from fruits and vegetables, and daily fiber intake was between 20 and 35 g/day.

A low-fat, high-fiber diet is now highly recommended in Western countries,[13] as this diet should reduce the prevalence of atherosclerosis and some types of cancer, as suggested by several epidemiological studies worldwide.[8,14] Although the effects of a saturated fat-rich diet on serum cholesterol level were already known the in mid-1960s, the favorable effect of olive oil on lipoprotein profile has only been recognized in the last decade, as well as the protective effects of n-3 fatty acids. More recently, the preventive effect of antioxidant vitamins and bioflavonoids, largely supplied in the Mediterranean diet, have been outlined. Olive oil, rich in tyrosol, a powerful antioxidant bioflavonoid, seems very useful in the prevention of LDL oxidation. The antioxidant compounds, abundant in the Mediterranean diet, also have a protective effect against cancers (colon, breast, and prostate), in association with low-fat and low-caloric intake, and with a high-fiber intake.[15]

There are modifications in southern Italy related to a change in Italian lifestyle from a rural model toward a developed-country model (including also dietary habits), with a relevant increase of global income. In southern Italy the lifestyle modifications were more relevant, as northern Italy was already a fairly developed area, with dietary habits closer to the central European models. In Calabria, (a rural region, without large cities and with the population living mostly in villages or small towns) in the last two decades, a progressive shift from a low-fat, high-fiber, Mediterranean diet toward a Western-style diet has been shown by the modifications of average intakes of pasta, bread, and meat, evaluated by total expenditure per year (accounting for inflation).

The aim of the present study was to investigate the relationship, if any, between diet and cancer incidence rates in Calabria and to compare the food intake in Nicotera (a small town), as assessed in 1990,[16] to the food intake assessed in 1996 in the same village.

METHODS AND SUBJECTS

In 1996, 80 Nicotera subjects, 37 females and 43 males, 40 to 60 years old, were studied. Nicotera was a town in the Seven Countries Study. The food intake of the 1996 study participants was assessed by a semiquantitative questionnaire of food frequency, using the "Questionario di frequenza dei consumi alimentari," (food frequency consumption questionnaire), proposed and validated for the Italian population.[17] The foods most common in Italy were depicted in colored pictures (61 different foods), each of them in three different-sized servings, and the frequency of consumption was reported by the participants, in a range between "each day" and "six times a month" (self-administered questionnaire). For the 1960 food intake of Nicotera, a sample was calculated from the results of Fidanza's papers.[12] A descriptive analysis and plot were performed using an SPSS/PC for Windows program.

From 1974 to 1996, the total consumption of pasta and bread (evaluated cumulatively), and meat (total meat consumption and bovine meat only) were evaluated from total expenditure per year (accounting for inflation). Mortality rates for cancers at different sites (colon, breast, and pancreas) were recorded and expressed as deaths per year per 10^{11} inhabitants (interpolated data, FIG. 2). The autoregression trend (AMIRA) between the consumption rates and the rates of mortality for the cancers on study was performed, using an SPSS/PC for Windows program.

RESULTS

In FIGURE 1 daily intake values of nutrients for the 1960 and 1996 samples are reported: the values for carbohydrates, proteins, and total lipids. Total protein and lipid values were also divided into animal and vegetable ones. In 1996 the total ca-

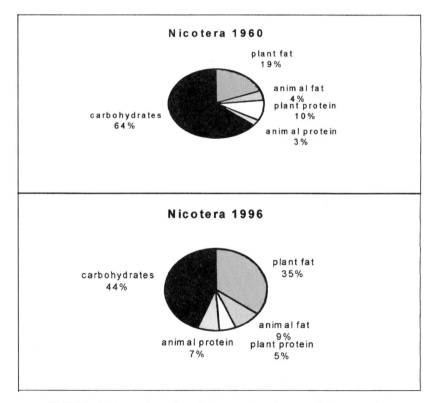

FIGURE 1. Comparison of nutrient percentages between the two samples.

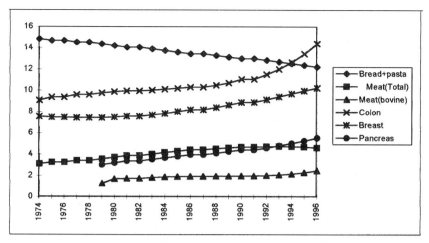

FIGURE 2. Consumption ×10^{11} kg/year and cancer mortality/10^{11}. Interpolated data.

loric intake was 2600 kcal/day: 1149 kcal from carbohydrates (44.2%), 317 kcal (12.2%) from proteins, and 1133 kcal from lipids (43.6%). Furthermore, cholesterol, fiber, and alcohol were analyzed. Calories from alcohol (287 kcal/day) were not included in the total caloric intake, but cholesterol and fiber values are lacking, because their calculation from available data (Fidanza's tables) was impossible. In 1960 the total caloric intake was 2144 kcal, 64.1% from carbohydrates, 12% from proteins, and 23.3% from lipids, a diet very close to the Mediterranean tradition.[1]

In the Nicotera 1960 sample, the diet was very close to the Italian Mediterranean diet, whereas an excess intake of lipids was found in the 1996 sample, and the carbohydrate intake was lower than the recommended dietary allowance.

From 1974 to 1996 the consumption of bread and pasta fell from 150.4 × 10^{11} (kg per year) to 125.9 × 10^{11}, whereas meat consumption (evaluated cumulatively) rose from 31.8 × 10^{11} to 48.8 × 10^{11}. From 1974 to 1996 bovine meat consumption increased from 13.3 × 10^{11} to 22.6 × 10^{11}. In the same years, the incidence of colon, breast, and pancreatic cancer mortality increased.

For the colon cancer mortality rate, a strong negative correlation (linear correlation: $r = 0.91613$) with bread and pasta consumption was observed; a weak positive correlation ($r = 0.73875$) with meat intake was observed. For the breast cancer mortality rate, a strong negative correlation ($r = 0.9544$) with bread and pasta consumption and positive correlation with meat consumption ($r = 0.81715$) were observed. For the pancreatic cancer mortality rate, a significant positive correlation with meat intake was observed ($r = 0.8761$), as well as a strong positive correlation with bovine meat consumption ($r = 0.9255$) (Fig. 2).

CONCLUSION

The results obtained in our study on food intake in Nicotera in 1996 are very close to the results obtained in a food consumption survey on the Italian population in

1991.[18] Thus, whereas in 1960 inhabitants of Nicotera followed a "reference Mediterranean Italian diet," [1,11] in 1996 the Nicotera diet was very close to the average Italian diet, which is no longer a Mediterranean diet, because of a striking increase in the use of animal products, like meat, milk, dairy products, animal fat, with a net decrease of bread and pasta consumption. According to our study, in Nicotera in almost 40 years, the lipid intake was increased to 43.6% of calories, whereas the carbohydrate intake was decreased to 44.2 percent. The protein intake was almost unmodified, but meat proteins are preferred today. The total caloric intake was increased by 20%, when physical activity was decreased (data not showed). As expected, many people were overweight (data not showed). The same trend was observed in most Mediterranean countries, suggesting that the Mediterranean diet should be adopted, especially in southern Italy and in most developed Mediterranean areas.[11,15] The most relevant finding is a strong negative correlation between bread and pasta consumption and colon and breast cancer mortality, never reported before.

Modifications to dietary habits may increase the risk of cancer in the general population: in our study, a close relationship was demonstrated between the modifications of food consumption patterns and cancer mortality at different sites (colon, breast, and pancreas). Calabrian people gave up the safe Mediterranean diet to adopt the less safe Western diet, with an increase of cancer risk, whereas in western developed countries an increase in the consumption of starch, and fresh fruits and vegetables (which are the main components of the Mediterranean diet) is being ever more strongly advised, with a proportionate diminution in meat and animal fat consumption. Therefore, these dietary trends in Calabria should be rapidly reversed. Future intervention to improve the health and nutritional status of our nation's children and adults and a return to the Mediterranean diet are culturally appropriate; changes need to be implemented at the individual, family, and community levels.

REFERENCES

1. NESTLE, M. 1995. Mediterranean diets: Historical and research overview. Am. J. Clin. Nutr. **61**(6): 1313S–1320S.
2. HUIJBREGTS, P.P., E.J. FESKENS, L. RASANEN, F. FIDANZA, A. NISSINEN, A. MENOTTI & D. KROMHOUT. 1997. Dietary pattern and 20 year mortality in elderly men in Finland, Italy, and The Netherlands : Longitudinal cohort study. Br. Med. J. **315** (7099): 13–7.
3. PETERS, E.T., J.C. SEIDELL, A. MENOTTI, C. ARAYANIS, A. DONTAS, F. FIDANZA, M. KARVONEN, S. NEDELJKOVIC, A. NISSINEN, R. BUZINA et al. 1995. Changes in body weight in relation to mortality in 6441 European middle-age men: The Seven Countries Study. Int. J. Obes. Relat. Metab. Disord. **19**(12): 862–868.
4. HUIJBREGTS, P.P., E.J. FESKENS, L. RASANEN, A. ALBERTI-FIDANZA, M. MUTANEN, F. FIDANZA & D. KROMHOUT. 1995. Dietary intake in five ageing cohorts of men in Finland, Italy and The Netherlands. Eur. J. Clin. Nutr. **49**(11): 852–860.
5. OCKE, M.C., D. KROMHOUT, A. MENOTTI, C. ARAVANIS, H. BLACKBURN, R. BUZINA, F. FIDANZA, A. JANSEN, S. NEDELJKOVIC, A. NISSIENEN et al. 1995. Average intake of anti-oxidant (pro)vitamins and subsequent cancer mortality in the 16 cohorts of the Seven Countries Study. Int. J. Cancer **61**(14): 480–484.
6. HERTOG, M.G., D. KROMHOUT, C. ARAVANIS, H. BLACKBURN, R. BUZINA, F. FIDANZA, S. GIAMPAOLI, A. JANSEN, A. MENOTTI, S. NEDELJKOVIC et al. 1995. Flavonoid intake and long-term risk of coronary heart disease and cancer in the Seven Countries Study. Arch. Intern. Med. **155**(11): 1184.

7. FARCHI, G., F. FIDANZA, S. MARIOTTI & A. MENOTTI. 1994. Is diet an independent risk factor for mortality? 20 year mortality in the Italian rural cohorts of the Seven Countries Study. Eur. J. Clin. Nutr. **48**(1): 19–29.
8. DOLL, R. 1992. The lessons of life: Keynote address to the nutrition and cancer conference. Cancer Res. (Suppl.) **52:** 22024s–22029s.
9. BOLAND, C.R. 1991. Malignant tumors of the colon. *In* Textbook of Gastroenterology. T. Yamada *et al.* Eds.: 1105. J.B. Lippincott Co. Philadelphia.
10. WILLETT, W.C., M.J. STAMPER, G.A. COLDITZ, B.A. ROSNER & E. SPEIZER. 1990. Relation of meat fat and fiber intake to the risk of colon cancer in a prospective study among women. N. Engl. J. Med. **323:** 1664–1672.
11. SASSO, G.F., L. IACOPINO, A. ANDREOLI, C. CARLOMUSTO & A. DE LORENZO. 1995. Consumo di alcol e carcinoma pancreatico. Alcologia **7**(2): 71.
12. FIDANZA, R. 1991. The Mediterranean Italian diet: Keys to contemporary thinking. Proc. Nutr. Soc. **50:** 519–526.
13. USDA-USDHHS NUTRITION AND YOUR HEALTH. 1990. Dietary Guidelines for Americans. 3rd ed. US Government Printing Office. Washington, DC.
14. LA VECCHIA, C. 1993. Dietary fat and cancer in Italy. Eur. J. Clin. Nutr. (Suppl.) **47:** 35s–38s.
15. GHISELLI, A. A. D'AMICIS & A. GIACOSA. 1997. The antioxidant potential of the Mediterranean diet. Eur. J. Cancer Prev. **6** (suppl 1): 15s–19s.
16. FIDANZA, F. & A. FIDANZA. 1971. Rilevamento dei consumi alimentari di alcune famiglie in tre zone agricole d'Italia. Quaderni della Nutrizione **31:** 139–188.
17. FIDANZA, F., M. PORRINI & M.G. GENTILE. 1995. Biochemical validation of a self-administered semi-quantitative food-frequency questionnaire. Br. J. Nutr. **74:** 323–333.
18. TICCA, M. 1992. Il modello alimentare mediterraneo. La salute a tavola ariva dalla tradizione. Ist. Naz. Nutrizione.

Season-specific Correlation between Dietary Intake of Fruits and Vegetables and Levels of Serum Biomarkers among Chinese Tin Miners at High Risk for Lung Cancer

M.R. FORMAN,[a,h] J. ZHANG,[b] E. GUNTER,[c] S.X. YAO,[b] M. GROSS,[d] Y.L. QIAO,[e] B.I. GRAUBARD,[f] P.R. TAYLOR,[a] S. KEITH,[g] AND M. MAHER[a]

[a]Cancer Prevention Studies Branch, Division of Clinical Sciences, National Cancer Institute, Bethesda, Maryland 20892-7058, USA

[b]Labor Protection Institute, Yunnan Tin Mine Corporation, Gejiu, Yunnan, PR China

[c]NHANES Laboratory of Biochemical Analyses, Centers for Disease Prevention and Control, Atlanta, Georgia, USA

[d]Department of Epidemiology, School of Public Health, University of Minnesota, Minneapolis, Minnesota, USA

[e]Department of Cancer Epidemiology, Cancer Institute, Chinese Academy of Medical Sciences, Beijing 100002 1, PR China

[f]Biostatistics Branch, Division of Cancer Epidemiology and Genetics, National Cancer Institute, Bethesda, Maryland 20892, USA

[g]Informaiton Management Sciences, Silver Spring, Maryland, USA

INTRODUCTION

Tin miners have been at an increased risk of lung cancer by virtue of their occupational exposures to arsenic and radon.[1,2,35] In the early 1990s, the lung cancer mortality rate among Yunnan Tin Corporation (YTC) miners in southern China was 487/100,000 compared with a rate of 30/100,00 in Chinese men.[3] In an incident case-control study of the YTC miners, dietary intakes of specific fruits and vegetables were inversely associated with the odds ratio of lung cancer, after adjustment for occupational and smoking histories.[4]

High intakes of fruits and vegetables and elevated blood levels of β-carotene have been consistently associated with a reduced risk of lung cancer.[5,6] Dietary intake of fruits and vegetables has been positively correlated with blood levels of carotenoids and vitamin C as well as urinary flavonoid metabolites.[7-10] The magnitude of these correlations varied by gender, age, and season.[10-12] Smoking status, alcohol intake, body weight, and intakes of fat and fiber have confounded the diet-biochemical correlation.[11-16]

[h]Address for communication: Michele R. Forman, Ph.D., Senior Investigator, Cancer Prevention Studies Branch, Division of Clinical Sciences, National Cancer Institute, 6006 Executive Boulevard, Suite 321, MSC 7058, Bethesda MD 20892-7058. Voice: 301-594-2938; fax: 301-435-8645.

e-mail: mf63p@nih.gov

As part of a large-scale prospective cohort study of lung cancer among the YTC miners, a diet-biochemical validation study (DBVS) was conducted in 1995 and 1996. The objective of this paper is to examine the season-specific correlation between intakes of fruits and vegetables and serum biomarker levels, before and after adjustment for covariates.

MATERIAL AND METHODS

Study Population

Over 7,000 miners, who were aged ≥ 40 y, had ≥ 10 y of underground mining experience, and who were free of all cancer except nonmelanoma skin cancer, were enrolled prospectively as the high-risk cohort for lung cancer beginning in 1992 and followed annually to the present.[1] The DBVS miners (N = 128) were randomly selected from workers in four mine units who were similar by demographic and occupational characteristics to all YTC miners. Fifteen of the 128 were excluded from analysis because of incomplete dietary data or a diagnosis of a chronic disease in 1995–1996.

Dietary Data

Seven consecutive days of 24-hour food recalls were collected once during each of four seasons, beginning in the spring of 1995 and ending in the winter of 1996, for a total of 28 days of food recalls in one year. Trained interviewers administered food recalls at the same time daily in the miner's home. The interviewer asked about intake of each food item in a mixed dish or eaten individually by time of day, food preparation technique, gram amount, and place of consumption.[17]

Blood Sample Collection

In the morning of food recall day seven in the spring, blood was drawn from each miner after 12 hours in the fasting state. Because of cultural taboos about blood, subsequent blood collection was limited. One third of the DBVS sample was randomly selected for a blood drawing on food recall day seven during one of the remaining three seasons, for a total of two blood drawings from each participant.

Blood to measure red blood cell (RBC) folate; vitamins A, E, and C; as well as the carotenoids was collected in 6-mL serum separator tubes (SST®) and 3-mL K$_3$EDTA Vacutainers® (Becton-Dickenson, Franklin Lakes, NJ), protected from light by aluminum foil wrapping, and kept in ice until delivery to the clinic. Blood was centrifuged for 15 minutes at 2400–2500 rpm ($1500 \times g$). A 250 µL of serum was placed into a cryovial (Nalge, Rochester, NY) with 1.0 mL of 6 g/dL metaphosphoric acid preservative added for the vitamin C sample; 0.5 mL of the EDTA tube for the carotenoids was removed for hematocrit measurement, and 100 µL of the whole blood was added to 1.0 mL of 1 g/dL ascorbic acid to preserve the RBC folate sample. All samples were stored at $-70°$C until shipment to the Centers for Disease Control and Prevention for laboratory analysis.

Serum levels of vitamin C (ascorbic acid), vitamin A (retinol), vitamin E (α-to-copherol), retinyl esters, and five carotenoid peaks (α- and β-carotene, β-cryptoxanthin, lutein/zeaxanthin (referred to as lutein), and lycopene) were measured by C-18 reverse-phase column using high-performance liquid chromatography (HPLC).[18,19] Quantitation was by peak height and based on a standard curve generated from external standards as part of the NIST Round Robin Program. RBC folate was measured using the Bio-Rad Laboratories Quantaphase II^{125}/I^{57} Co radioassay (Hercules, CA).[20]

Body mass index (BMI) was calculated from weight measured to the nearest kilogram in 1995 and from height measured to the nearest centimeter at the baseline exam in 1992.

Statistical Analysis

The statistical analysis involved two phases. In phase one, 223 foods, that were coded from the food recalls, were classified into food groups, including fruits and vegetables. The total gram intake of each food was calculated from its intake over the seven days in each season, followed by a calculation of the percentage that the food contributed to the food group intake in each season. The seasons were defined: spring (March–May), summer (June–August), fall (September–November), and winter (December–February). To test for seasonal differences in dietary intake of fruits and vegetables and for seasonal differences in biochemical levels, analysis of variance (ANOVA) was performed, with statistical significance set at a two-tailed p value of ≤ 0.05.

In phase two, season-specific Spearman Rank partial correlation coefficients were calculated between intakes of all fruits, of all vegetables, and of all fruits and vegetables and serum biomarker levels. Alcohol intake (g/d), smoking (number of cigarettes/d), BMI (kg/m^2), age, and income were adjusted in the ANOVA and in the correlation analyses, because each variable met one or both of two conditions. Notably, age, income, alcohol intake, and smoking were statistically significantly related to the mean serum levels in the ANOVAs in phase one, and/or they were recognized confounding factors of the diet-biochemical relationship in earlier studies.[10–12,15,21,22]

RESULTS

Total fruit intake was higher in the spring and summer than in the fall and winter; whereas total vegetable intake was higher in the summer than in the spring (TABLE 1). Over 70% of the miners smoked cigarettes, and 60% drank alcohol (grain liquor) in fairly heavy amounts daily. Serum α-carotene levels were higher in the fall than in the spring and summer. β-carotene levels were higher in the winter than in all other seasons and also were higher in the spring and fall than in the summer. Lutein levels were lower in the summer than in the spring and winter. Serum lycopene and RBC folate levels were higher in the spring than in any other season. From 3 to 13% of the miners were folate deficient (RBC folate < 85 ng/mL) in one of the seasons. Serum vitamin C levels were lower in the spring and summer than in the fall and winter. The seasonal peaks of fruit and vegetable intake and of serum biomarker levels remained after adjustment for smoking, alcohol intake, BMI, age, and income.

TABLE 1. Mean (±SD) demographic characteristics; dietary intake of fruits, vegetables, and alcohol; and mean (±SE) serum biomarker levels by season: DBVS

Characteristic	Spring (n = 113)	Summer (n = 35)	Fall (n=31)	Winter (n = 32)
Age at interview (yr)	52 (9)	52 (9)	50 (9)	51 (8)
BMI	23 (3)	22 (3)	23 (3)	22 (3)
Income (Yuan/mo)	554 (552)	535 (195)	598 (195)	565 (223)
Education	5 (4)	6 (4)	6 (3)	6 (5)
Percent Current Smokers	75	77	72	74
Alcohol (g/d)	104 (115)	81 (117)	68 (100)	66 (105)
Fruit Intake (g/d)	56 $(10.1)^{b,\#,c,*}$	53 $(4.7)^{d,*,e,*}$	32 (5.5)	23 (9.9)
Vegetable Intake (g/d)	263 $(10.2)^{a,\#}$	296 (12.3)	275 (10.7)	281 (11.4)
Serum (mg/dL)				
α-carotene	3 (0.2)	2 (0.2)	4 $(0.3)^{b,\#,d,*}$	3 (0.3)
β-carotene	23 $(1.3)^{a,+}$	15 (0.9)	22 $(1.5)^{d,+}$	31 $(2.0)^{c,\#,e,+,f,*}$
Lutein/Zeaxanthin	66 (2.5)	57 $(2.3)^{a,+,e,*}$	59 (2.2)	68 (2.1)
Lycopene	8 $(0.5)^{a,+,b,+,c,+}$	2 $(0.2)^{e,+}$	2 $(0.2)^{f,*}$	1 (0.1)
RBC Folate (ng/mL)	165 $(5.5)^{a,+,b,\#,c,*}$	149 (5.7)	130 (4.1)	153 (5.0)
Vitamin C	0.6 $(0.03)^{b,\#,c,+}$	0.7 $(0.03)^{d,*,e,\#}$	0.8 (0.04)	0.8 (0.03)

[a]Spring vs. Summer. [b]Spring vs. Fall. [c]Spring vs. Winter. [d]Summer vs. Fall. [e]Summer vs. Winter. [f]Fall vs. Winter.
*$p \leq 0.05$. #$p \leq 0.01$. +$p \leq 0.001$.

Seasonal patterns of the major contributors (by at least 1%) to fruit intake included watermelon, bananas, and peaches in the spring; and bananas, peaches, pomegranates, pears, and apples in the summer (FIG. 1). By fall, apples as well as oranges and tangerines were the highest contributors, with bananas, pineapples, and persimmons adding another 6% each. Finally, in the winter, oranges and tangerines, apples, and bananas were the major contributors to fruit intake. Seasonal patterns of the major contributors to vegetable intake included a variety of fresh and pickled/salty green vegetables, scallions and leeks, white vegetables such as potato and radish root, and occasionally tomatoes (FIG. 2).

The significant diet-biochemical associations were positively correlated (TABLE 2). Serum α-carotene levels were correlated with fruit intake in the spring. During the summer, levels of α-carotene, lycopene, and RBC folate were correlated with fruit intake; serum lutein and vitamin C levels were correlated with vegetable intake; and RBC folate, serum α-carotene, lutein, and vitamin C levels were correlated with fruit and vegetable intake. During the fall, RBC folate was correlated with fruit intake; levels of α- and β-carotene, lutein, and vitamin C were correlated with vegetable intake; whereas α- and β-carotene, lutein, vitamin C, and RBC folate levels were correlated with fruit and vegetable intake. During the winter, vitamin C levels were correlated with vegetable intake and both fruit and vegetable intake.

In an analysis of fruit consumers (n = 56 in spring; n = 24 in summer; n = 14 in fall; n = 11 in winter), the following diet-biochemical correlations changed: fruit intake in spring and serum α-carotene (r = 0.19); fruit intake in summer and serum α-

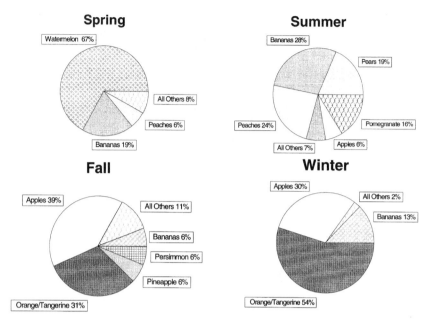

FIGURE 1. Percent contribution of individual fruits to fruit intake: DBVS.

carotene (r = 0.34), β-carotene (r = 0.46, $p \leq 0.05$), and RBC folate (r = 0.66, $p \leq$ 0.01); fruit intake in fall and RBC folate (r = 0.74, $p \leq 0.01$); fruit intake in winter and β-carotene (r = 0.71, $p \leq 0.01$). By and large, the correlation between the dietary intake of fruits and serum biomarker levels increased in the analysis of fruit consumers, with the exceptions of the relationship between fruit intake and serum α-carotene levels.

DISCUSSION

Based on seven days of food recalls and serum biomarker levels in each of four seasons of a year, miners experienced peak fruit intake in the spring; peak vegetable intake in the summer; and peak levels of α-carotene in the fall, β-carotene and lutein in the winter, lycopene and RBC folate in the spring, and higher vitamin C levels in the fall and winter than in the spring and summer. The magnitude of the correlation between fruit and vegetable intake and biomarker levels varied by season, with most significant correlations appearing in the summer and fall.

Individual foods contributing to fruit intake varied by season; only bananas were eaten in every season. Although bananas contain folate, only peaches are rich in β-carotene, and oranges and tangerines have β-cryptozanthin. Likewise individual foods contributing to vegetable intake varied by season. Potatoes, Chinese cabbage, green beans, and scallions plus leeks were eaten in every season. Whereas all the fresh and pickled dark green vegetables are rich in folate and lutein and to some ex-

TABLE 2. Spearman correlations^a between dietary fruit and/or vegetable intake and serum biomarkers by season: DBVS, YTC

Season	α-Carotene	β-Carotene	Lutein	Lycopene	RBC Folate	Vitamin C
			Biomarkers			
Spring						
Fruit	0.32*	0.14	0.08	0.19	0.08	0.13
Vegetables	0.07	0.12	0.07	0.01	0.02	0.05
Fruits and Vegetables	0.19	0.11	0.09	0.05	0.03	0.07
Summer						
Fruit	0.47#	0.27	0.18	0.38*	0.46*	0.35
Vegetables	0.33	0.27	0.45*	0.16	0.23	0.44*
Fruits and Vegetables	0.41*	0.33	0.46*	0.24	0.39*	0.51#
Fall						
Fruit	0.01	0.07	0.04	0.12	0.71+	0.28
Vegetables	0.51*	0.62#	0.52*	0.23	0.34	0.58#
Fruits and Vegetables	0.45*	0.61#	0.55#	0.21	0.61#	0.74+
Winter						
Fruit	−0.10	−0.03	−0.22	0.33	0.05	−0.10
Vegetable	0.08	0.33	0.32	0.20	−0.06	0.48*
Fruits and Vegetables	0.11	0.29	0.20	0.35	−0.03	0.47*

^{a} With adjustment for age, income, alcohol, smoking, and body mass index.
*$p = < 0.05$. #$p = < 0.01$. +$p = < 0.001$.

tent β-carotene, raw tomatoes provide lower levels of lycopene than tomato products. Among the vegetables in the "other" category, limited orange and yellow vegetables were eaten to add to α-carotene and β-carotene intake.

The range in fruit intake over the four seasons of the DBVS was from one tenth of a cup to a little over one quarter of a cup each day, when one half a cup of raw fruit per day is equivalent to a serving based on the National Cancer Institute's (NCI) 5-A-Day Program. The range in vegetable intake was from one and one quarter cup to one and one half cup a day over the year, when one cup of leafy green vegetables or one half a cup of raw vegetables is equivalent to a serving in the NCI 5-A-Day Program. Therefore fruits and vegetables were consumed in very small amounts daily, with a minimal range in intake from the lowest to the peak seasons.

The seasonal peak of fruit and vegetable intake did not correspond with the biochemical peaks of the serum markers because the major contributors to fruit intake did not frequently have high concentrations of the same micronutrients as the serum markers. The amount of fruit and vegetable intake across the seasons did not vary appreciably, even though the seasonal differences in intake were statistically significant (see above). Fat intake was in the form of lard used in food preparation (13g/d),

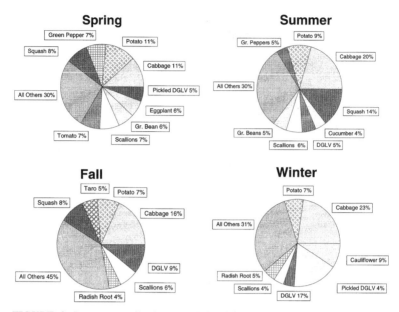

FIGURE 2. Percent contribution of individual foods to vegetable intake: DBVS.

and therefore uptake of lipid soluble micronutrients might have been hindered by the low-fat intake. Finally, alcohol intake was high and altered levels of serum lipoproteins, which transport the carotenoids.

Seasonal differences in dietary intake of fruits and vegetables and in serum biomarker levels have been reported across cultures, including the northern province of Linxian, China,[23] the Gambia,[24] Spain,[25] Finland,[26] Britain,[16,27] and Hawaii.[28] Seasonal patterns of fruit and vegetable intake might be due to market availability, cost, and accessibility as well as refrigeration, whereas seasonal variation in blood levels might be associated with the level of fruit and vegetable intake, underlying health status, and lifestyle characteristics.

Serum lycopene and α-carotene levels of the miners were lower than other populations, except for other Chinese.[10,16,23,27,29] β-carotene levels were similar to[27] or were slightly higher than other male smokers[10,29] and higher than other Chinese.[23] Vitamin C levels were comparable to other smoking populations,[27,30] whereas lutein levels were much higher than others.[27]

In the DBVS, the magnitude of the diet-biochemical correlation varied by season. The larger values and higher frequency of correlations typically appeared in the summer and fall, and the lower ones appeared in the spring and winter. Diet-lycopene levels were not significantly correlated in any season, except for one in summer that could be due to chance. Likewise, total fruit and vegetable intake among American women was the most significant determinant of each carotenoid except for lycopene.[31]

One factor that could potentially influence the magnitude of the diet-biochemical correlation was the number of food recall days that were averaged to reflect dietary intake. In this paper, seven consecutive days of food recalls were averaged because the blood was collected on day seven. Earlier clinical nutrition research in men has demonstrated that the carotenoids appeared in the blood from two to seven days after dietary intake.[32-34] In a separate analysis, two days (food recall days 5 and 6) were averaged and then the diet-biochemical correlations were computed. No appreciable difference in the magnitude or the direction of these diet-biochemical correlations apeared using the two-day versus the seven-day averaged intakes. Our findings might not reflect earlier studies because of the differences in the diet and alcohol intakes as well as the smoking habits of the miners in contrast with healthy, nonsmoking male volunteers in the United States.

In summary, miners experienced peak seasons of fruit and vegetable intake and of serum biomarker levels. The magnitude of the diet-biochemcial correlation varied by season with most correlations appearing in the summer and fall. Future research in the relationship between diet and/or biochemical parameters and lung cancer risk needs to take into account the seasonal patterns of diet and serum biochemical markers.

ACKNOWLEDGMENTS

The authors would like to gratefully acknowledge the support of the staff of the NHANES Laboratory of Biochemical Analyses at the Centers for Disease Prevention and Control, Atlanta, GA.

REFERENCES

1. QIAO, Y.L., P.R. TAYLOR, S.X. YAO, Y.S. EROZAN, X.C. LUO, M.J. BARRETT, Q.Y. YAN, C.A. GIFFEN, S.Q. HUANG, M.M. MAHER, M.R. FORMAN & M.S. TOCKMAN. 1997. Risk factors and early detection of lung cancer in a cohort of Chinese tin miners. Ann. Epidemiol. **7:** 533–541.
2. TAYLOR, P.R., Y.L. QIAO, A. SCHATZKIN, S.X. YAO, J. LUBIN, B.L. MAO, J.Y. RAO, X.Z. XUAN, J.Y. LI & M. MCADAMS. 1989. Relation of arsenic exposure to lung cancer among tin miners in Yunnan Province, China. Br. J. Ind. Med. **46:** 881–886.
3. LI, L., F. LU & S. ZHANG. 1996. [Analysis of cancer mortality and distribution in China from year 1990 through 1992—An epidemiologic study]. Chung Hua Chung Liu Tsa Chih (Chin. J. Oncol.) **18**(6): 403–407.
4. FORMAN, M.R., S.X. YAO, B.I. GRAUBARD, Y.L. QIAO, M. MCADAMS, B.L. MAO & P.R. TAYLOR. 1992. The effect of dietary intake of fruits and vegetables on the odds ratio of lung cancer among Yunnan tin miners. Int. J. Epidemiol. **21:** 437–441.
5. ZIEGLER, R.G., A.F. SUBAR, N.E. CRAFT, G. URSIN, B.H. PATTERSON & B.I. GRAUBARD. 1992. Does β-carotene explain why reduced cancer risk is associated with vegetable and fruit intake. Cancer Res. (Suppl.) **52:** 2060s–2066s.
6. STEINMETZ, K.A. & J.D. POTTER. 1996. Vegetables, fruit, and cancer prevention: A review. J. Am. Diet. Assoc. **96:** 1027–1039.
7. MICHAUD, D.S., E.L. GIOVANNUCCI, A. ASCHERIO, E.B. RIMM, M.R. FORMAN, L. SAMPSON & W.C. WILLETT. 1998. Associations of plasma carotenoid concentrations and dietary intake of specific carotenoids in samples of two prospective cohort studies using a new carotenoid database. Cancer Epidemiol. Biomarkers Prev. **7:** 283–290.
8. HUNTER, D. 1998. Biochemical indicators of dietary intake in Nutritional Epidemiology. W. Willett, Ed.: 174–243. Oxford University Press. Oxford.

9. GROSS, M., M. PFEIFFER, M. MARTINI, D. CAMPBELL, J. SLAVIN & J. POTTER. 1996. The quantitation of metabolites of quercetin flavonols in human urine. Cancer Epidemiol. Biomarkers Prev. **5:** 711–720.

10. ITO, Y., Y. SHIMA, J. OCHIAI, M. OTANI, R. SASAKI, S. SUZUKI, N. HAMAJIMA, H. OGAWA & K. AOKI. 1991. Effects of the consumption of cigarettes, alcohol and foods on serum concentrations of carotenoids, retinol, and tocopherols in healthy inhabitants living in a rural area of Hokkaido. Nippon Eiseigaku Zasshi **46:** 874–882.

11. SHIBATA, A., R. SASAKI, Y. ITO, N. HAMAJIMA, S. SUZUKI, M. OHTANI & K. AOKI. 1989. Serum concentration of beta-carotene and intake frequency of green-yellow vegetables among healthy inhabitants of Japan. Int. J. Cancer **44:** 48–52.

12. SCOTT, K.J., D.I. THURNHAM, D.J. HART, S.A. BINGHAM & K. DAY. 1996. The correlation between the intake of lutein, lycopene, and β carotene from vegetables and fruits, and blood plasma concentrations in a group of women aged 50–65 years in the UK. Br. J. Nutr. **75:** 409–418.

13. DREWNOWSKI, A., C.L. ROCK, S.A. HENDERSON, A.B. SHORE, C. FISCHLER, P. GALAN, P. PREZIOSI & S. HERCBERG. 1997. Serum β-carotene and vitamin C as biomarkers of vegetable and fruit intakes in a community based sample of French adults. Am. J. Clin. Nutr. **65:** 1796–1802.

14. ERDMAN, J.W., T.L. BIERER & E.T. GUGGER. 1993. Absorption and transport of carotenoids. *In* Carotenoids in Human Health. L.M. Canfield, N.I. Krinsky & J.A. Olson, Eds.: **691:** 76–85. The New York Academy of Sciences. New York.

15. RIMM, E. & G. COLDITZ. 1993. Smoking, alcohol, and plasma levels of carotenes and vitamin E. Ann. N.Y. Acad. Sci. **686:** 323–334.

16. HOWARD, A.N., N.R. WILLIAMS, C.R. PALMER, J.P. CAMBOU, A.E. EVANS, J.W. FOOTE, P. MARQUES-VIDAL, E.E. MCCRUM, J.B. RUIDAVETS, S.V. NIGDIKAR, J. RAJPUT-WILLIAMS & D.I. THURNHAM. 1996. Do hydroxy-carotenoids prevent coronary heart disease? A comparison between Belfast and Toulouse. Int. J. Vitam. Nutr. Res. **66:** 113–118.

17. FORMAN, M.R., J. ZHANG, L. NEBELING, S-X. YAO, M.J. SLESINSKI, Y-L. QAIO, S. ROSS, S. KEITH, M. MAHER, C. GIFFIN, M. BARRETT, P.R. TAYLOR & B.I. GRAUBARD. 1999. Relative validity of a food frequency questionnaire among tin miners in China: 1992–1993 and 1995–1996 Diet validation studies. Public Health Nutr. **2:** 301–315.

18. SOWELL, A.L., D.L. HUFF, P.R. YEAGER, S.P. CAUDILL & E.W. GUNTER. 1994. Retinol, α-tocopherol, β-cryptoxanthin, lycopene, α-carotene, trans-β-carotene, and four retinyl esters in serum determined simultaneously by reversed-phase HPLC with multi-wavelength detection. Clin. Chem. **40:** 411–416.

19. HERMANN, H.H., K. WIMALASENA, L.C. FOWLER, C.A. BEARD & S.W. MAY. 1988. Demonstration of the ascorbate dependence of membrane-bound dopamine β-monooxygenase in adrenal chromaffin granule ghosts. J. Biol. Chem. **263:** 666–672.

20. GUNTER, E.W., B.L. LEWIS & S.M. KONCIKOWSKI. 1996. Laboratory methods used for the Third National Health and Nutrition Examination Survey (NHANES III), 1988–1994. Centers for Disease Control and Prevention, Hyattsville, MD. VII-D-1 to VII D-7.

21. FORMAN, M.R., G.R. BEECHER, E. LANZA, M.E. REICHMAN, B.I. GRAUBARD, W. CAMPBELL, T. MARR, C.Y. LEE, J.T. JUDD & P.R. TAYLOR. 1995. Effect of alcohol consumption on plasma carotenoid concentrations in premenopausal women: A controlled dietary study. Am. J. Clin. Nutr. **62:** 131–135.

22. ASCHERIO, A., M.J. STAMPFER, G.A. COLDITZ, E.B. RIMM, L. LITIN & W.C. WILLETT. 1992. Correlations of vitamin A and E intakes with the plasma concentrations of

carotenoids and tocopherols among American men and women. J. Nutr. **122:** 1792–1801.

23. ZHENG, S., A.G. ERSHOW, C.S. YANG, G. LI, R. LI, H. LI, X. ZOU, L. SONG, Q. QING, Q. YANG, Y. SUN, J. LI & W. J. BLOT. 1989. Nutritional status in Linxian, China: Effects of season and supplementation. Int. J. Vitam. Nutr. Res. **59:** 190–199.

24. BATES, C.J., L. VILLARD, A.M. PRENTICE, A.A. PAUL & R.G. WHITEHEAD. 1984. Seasonal variations in plasma retinol and carotenoid levels in rural Gambian women. Trans. R. Soc. Trop. Med. Hyg. **78:** 814–817.

25. OLMEDILLA, B., F. GRANDO, I. BLANCO & E. ROJAS-HIDALGO. 1994. Seasonal and sex-related variations in six serum carotenoids, retinol, and α-tocopherol. Am. J. Clin. Nutr. **60:** 106–110.

26. RAUTALAHTI, M., D. D. ALBANES, J. HAUKKA, E. ROOS, C-G. GREF & J. VIRTAMO. 1993. Seasonal variation of serum concentrations of β-carotene and α-tocopherol. Am. J. Clin. Nutr. **57:** 1–6.

27. ROSS, M.A., K.M. CROSLEY, S.J. DUTHIE, A.C. COLLINS, A.C. ARTHUR & G.G. DUTHIE. 1995. Plasma concentrations of carotenoids and antioxidant vitamins in Scottish males: Influences of smoking. Eur. J. Clin. Nutr. **49:** 861–865.

28. COONEY, R.V., A.A. FRANKE, J.H. HANKIN, L.J. CUSTER, L.R. WILKENS, P.J. HARWOOD & L. LEMARCHAND. 1995. Seasonal variations in plasma micronutrients and antioxidants. Cancer Epidemiol. Biomarkers Prev. **4:** 207–215.

29. STRYKER, W.S., L.A. KAPLAN, E.A. STEIN, M.J. STAMPFER, A. SOBER & W. C. WILLETT. 1988. The relation of diet, cigarette smoking, and alcohol consumption to plasma β-carotene and α-tocopherol levels. Am. J. Epidemiol. **127:** 283–296.

30. CHOW, C.K., R.R. THACKER, C. CHANGCHIT, R.B. BRIDGES, S.R. REHM, J. HUMBLE & J. TURBEK. 1986. Lower levels of vitamin C and carotenes in plasma of cigarette smokers. J. Am. Coll. Nutr. **5:** 305–312.

31. CAMPBELL, D.R., M.D. GROSS, M.C. MARTINI, G.A. GRANDITS, J.L. SLAVIN & J.D. POTTER. 1994. Plasma carotenoids as biomarkers of vegetable and fruit intake. Cancer Epidemiol. Biomarkers Prev. **3:** 493–500.

32. FORMAN, M.R., E. LANZA, L-C. YONG, J.M. HOLDEN, B.I. GRAUBARD, G.R. BEECHER, M. MELITZ, E.D. BROWN & J.C. SMITH. 1993. The correlation between two dietary assessments of carotenoid intake and plasma carotenoid concentrations: Application of a cartenoid food-composition database. Am. J. Clin. Nutr. **58:** 519–524.

33. BROWN, E.D., A. ROSE, N. CRAFT, K.E. SEIDEL & J.C. SMITH. 1989. Concentrations of carotenoids, retinol, and tocopherol in plasma in response to ingestion of a meal. Clin. Chem. **35:** 310–312.

34. KIM, H., K.L. SIMPSON & L.E. GERBER. 1988. Serum carotenoids and retinol of human subjects consuming carrot juice. Nutr. Res. **8:** 1119–1127.

35. GUIDOTTI, T.L. 1997. Occupational epidemiology in China comes of age. Ann. Epidemiol. **7:** 530–532.

BRCA 1/2 Gene Mutation Testing–based Cancer Prevention and the Moral Concerns of Different Types of Patients

GUIDO GOELEN,[a] ADELHEID RIGO,[b] MARYSE BONDUELLE,[c] AND JACQUES DE GRÈVE[a,d,e]

Departments of [a]Cancer Prevention, [b]Philosophy and Moral Sciences, [c]Medical Genetics, and [d]Medical Oncology, Vrije Universiteit Brussels, B-1090 Brussels, Belgium

INTRODUCTION

Predictive genetic testing can be part of a comprehensive cancer prevention program. The *BRCA1* and *BRCA2* gene mutation analysis–based testing, for the familial susceptibility to breast and ovarian cancer, may be a quantitatively important example of such testing.[1] The possibilities of identifying the predisposing mutation, in a family with a documented inherited breast cancer history, were greatly enhanced by the sequencing of the genes *BRCA1* and *BRCA2*, in 1994 and 1995, respectively.[2,3] However, the widespread implementation of this new diagnostic tool may raise specific ethical problems.[4,5] Some health care providers, including genetic counselors, reported their position in this matter.[6,7] This report concerns the results of a study that was dominated by the doctrine that a discussion of the ethical aspects of *BRCA 1/2* gene mutation testing would benefit from a contribution from the patient's perspective. The object of the study was to determine the moral concerns of the patients attending a familial cancer clinic for *BRCA 1/2* gene mutation testing–based genetic counseling.

PATIENTS AND METHODS

Patients

The patients in the study sample are members of a consecutive series of 100 families who attended a familial cancer clinic. The recruiting period started in September 1994 and lasted two years. A *BRCA 1/2* gene mutation screen was initiated if there was a request for testing from at least one family member, if there was a sample of a symptomatic individual available for analysis, and if the family history was compatible with the segregation of a *BRCA1* or a *BRCA2* gene mutation. This was considered to be the case if there were two first-degree relatives, one affected with

[e]Address for communication: Department of Medical Oncology, Department of Cancer Prevention, Vrije Universiteit Brussels, Laarbeeklaan 101, B-1090 Brussels, Belgium. Voice: +32 2 477 54 51; fax: +32 2 477 62 10.
e-mail: ongdgej@az.vub.ac.be

breast cancer and one with ovarian cancer; or two first-degree relatives affected with breast cancer if one of these was diagnosed before the age of fifty. Intermediate male family members were ignored in determining the degree of kinship.

Accordingly, a *BRCA 1/2* gene mutation screen was initiated in 42 families in the study sample. Ten *BRCA1* and 4 *BRCA2* gene mutations were found in symptomatic family members and confirmed by sequencing.[8] Fourteen of the 52 eligible pre-symptomatic women requested testing, as did 8 of the 46 eligible men.

METHODS

The counseling sessions for familial cancer were tape-recorded as a matter of routine. All counselors consented to this procedure, as did the patients, bar two. An attempt was made to identify the moral concerns of the patients by analysis of the verbal transcripts of the counseling sessions. The grounded theory approach was used in the qualitative analysis of these data.[9,10] Counseling sessions were selected for transcription and analysis in accordance with the theoretical sampling process of grounded theory. The analysis of 30 counseling sessions allowed for the 87 candidate categories of moral concerns of patients initially identified to be reduced to 4 core categories of moral concerns. Unexpectedly, these core categories could be linked to the carrier status of the patients. A final batch of 15 counseling sessions was selected for transcription and analysis according to the carrier status of the patients, bringing the total of sessions transcribed and analyzed to 45. The quotes subsequently to be found in this report are the author's (Goelen) translations of colloquial Flemish sentences. Names and nonessential details have been omitted.

RESULTS

The knowledge of a specific *BRCA1* or *BRCA2* mutation segregating in the family, and the subsequent genetic testing, divides family members into clinically relevant categories. An individual in a *BRCA* family affected by breast or ovarian cancer is probably a mutation carrier. These individuals can be thought of as belonging to a category of probable carriers, and their moral concerns relate to their being instrumental in the detection of the specific mutation segregating in the family. They value the opportunity to make a contribution towards the well-being of their relatives (*So my getting cancer is good for something after all*), but facing the fact that one is a carrier can be painful (*Yes that was not a good day. I can honestly say that.*).

The first or second degree relatives of a known mutation carrier in our sample were eligible for testing. Moral dilemma's can be created for these possible carriers when a course of action that is perceived as beneficial to others, such as one's children, clashes with one's personal preferences (*Yes, it means a lot to my children, I cannot pass it on to my children. I find that that was my only worry, that I could pass it on to my children, so to speak. That is actually the only reason I had the tests done*).

The patients who are found to harbor the mutant *BRCA* gene become proven carriers. Their moral concerns have mainly to do with privacy and confidentiality. Problems arose when patients wanted to keep the test result secret from their own family. The fact that one shares the responsibility for any children with the other parent can complicate matters. (*I think they agreed to tell each other but to keep it in the family, so that the entire village would not know. But a person who had himself been tested would tell his wife, and the wife maybe would tell her mother, and so on.*)

The moral preoccupations of the patients who tested negative, becoming proven noncarriers, relate to their wanting to help other family members, in most cases their siblings. Regarding deciding on testing, as well as in the matter of deciding on preventive options, first-degree relatives seem to want to help each other make the right choice while respecting each other's preferences. (*We talked about it very openly; we are all very open about such things. I knew about the testing. I could have done it also, and when I asked them, "What do you think I should do? I am still very young," all three* [her mother and two aunts] *gave me the same answer: "You have to decide for yourself." Right up to the end, even my own mother said, "No I am not going to answer that question for you."*)

The descendants of proven noncarriers are obligatory noncarriers. As such, they had no reason to come for counseling, but there was no evidence of these individuals having particular moral concerns to be found in the transcripts of the counseling sessions with their relatives.

The last category of family member, the in-laws, can be called "partners." Their moral concerns, as far as they could be deduced from the transcripts, are reminiscent of the moral concerns of proven noncarriers. (*No, I leave that totally up to her* [referring to his wife deciding for or against prophylactic mastectomy]. *She has to decide for herself; I will not influence her. There are just a few questions that I would ask if I were her.*)

DISCUSSION

Sub hoc signo[11],f

The fact that the *BRCA1/2* gene mutation carrier status of a patient turns out to be the best fit for correlation with his or her moral concerns may be an intriguing aspect of these results. The study has several limitations, such as the data being gathered in the context of one familial cancer clinic, but it will be interesting to compare these results with the results of future research in this area. At the moment there seem to be no empirical data on the moral concerns of patients in the context of predictive genetic testing for adult-onset diseases available for comparison.

Tiresias' Future[12],g

Health care providers have their own moral concerns in the matter of providing *BRCA 1/2* gene mutation testing. The results of this study may help care providers,

---

[f]The Christian Emperor Constantine I had the motto 'In hoc signo vinces' inscribed on the cross. Nietzsche has changed the prefix and left out the verb.

[g]Tiresias realizes the full horror of the secret that he holds when he is in the presence of Oedipus. 'Alas, how dreadful to have wisdom where it profits not the wise!' (The authors preferred the spelling Tiresias over Teiresias, which was used by Jebb.)

who think medicine should be patient centered, to be aware of the moral preoccupations of their own patients.

In view of the increasing number of predictive diagnostic tests that will become available in the near future, and the role they may play in cancer prevention, more research on the moral concerns of the patients may be appropriate. We expect a variety of research methods to prove useful for this purpose.

ACKNOWLEDGMENTS

The Department of Cancer Prevention is supported by Grants from Ms. Wivina Demeester, the Flemish Minister of Finance, Budget and Health Policy. We gratefully acknowledge the cooperation of the patients who agreed to be tape-recording and the other members of the oncogenetic team: E. Teugels, Ph.D.; Bart Neyns, M.D.; Robert Sacré, M.D.; Ph. De Sutter, M.D.; Sabine Bauwens, licensed psychologist; Paul Wylock, M.D.; and Mr. Patrick Cousin for the typing of the verbal transcripts.

REFERENCES

1. BURKE, W., M. DALY, J. GARBER, J. BOTKIN, M.J.E. KAHN, P. LYNCH *et al.* 1997. Recommendations for follow-up care of individuals with an inherited predisposition to cancer II. *BRCA1* and *BRCA2*. J. Am. Med. Assoc. **277:** 997–1003.
2. MIKI, Y., J. SWENSEN, D. SHATTUCK-EIDENS, P.A. FUTREAL, K. HARSHMAN, S. TAVTIGIAN *et al.* 1994. A strong candidate for the breast and ovarian cancer susceptibility gene BRCA1. Science **266:** 66–71.
3. WOOSTER, R., G. BIGNELL, J. LANCASTER, S. SWIFT, S. SEAL, J. MANGLON *et al.* 1995. Identification of the breast cancer susceptibility gene BRCA2. Nature **378:** 789–792.
4. JONSEN, A.R, S.J. DURFY, W. BURKE & A.G. MOTULSKY. 1996. The advent of the 'unpatients.' Nature Med. **2:** 622–624.
5. PARKER L.S. 1995. Breast cancer genetic screening and critical bioethics' gaze. J. Med. Philos. **20:** 313–337.
6. NATIONAL ADVISORY COUNCIL FOR HUMAN GENOME RESEARCH. Statement on Use of DNA Testing for Presymptomatic Identification of Cancer Risk. 1994. J. Am. Med. Assoc. **271:** 785.
7. PREDISPOSITION GENETIC TESTING FOR LATE-ONSET DISORDERS IN ADULTS. 1997. A position paper of the National Society of Genetic Counselors. J. Am. Med. Assoc. **278:** 1217–1220.
8. GOELEN, G., E. TEUGELS, M. BONDUELLE, B. NEYNS & J. DE GRÈVE. 1999. High frequency of *BRCA 1/2* germline mutations in 42 Belgian families with a small number of symptomatic individuals. J. Med. Genet. **36:** 304–308.
9. GLASER, B.G. & A.L. STRAUSS. 1967. The discovery of grounded theory: Strategies for qualitative research. Aldine De Gruyter. New York.
10. STRAUSS, A.L. 1987. Qualitative Analysis for Social Scientists. Camridge University Press. Cambridge.
11. NIETZSCHE, F. 1997. Zur Genealogie der Moral. Philipp Reclam. Stuttgart. p. 25. SOPHOCLES. The Plays and Fragments. Part I. The Oedipus Tyrannus. R.C. Jebb, Ed. Cambridge University Press, 1914. Reprint of the edition. 1966. Adolf M. Hakkert. Amsterdam. p. 53.
12. SOPHOCLES. The Play and Fragments. Part I. The Oedipus Tyrannus. R.C. Jebb, Ed. Reprint of the 1914 Cambridge University Press Edition. 1966. Adolf M. Hakkert. Amsterdam. p. 53.

Cohort Analysis of Etiological Factors for Colorectal Cancer following Endoscopic Resection of Colorectal Tumors

HIDEKI ISHIKAWA,[a,c] KENICHIRO MITANI,[a] IKUKO AKEDO,[a] KAZUSHIGE ISEKI,[a] TAKAICHIRO SUZUKI,[a] TATSUYA IOKA,[a] ITARU KAJI,[b] HIROYUKI NARAHARA,[b] AND TORU OTANI[b]

[a]Department of Cancer Epidemiology, Research Institute, and [b]Department of Gastroenterology, Osaka Medical Center for Cancer and Cardiovascular Diseases, Osaka, Japan

INTRODUCTION

In Japan, it is estimated that colorectal cancer is the second most commonly diagnosed cancer in both men and women.[1] Therefore we planned a randomized controlled trial (RCT) in a high-risk group of colorectal cancer to study preventive methods against cancer and formulated a practical protocol.[2] This protocol has been in progress as scheduled for six years since its beginning. In this report, the protocol that we formulated is explained, as is the cohort analysis of etiological factors for colorectal cancer following endoscopic resection of colorectal tumors, using colonoscopy results at two years in our intervention trial subjects.

METHODS

The subjects are patients with multiple colorectal tumors, who are in a high-risk group for colorectal cancer. They are limited to those in whom two or more colorectal lesions have been diagnosed histologically by endoscopic examination to be carcinoma or adenoma; all these tumors have been resected radically by endoscopic procedures. They are 40–65 years of age; have no history of intestinal resection, except appendectomy; are presently free of malignant diseases; and have no serious complications.

Two regimens were established for prevention of colorectal tumors based on dietary guidance and regular intake of wheat bran (WB) biscuits. The first regimen (regimen I) is dietary guidance alone, and the second regimen (regimen II) consists of dietary guidance and intake of WB biscuits. A regimen is assigned at random for each week in advance. All patients who have received endoscopic treatment, have been examined by a doctor of our group, and have fulfilled the entry criteria are recruited. Consent to participate in the trial must be obtained by the patient's free will, and the record of the consent is on a informed consent form.

[c]Address for communication: Hideki Ishikawa, M.D., Department of Cancer Epidemiology, Research Institute, Osaka Medical Center for Cancer and Cardiovascular Diseases, 3-3, Nakamichi 1-chome, Higashinari-ku, Osaka 537-8511, Japan. Voice: +81-6-6972-1181; fax: +81-6-6981-3000.
e-mail: cancer@gol.com

The core of the dietary guidance is to restrict energy intake from oil and fat to 18–22% of the total energy intake. The contents of meals for three consecutive days before the examination are recorded on diet record forms, a nutritionist interviews the patient on the basis of this record, and the total energy intake and the intake of fat and oil are estimated. For nutritional guidance, the patient is requested to visit the hospital with the family, and instructions about the intake of oil and fat are given individually for about one hour by a nutritionist assigned exclusively to this project, using a "Pamphlet for Guidance of Oil and Fat Intake" prepared especially for this trial. On a later day, the mean daily intake of each nutrient from the date of the dietary investigation is calculated using a computer, and the results are returned by mail to the patients with comments by the nutritionist. Follow-up dietary investigations are made after three months and one year to examine the effects of the dietary guidance, and, if necessary, guidance is given again.

The WB biscuits that we developed have a wheat bran content of about 30% by weight. The patients are instructed to eat 25 g of WB biscuits (7.5 g as wheat bran) daily before each meal. The regimen is continued for four years.

The main end point of the trial is examination of the presence or absence, or recurrence of colorectal tumors. Colorectal endoscopy is performed two and four years after the beginning of the regimen to examine for the recurrence of colorectal tumors. A video colonoscope system (Olympus EIVS 200), which shows real-time endoscopic images on cathode ray tubes, so that two or more doctors can study the images simultaneously, is used for the examination. Examination is always done by two or more doctors to detect new lesions. All lesions observed are biopsied and examined histologically without the knowledge of which group the patient belongs to. The cell proliferation in ascending and sigmoid color biopsy specimens is also studied by the immunohistochemical technique, and this examination is also done without the knowledge of which group the patient belongs to.

The tolerability of the biscuits is assessed by examining compliance through a questionnaire. The compliance with the dietary guidance is evaluated according to the percentage of oil and fat in the total energy intake at follow-up dietary investigations three months and one year after the beginning of the regimen.

The target number of patients is 200, namely 100 for each group. How to estimate the necessary number of subjects was as follows. We expect that the recurrence rate for colorectal tumors that has been determined by endoscopic examination after two years in regimen I (dietary guidance alone) is 60%; the recurrence rate for colorectal tumors in regimen II (dietary guidance plus eating wheat bran biscuits) is 40 percent. To establish a significant difference in the number of subjects who have been recruited between the two regimens, to fix for α error to be 5% and for β error to be 80%, 97 patients are needed for each group. The necessary number of subjects is 100 for each group.

This plan was approved by the Ethics Committee, Osaka Medical Center for Cancer and Cardiovascular Diseases in March1993, and entry of subjects was started in June 1993.

RESULTS

Recruiting of subjects was started in June 1993 and was finished in September 1997; 100 (90%) of 115 patients recruited for regimen I and 100 (88%) of 116 pa-

TABLE 1. Characteristics at entry and two years after treatment

Characteristics	New Tumor at 2 Years		Relative Risk
	$0-1$	$1<$	(95% confidence interval)
Number of tumors			
2–5	60 (79%)	16 (21%)	2.31
5<	19 (51%)	18 (49%)	(1.18–4.53)
Diameter of largest tumor (mm)			
1–9	53 (80%)	13 (20%)	2.27
10<	27 (56%)	21 (44%)	(1.14–4.53)
Family history of colorectal cancer			
Absence	71 (32%)	28 (28%)	1.51
Presence	8 (57%)	6 (43%)	(0.63–3.66)
Body mass index[a]			
<24	45 (70%)	19 (30%)	1.03
24 or 24<	34 (69%)	15 (31%)	(0.52–2.03)
Smoking status			
Nonsmokers	39 (78%)	11 (22%)	1.68
Current smokers	29 (63%)	17 (37%)	(0.79–3.59)

[a]The body mass index is weight in kilograms divided by the square of the height in meters.

tients recruited for regimen II consented to participate in the trial. No severe adverse effects have been reported, and the trial is progressing well. The trial will be completed in September 2001, when the four-year follow-up of the last patient will be complete.

At the time of writing, 115 subjects are due for their two-year colonoscopy, of whom 113 (98%) have undergone examination of the entire colon. At the two-year colonoscopy, no colorectal tumor was seen in 42 subjects (37%), a single tumor was found in 37, two were found in 19, and three or more tumors were found in 15 cases. Two or more tumors were seen at two years in 28/99 (28%) of subjects without a family history of colorectal cancer and in 6/14 (43%) with a positive family history; 16/76 (21%) of subjects had five or fewer tumors before the time of entry; 18/37 (49%) had six or more; 13/66 (20%) of subjects had tumor diameters no greater than 9 mm; and 21/48 (44%) had tumors larger than 10 mm (TABLE 1). New tumors were seen more frequently at two years in subjects with a large number of lesions initially, or those who had the largest tumor diameters.

REFERENCES

1. THE RESEARCH GROUP FOR POPULATION-BASED CANCER REGISTRATION IN JAPAN. 1998. Cancer Incidence in Japan in 1991: Estimates based on data from population-based cancer registries. Jpn. J. Clin. Oncol. **28:** 574–577.
2. ISHIKAWA, H., I. AKEDO, T. SUZUKI, T. OTANI & T. SOBUE. 1995. Interventional trial for colorectal cancer prevention in Osaka: An introduction to the protocol. Jpn. J. Cancer Res. **86:** 707–710.

Negative Growth Regulation of Oncogene-transformed Human Breast Epithelial Cells by Phytochemicals

Role of Apoptosis

MEENA KATDARE, HIROMITSU JINNO, MICHAEL P. OSBORNE, AND NITIN T. TELANG[a]

Carcinogenesis and Prevention Laboratory, Strang Cancer Prevention Center, New York, New York 10021, USA

INTRODUCTION

Evidence from epidemiological investigations and from experiments on animal models supports the concept that natural phytochemicals present in fresh fruits, vegetables, and grain products may offer protection against human organ-site carcinogenesis.[1–5] Such phytochemicals as phytoalexins, terpenoids, flavanoids, and retinoids, either as single agents or as adjuvants, may represent valuable lead compounds for preventive/therapeutic intervention. Clinically relevant mechanistic evidence for the efficacy of phytochemicals, at present, is largely dependent on extrapolation and is therefore equivocal.

Human tissue–derived *in vitro* models and mechanistic end point biomarkers provide an innovative approach for reducing a need for extrapolation of basic research data for their clinical relevance. Our earlier studies have sought to develop reliable models from explant and cell cultures of noncancerous breast tissue, wherein induction and modulation of chemical carcinogen- or oncogene-induced preneoplastic transformation is quantified at molecular, biochemical, and cellular levels using a spectrum of mechanistic biomarker assays.[6–11]

In the multistep process of human breast carcinogenesis, transformation of target epithelial tissue from the terminal duct lobular unit (TDLU) to simple hyperplasia, atypical hyperplasia, lobular carcinoma *in situ,* and ductal carcinoma *in situ* exhibits progressively increased risk for developing aggressive breast cancer.[12] Furthermore, the comedo type of ductal carcinoma *in situ* that lacks estrogen receptor (ER) frequently overexpresses HER-2/neu, mutant p53, and epidermal growth factor receptor (EGFR). These lesions are at higher risk for developing drug-resistant, invasive breast cancer.[13–15] A cell culture model exhibiting these characteristics represents a valuable experimental system for clinically relevant translational research. To this end, efforts are focused to establish epithelial cell cultures from reduction mammoplasty-derived normal breast tissue, and proliferative disease without atypia, atypical

[a]Address for communication: Strang Cancer Research Laboratory, The Rockefeller University, Box 231, 1230 York Avenue, New York, NY 10021. Voice: 212-734-0567 ext. 213; fax: 212-472-9471.

e-mail: telangn@rockvax.rockefeller.edu

hyperplasia, fibrocystic disease, fibroadenoma, ductal carcinoma *in situ*, lobular carcinoma *in situ,* and invasive cancer. These cultures will provide models for a systematic analysis of progressive pathogenic changes that represent critical events in the multistep carcinogenic process, and to examine whether downregulation of these events leads to effective prevention of carcinogenesis.

Experiments in the present study have used HER-2/neu expressing the $ER^-/EGFR^+$ preneoplastic human breast epithelial 184-B5/HER cell line as a preclinical model for human breast cancer to (1) examine whether selected natural phytochemicals (phytoalexins, terpenoids, flavanoids, and retinoids) inhibit HER-2/neu-mediated aberrant proliferation and (2) identify mechanisms responsible for the inhibitory effects of the phytochemicals.

MATERIAL AND METHODS

184-B5/HER Cell Line

The HER-2/neu oncogene expressing preneoplastic human breast epithelial 184-B5/HER cell line[16] was routinely maintained in serum-free KBM/MEM medium supplemented with 10 µg/mL insulin, 10 ng/mL epidermal growth factor, 0.5 µg/mL hydrocortisone, 5 µg/mL gentamycin, and 200 µg/mL geneticin, as described.[10,11]

Phytochemicals

The stock solutions ($\times$ 1000) of phytoalexins, terpenoids, flavonoids, and retinoids were made up in appropriate solvents and were diluted in the KBM/MEM medium to identify the IC_{90} and IC_{20} concentrations using a seven-day growth assay.[10,11] The IC_{90} concentrations were used in cell cycle, apoptosis, and gene-product expression assays, whereas IC_{20} concentrations were used in an anchorage-dependent colony formation assay. The cytostatic nature of the phytochemicals at IC_{90} concentration was determined by examining the reversible growth arrest upon withdrawal of the test compounds.

Biomarker Assays

Fluorescence-assisted cell sorting was used to monitor cell cycle progression, apoptosis, and immunoreactivity to specific gene products, as described.[11] Commercially available fluorescein isothiocyanate– (FITC) labeled antibodies were used at previously optimized dilutions. The data were corrected for nonspecific FITC-IgG staining and expressed as arbitrary fluorescence units (FITC-AFU).

RESULTS AND DISCUSSION

Modulation of Cell Cycle Progression

A comparison of the status of cell cycle progression in noncancerous 184-B5, preneoplastic 184-B5/HER, and carcinoma-derived MDA-MB-231 cells revealed progressive increase in the proliferative (P = S + G/M) population, with a concomi-

TABLE 1. Modulation of cell cycle progression by chemopreventive test compounds in preneoplastic human mammary 184-B5/HER cells

Test Compound[a]	IC$_{90}$ μM	Cell Cycle Modulation ($\times$ control)[b]			
		Q/P	Sub G$_0$/G$_1$	S	G$_2$/M
Phytoalexin					
I3C	100	2.5	9.1	0.2	0.3
RES	100	2.2	6.4	0.3	0.3
Terpenoid					
CA	10	1.5	ND	0.4	2.7
CSOL	10	1.5	ND	0.3	2.2
Flavanoid					
EGCG	20	2.1	11.6	0.3	0.7
GEN	10	4.2	18.1	0.5	0.8
Retinoid					
ATRA	2	2.5	4.0	0.2	0.1
9-cis RA	3	5.2	3.1	0.5	1.9

[a]I3C: Indole-3-carbinol; RES: Resveratrol; CA: Carnosic acid; CSOL: Carnasol; EGCG: (−)epi-gallocatechin gallate; GEN: genistein; ATRA: all-*trans* retinoic acid; 9-cisRA: 9-*cis* retinoic acid. Duration of exposure, 24 hr.
[b] Solvent controls treated with 0.1% DMSO for 24 hr.
ND, not detected.

tant decrease in the quiescent (Q = G$_0$/G$_1$) population. Furthermore, the relative extent of cellular apoptosis exhibited an inverse correlation with the extent of transformation. Thus, the homeostatic growth control appeared to be impaired in the preneoplastic and carcinoma cells relative to that observed in the noncancerous cells. This impairment was in part due to enhanced aberrant proliferation and downregulated apoptosis.[10,11]

The effect of phytochemicals on cell cycle progression in 184-B5/HER cells is shown in TABLE 1. The phytoalexins, flavonoids, and retinoids at cytostatic dose levels exhibited a 2.1-fold to 5.2-fold increase in the ratio of quiescent (Q = G$_0$/G$_1$) to proliferative (P = S + G$_2$/M) cell population. This alteration was mainly due to inhibited S and/or G$_2$/M phases of the cell cycle. In addition, these phytochemicals induced a 3.1-fold to 18.1-fold increase in the sub G$_0$/G$_1$ (apoptotic) cells population. By contrast, two terpenoids tested induced a 2.2-fold to 2.7-fold increase in cells in the G$_2$/M phase of the cell cycle. These data taken together suggest that mechanistically distinct classes of chemopreventive test compounds affect distinct phases of the cell cycle to inhibit aberrant proliferation.

Modulation of Cell Cycle Regulatory Proteins

The experiment designed to identify cellular targets responsible for preventive efficacy of phytochemicals is presented in TABLE 2. The data generated from this experiment demonstrate that the chemopreventive compounds at cytostatic dose levels induced a 31.0% to 87.1% decrease in immunoreactivity to tyrosine kinase–specific antibody, and a 29.8% to 94.5% increase in immunoreactivity to the antibody spe-

TABLE 2. Modulation of cell cycle regulatory proteins by chemopreventive test compounds in preneoplastic human mammary 184-B5/HER cells

Test Compound	IC_{90} µM	Tyrosine kinase	cdki p16^{INK4}	Bcl-2	Bax
Phytoalexin					
I3C	100	−36.0	+89.4	−22.8	+22.5
RES	100	−44.0	+29.8	−61.5	+38.5
Terpenoid					
CA	10	−31.0	+94.5	−60.9	+40.9
CSOL	10	−33.0	+64.1	−62.8	+67.3
Flavanoid					
EGCG	20	−74.6	+79.4	−36.6	+32.4
GEN	10	−87.1	+75.1	−66.8	+65.8
Retinoid					
ATRA	2	−69.9	+52.1	−53.0	+25.8
9-cis RA	3	−60.5	+65.6	−58.8	+28.5

Fluorescence Intensity[a] (% of control)[b]

[a] Arbitrary fluorescence units corrected for FITC-IgG.
[b] Corrected value for 0.1% DMSO–treated solvent control = 100%. Duration of exposure 24 hr.

cific for cyclin-dependent kinase inhibitor p16^{INK4}. These data suggest that the phytochemicals may alter the growth of 184-B5/HER cells, in part, by inhibiting the positive regulatory effect of tyrosine kinase and by enhancing a negative growth regulatory effect of p16^{INK4}.[11,17–19]

The induction of apoptosis by the phytochemicals was associated with a 22.8% to 62.8% inhibition of immunoreactivity to antiapoptotic Bcl-2. This inhibition was associated with a 22.5% to 67.3% enhancement of immunoreactivity to proapoptotic Bax. It is noteworthy that the two terpenoids exhibited a 60.9% to 62.8% decrease in Bcl-2 immunoreactivity and a 40.9% to 67.3% increase in Bax immunoreactivity. This alteration in apoptosis-specific gene products was followed by a moderate increase in the sub-G_0/G_1 population at the 96-hr time point (data not shown). Factors responsible for the delay between expression of biochemical markers (Bcl-2/Bax) and of cellular marker (apoptosis) remain to be identified.

Inhibition of Anchorage-dependent Colony Formation

Interruption of administration of the chemopreventive agent leads to tumor regrowth.[20–22] In the present cell culture model retinoid-mediated growth arrest is reversible upon withdrawal of the compound.[23] Long-term preventive efficacy of the phytochemicals was therefore examined using the colony-forming assay that measured the colony-forming efficiency (CFE) after a continuous 21-day exposure to test compounds at IC_{20} levels. The phytochemicals tested induced a 63.8% to 82.0% inhibition of CFE relative to that seen in solvent-treated controls.

In conclusion, the data generated from this study indicate that cell cycle– and apoptosis-related biomarkers that are altered in response to HER-2/neu-mediated tumorigeneic transformation may represent mechanistic end points for evaluating preventive efficacy of natural dietary components. Thus, the present study validates a preclinical *in vitro* model for human breast cancer chemoprevention.

ACKNOWLEDGMENTS

This work was supported by Department of Defense Grant DAMD 17-94-J-4208, National Institutes of Health Grant P01CA29502, and the Anne Fisher Nutrition Center. The authors wish to acknowledge the expert technical assistance of Milan Zvanovec and excellent editorial assistance of Theresa Di Meola. The data generated were presented in part at the 88th American Association for Cancer Research (AACR) meeting, Abst. #1400, 1997; and at the 89th AACR meeting, Abst. #2446, 1998.

REFERENCES

1. STENMETZ, K.A. & J.D. POTTER. 1991. Vegetables, fruits and cancer. Int. J. Epidemiol. Cancer Causes Control **2:** 325–357.
2. VERHOEVEN, D.T.H. *et al.* 1996. Epidemiological studies on brassica vegetables. Cancer Epidemiol. Biomarkers Prev. **5:** 733–748.
3. BRADLOW, H.L. *et al.* 1991. Effect of dietary indole-3-carbinol on estradiol metabolism and spontaneous mammary tumorigenesis in mice. Carcinogenesis **12:** 1571–1574.
4. XU, Y. *et al.* 1992. Inhibition of tobacco specific nitrosamine induced lung tumorigenesis in A/J mice by green tea and its major polyphenols as antioxidants. Cancer Res. **52:** 3875–3879.
5. LAMARTINIERE, C.A. *et al.* 1995. Neonatal genistein chemoprevents mammary cancer. Proc. Soc. Exp. Biol. Med. **208:** 120–123.
6. TELANG, N.T. *et al.* 1992. Molecular and endocrine biomarkers in noninvolved breast: Relevance to cancer chemoprevention. J. Cell. Biochem. **16G:** 161–169.
7. TELANG, N.T. *et al.* 1991. Biotransformation of estradiol by explant cultures of human mammary tissue. Steroids **56:** 37–43.
8. TELANG, N.T. *et al.* 1990. Cellular ras protooncogene expression in human mammary explant cultures: A potential marker for chemical carcinogenesis. Ann. N.Y. Acad. Sci. **586:** 230–237.
9. TELANG, N.T. 1996. Oncogenes, estradiol biotransformation, and mammary carcinogenesis. Ann. N.Y. Acad. Sci. **784:** 277–287.
10. TELANG, N.T. *et al.* 1997. Inhibition of proliferation and modulation of estradiol metabolism: Novel mechanisms for breast cancer prevention by the phytochemical indole-3-carbinol. Proc. Soc. Exp. Biol. Med. **216:** 246–252.
11. KATDARE, M. *et al.* 1998. Inhibition of aberrant proliferation and induction of apoptosis in preneoplastic human mammary epithelial cells by natural phytochemicals. Oncol. Rep. **5:** 311–315.
12. BERARDO, M.D. *et al.* 1996. Biological characteristics of premalignant and preinvasive breast disease. *In* Hormone Dependent Cancer. J.R. Pasqualini & B.S. Katzene Ilenbogen, Eds.: 1–23. Marcel Dekker Inc. New York.
13. VAN DE VIJNER, M.J. *et al.* 1988. Neu protein overexpression in breast cancer: Association with comedo type ductal carcinoma *in situ* and limited prognostic value in stage II breast cancer. N. Engl. J. Med. **319:** 11239–11245.
14. FABIAN, C.J. *et al.* 1993. Biomarker and cytologic abnormalities in women at high and low risk of breast cancer. J. Cell. Biochem. **17G:** 153–160.
15. PEGRAM, M.D. *et al.* 1998. Phase II study of receptor enhanced chemosensitivity using recombinant humanized anti p185$^{HER2/neu}$ antibody plus cisplatin in patients

with HER-2/neu overexpressing metastatic breast cancer refractory to chemotherapy treatment. J. Clin. Oncol. **16:** 2659–2671.

16. ZHAI, Y.F. *et al.* 1993. Increased expression of specific tyrosine phosphatases in
human breast epithelial cells neoplastically transformed by the HER-2/neu onoc-
gene. Cancer Res. **53:** 2272–2278.

17. VAN DE VIJVER, M. & R. NUSSE. 1991. The molecular biology of breast cancer. Biochem. Biophys. Acta **1072:** 33–50.

18. PIERCE, J.H. *et al.* 1991. Oncogenic potential of erbB-2 in human breast epithelial
cells. Oncogene **6:**1189–1194.

19. HUSCHTSCHA, L.I. *et al.* 1998. Loss of p16^{INK4} by methylation is associated with life
span extension of human mammary epithelial cells. Cancer Res. **58:** 3508–3512.

20. COSTA, A. *et al.* 1994. Prospects of chemoprevention of human cancers with the synthetic retinoid Fenretinide. Cancer Res. **54** (Suppl.): 2032–2037.

21. MOON R.C. *et al.* 1992. Retinoids as chemopreventive agents for breast cancer. Cancer Detect. Prev. **16:** 73–79.

22. VERONESI, U. *et al.* 1992. Chemoprevention of breast cancer with retinoids. J. Natl.
Cancer Inst. Monogr. **12:** 93–97.

23. JINNO, H. *et al.* 1999. Inhibition of aberrant proliferation and induction of apoptosis
in HER-2/neu oncogene transformed human mammary epithelial cells by N-(4-
hydroxyphenyl) retinamide. Carcinogenesis **20:** 229–236.

Fecal pH from Patients with Colorectal Tumors

KENICHIRO MITANI, [a,c] HIDEKI ISHIKAWA,[a] IKUKO AKEDO,[a]
KAZUSHIGE ISEKI,[a] TAKAICHIRO SUZUKI,[a] TATSUYA IOKA,[a] ITARU KAJI,[b]
HIROYUKI NARAHARA,[b] AND TORU OTANI[b]

[a]Department of Cancer Epidemiology, Research Institute, and
[b]Department of Gastroenterology, Osaka Medical Center for
Cancer and Cardiovascular Diseases, Osaka, Japan

INTRODUCTION

It has been reported that the usual fecal pH in normal humans is neutral, becoming more alkaline with the ingestion of meat, and more acidic with the ingestion of large amounts of sugars or fats.[1–3] There have also been reports that fecal pH varies among races, with South African whites having a significantly lower fecal pH than Indians and other people of color, as well as a higher incidence of colorectal cancer.[2] However, it has also been reported that carcinogens are induced when fecal pH becomes alkaline,[3–5] so the relationship between fecal pH and the risk of colorectal cancer is unclear. In this study, we attempted to elucidate the relationship between fecal pH and colorectal cancer. We measured fecal pH in subjects with early colorectal cancer or colorectal adenomas, which are thought to be precancerous, and in subjects with no colorectal disease.

METHODS

Fecal samples were obtained from patients who had undergone colonoscopy at the Osaka Medical Center for Cancer and Cardiovascular Diseases and who had given their consent. There were 302 subjects with two or more adenomas, 115 subjects with early colorectal cancer, and 12 subjects with no abnormality as judged by colonoscopy. Fecal samples were obtained at least two months after the removal, at colonoscopy, of any lesions. Samples were collected by the subjects defecating directly into specially made containers. Immediately after collection, the samples were put in anaerobic conditions, packed in ice and sent to the hospital. Within half a day, measurements were made directly with the pH meter. A record was made of all meals eaten by the subjects for the three days preceding testing, and they underwent an interview with a dietitian on the day of collection. Using a dietary chart, the amounts ingested of each dietary component were calculated, using the method previously reported.[6] Amounts are expressed as mean ± SD.

[c]Address for communication; Hideki Ishikawa, M.D., Department of Cancer Epidemiology, Research Institute, Osaka Medical Center for Cancer and Cardiovascular Diseases, 3-3, Nakamichi 1-chome, Higashinari-ku, Osaka 537-8511, Japan. Voice: +81-6-6972-1181; fax: +81-6-6981-3000.
e-mail: cancer@gol.com

TABLE 1. Age, sex, and fecal pH values of this study population

	Control Group	Adenoma Group	Cancer Group
M : F	7 : 5 (12)	246 : 56 (302)	94 : 21 (115)
Age	59.9 ± 9.7	54.5 ± 6.3	55.5 ± 5.9
Fecal pH Total	6.26 ± 0.39	6.20 ± 0.46	6.37 ± 0.55
Sex M	6.09 ± 0.40(7)	6.17 ± 0.47(246)	6.24 ± 0.45(94)
F	6.49 ± 0.27(5)	6.31 ± 0.55(56)	6.67 ± 1.95(21)
Age ~50y	6.26 ± 0.18(3)	6.16 ± 0.42(81)	6.68 ± 1.87(22)
51~60y	6.14 ± 0.59(4)	6.19 ± 0.50(167)	6.23 ± 0.47(67)
61y~	6.34 ± 0.36(5)	6.30 ± 0.51(54)	6.22 ± 0.50(26)

TABLE 2. Consistency and fecal pH

	M : F	Fecal pH
Soft (67)	60 : 7	6.17 ± 0.54
Nomal (261)	218 : 43	6.20 ± 0.48
Hard (45)	28 : 17	6.63 ± 1.30

RESULTS

Male/female ratios, average ages, and fecal pH for the adenoma, cancer, and control groups are shown in TABLE 1. A tendency toward a higher fecal pH was seen in the cancer group. Fecal pH tended to be higher in males than in females. Of the subjects with cancer, fecal pH tended to be higher in those aged 50 or less than in those aged 51 or older. In the adenoma group, fecal pH for subjects with four or more adenomas (n = 147) was 6.15 ± 0.47, significantly lower ($p = 0.042$) than that of 6.29 ± 0.49 for subjects with three or fewer adenomas (n = 100). No correlation was found in the cancer and adenoma groups between fecal pH and lesion numbers or sites. Subjects whose usual feces were hard tended to have a higher fecal pH than those with normal or soft feces (TABLE 2). A direct correlation was seen between increasing amounts in the diet of animal protein, calcium, iron, or vitamin B_{12} and fecal pH ($p < 0.05$).

DISCUSSION

In this study, fecal pH tended to be higher in subjects with colorectal cancer than in those with adenomas or with no colorectal disease. This agrees with a number of previous reports.[4–6] Fecal pH tended to be higher in subjects whose feces were normally hard, but this was thought to possibly be due to a decrease in the amount of short-chain fatty acids with constipation.[3] The rise in fecal pH with increased dietary intake of calcium and iron was thought to be due to an increase in positive ions. We plan to monitor the progress of these subjects with colonoscopy and to determine the relationship between fecal pH and the development of colorectal tumors.

TABLE 3. Relationship between the contents of meals on three consecutive days and fecal pH

Item	Coefficient	P	(Adjusted for total energy) Coefficient	P
Total energy	−0.071	0.29		
Total protein	0.090	0.18	0.28	<0.0001
Animal protein	0.127	0.06	0.249	0.0002
Vegetable proten	−0.021	0.75	0.083	0.21
Fat	0.050	0.46	0.089	0.11
Suger	0.017	0.80	0.091	0.17
Calcium	0.174	<0.05	0.221	0.0009
Iron	0.109	0.10	0.200	0.0027
Carotin	0.065	0.33	0.087	0.19
Vitamin B_{12}	0.158	0.18	0.259	<0.0001
Vitamin C	0.143	0.03	0.171	<0.0099
Arachidonic acid	0.037	0.58	0.104	0.12
Docosahexaenoic acid	0.088	0.19	0.115	0.09
Water-soluble dietary fiber	0.021	0.75	0.104	0.12
Non-water-soluble dietary fiber	0.069	0.31	0.130	0.05
Total dietary fiber	0.057	0.39	0.130	0.05

REFERENCES

1. WRONG, O.M., C.J. EDMONDS & V.S. CHADWICK, Eds. 1981. The large intestine: Its role in mammalian nutrition and homeostasis. MTP Press Limited. Lancaster, England. pp. 96–97.
2. WALKER, A.R.P., B.F. WALKER & A.J. WALKER. 1986. Faecal pH, dietary fiber intake, and proneness to colon cancer in four South African populations. Br. J. Cancer **53:** 489–495.
3. HOVE, H., M.R. CLAUSEN & P.B. MORTENSEN. 1993. Lactate and pH in faeces from patients with colonic adenomas or cancer. Gut **34:** 625–629.
4. THORNTON, J.R. 1981. High colonic pH promotes colorectal cancer. Lancet **1:** 1081–1082.
5. VAN DOKKUM, W., B.C.J. DE BOER, A. VAN FAASSEN, N.A. PIKAAR & R.J.J. HERMUS. 1983. Diet, faecal pH and colorectal cancer. Br. J. Cancer **48:** 109–110.
6. ISHIKAWA, H., I. AKEDO, T. SUZUKI, T. OTANI & T. SOBUE. 1995. Interventional trial for colorectal cancer prevention in Osaka: An introduction to the protocol. Jpn. J. Cancer Res. **86:** 707–710.

Oncogenetic Information in the Hands of Physicians and the Preventive Options of Persons Who Are Not Their Patients

A. RIGO[a] AND J. STUY

Vrije Universiteit Brussel, Department of Philosophy and Moral Sciences,
1050 Brussels, Belgium

INTRODUCTION

In recent years there have been remarkable developments in the molecular genetics of familial breast and ovarian cancer. The *BRCA1* gene, conferring susceptibility to breast and ovarian cancer, was identified in October 1994.[1] A second gene, the *BRCA2* gene, was identified in 1995.[2] These advances have led to dramatic improvements in the diagnosis and understanding of familial breast and ovarian cancer. An estimated 5–10% of all breast cancers occur in a familial context, with an autosomal dominant pattern of inheritance. Genetic counseling, based on mutation analysis, is now possible in some of these families.

Women belonging to a family with a documented inherited breast cancer predisposition, and carrying the mutant gene, are believed to have a risk of up to 80% of developing breast cancer between the ages of 30 and 70. The efficacy of intensive screening in this high-risk group is still unknown. There are no prospective data on the efficacy of prophylactic mastectomy. Male as well as female mutation carriers can transmit the mutated gene to their children.

Oncogenetic counseling, starting from this new knowledge and technology in the molecular genetics of familial breast and ovarian cancer, raises new ethical questions. Oncogenetic information, as all genetic information, has a predictive as well as a familial character. This last feature is unique: genetic risk information about a particular individual also has implications for her or his close relatives. Parents and children share half of their genes. Cousins have one eighth of their genes in common. Family bonds especially raise issues of confidentiality. The acquisition and disclosure of genetic information confronts individuals with new moral obligations to relatives. Have relatives an obligation to communicate genetic knowledge to one another? And what are the responsibilities of counselors or genetic institutions to family members who are not their patients? Questions also arise when a relative refuses collaboration to a diagnosis that might be important for the patient. Have individuals a moral right to pursue their own goals without contributing to their family's genetic history?

Not only the private family circle is interested in the genetic makeup of a patient. In the public sphere, employers, insurers, loan companies, adoption agencies, and

---

[a]Address for correspondence: Vrije Universiteit Brussel, Department of Philosophy and Moral Sciences, Pleinlaan 2, 1050 Brussels, Belgium. Voice: 32 2 767 26 48; fax: 32 2 477 62 10.
e-mail: johan.stuy@vub.ac.be

maybe even the government, to make its health policy more efficient, might be interested.

The ethical problems regarding the confidentiality of genetic information are many and diverse. In this short article, only one problematic situation will be considered. An individual belonging to a breast cancer family has provided the sample that permitted the identification of the *BRCA1* or *BRCA2* gene mutation segregating in her family. This information is important for her relatives. It confirms any suspicions they may have that an increased risk for breast cancer runs in the family. Moreover they can now opt to be tested for carriership of this particular mutation. However, this particular patient refuses to inform her relatives. In addition to this, she refuses to grant the counselor permission to pass on any information to other family members. In such circumstances genetic counselors experience conflicting obligations: on the one side they have a duty to protect the confidentiality of the patients' medical information; on the other hand they want to protect relatives from harm by informing them about their genetic risk.

MATERIAL AND METHODS

The Point of View of Genetic Counselors

Genetic counselors in the four Dutch-speaking Centers for Human Genetics in Belgium consented to a semistructured interview with open questions. These interviews were transcribed and analyzed. Some questions probed into the dilemma between keeping genetic information confidential (when this is the wish of the patient) and the doctor's obligation of beneficence (towards relatives at risk).

The Point of View of Bioethicists

To place the attitudes of the interviewed Belgian counselors in a wider perspective and to clarify this dilemma, now revived in the oncogenetic counseling, we searched in the international ethical literature. We looked to more theoretically (bioethicists) as well as to more practical (e.g., ethical committee or commission) orientated literature. We report our findings by classifying the most representative standpoints in three main categories (A, B, and C).

RESULTS

The Point of View of Genetic Counselors

None of the interviewed genetic counselors agreed with the view that "genetic information is family property and that the confidentiality of the doctor–patient relation can be breached to help family members." Flemish genetic counselors felt a "conflict in duties" when a patient refused to inform relatives of important risks for themselves or for their (potential) offspring. Nevertheless they never informed family members over their patient's refusal. The Flemish genetic counselors did not welcome a legal obligation to inform relatives over their patient's refusal.

The Point of View of Bioethicists

The standpoints in the literature are very diverse. They range from no limits for counselors to communicate genetic information to relatives to an absolute protection of medical information:

(A) The first standpoint is that of the advocates of breaching confidentiality of genetic information for relatives. They argue that individuals share their genes with their relatives. This way, genetic information is by its nature not only information about individuals but also about their relatives. Genetic information should be treated as family property to ensure access to the genetic information by family members.

Representatives of this standpoint are Wertz and Fletcher. They state that "it is the patient's ethical responsibility to inform relatives at genetic risk of the relevant medical facts, and it is the geneticist's ethical responsibility to remind patients of this responsibility. If parents will not fulfill their responsibility, doctors should be legally permitted to fulfill it for them."[4]

As in more communitarian approaches to ethics, the emphasis on individual rights, as the traditional "right to know," is replaced by considerations of individual responsibility.[5] In this same line of reasoning, the Royal College of Physicians (1991) suggests that not only is there a right to make reproductive decisions on the basis of as much information but also a duty to do so.[6] Kielstein and Sass[7] for example, speak of a "duty to know," based on a concept of "responsible parenthood." Arguments to base such a duty on include the welfare of as yet unborn generations and/or the need to reduce costs to society. A central value underlying this discourse is solidarity.

Some authors[8] see a possible parallel with notifiable, contagious diseases. In order to prevent the spread of the disease among the population, thus preventing great harm, it is justifiable to require that information about people who have the disease be made known. Overriding confidentiality is then justified on the grounds of trying to prevent great harm. The prima facie reason for overriding confidentiality, preventing great harm, also allows genetic information to be seen from the perspective of public population policy. In that perspective, steps to prevent the incidence of a genetic disorder in the population can consist not only of ensuring that individuals do not acquire the disorder but also of preventing the birth of individuals with that disorder.

Like Boddington,[9] one can ask oneself whether the analogy with an outside disease entity is not limited in the case of a genetic disorder? In the case of our genetic makeup the alleged danger, harm, or threats comes not from the outside but from inside, from our own natures.

(B) A more moderated standpoint can be found in the conclusions of the President's Commission for the Study of Ethical Problems in Medicine and Biomedical Research.[10] They state that confidentiality can be breached under some well-described conditions. To the question, "Can a doctor contact a relative in the face of the patient's refusal?" they recommended that disclosure be made only if (1) reasonable attempts to elicit voluntary disclosure are unsuccessful, (2) there is a high probability of serious (e.g., irreversible or fatal) harm to an identifiable relative, (3) there is reason to believe that disclosure of the information will prevent harm to the relative, and (4) the disclosure is limited to the information necessary for diagnosis or treatment of the relative.

The President's Commission did not conclude that there was a duty of disclosure, only that health professionals could ethically disclose such information. Previous legal cases (in the USA) regarding the duty to provide genetic information have all involved a health care provider in a professional relationship with the person to be informed (in this case, the relative). An infectious disease provides a precedent for warning strangers about potential risks.[11] As aforesaid, however, genetic diseases are different from infectious diseases. Quoting the above-mentioned conditions, the Committee On Assessing Genetic Risks[11] believes that the "only potential argument that the health care professional could make for contacting the relative is that through the diagnosis of the patient, the health care professional has reason to believe that the relative is at a higher risk then the general population of being affected by a genetic disorder." The committee determined that the disadvantages of informing relatives over the patient's refusal generally outweigh the advantages, except in rare instances. An example of such an instance is the dominantly inherited disorder malignant hyperthermia in which affected individuals are at high risk of dying from exposure to certain types of general anesthesia. The diagnosis of this condition should immediately be conveyed to relatives.

(C) The third and last standpoint states that confidentiality can never be breached. A doctor may never contact family members over the patient's refusal. Representative for this view is the report of the Danish Council of Ethics.[12] They state that "the next-of-kin must not be approached unsolicited by the genetic institution …. Such an initiative must come from the person who has had the hereditary disease diagnosed—the problem must be mutually resolved between the relevant family members. This should also be the case even in some situations where it can have serious consequences, e.g., where the next-of-kin has not been informed about the hereditary disease diagnosed and that relative gives birth to a child with the same disease."

The Danish Council of Ethics agrees that giving genetic information can empower people, can give them a "scope for action," but there may come a point at which so much information is forthcoming that it may become an intrusion into the inviolability of the private sphere. Widmer[13] speaks of the right to "adopt and maintain a subjective image of oneself, which may be objectively false." A woman who has a genetic predisposition to develop breast cancer in later life may have a self-image that is incompatible with this as a possible future. Is it justifiable to intrude on this woman's self-perception? Does her "right not to know" takes priority over other considerations?

A similar standpoint can be found in the report of the "Gezondheidsraad Nederland."[14] A former suggested solution for the conflicting obligations of the counselor was that the patient, before testing, is informed that testing always includes relatives at risk to be informed, even when he refuses. The Gezondheidsraad rejects this plan because seeking help becomes dependent on one's readiness to help relatives. Finally they are apprehensive that not more but fewer people will be helped.

CONCLUSION

The ethical problems regarding genetic information reopen the debate of medical confidentiality itself. Arguments for compromising the confidentiality of genetic information are illustrated with the striking case of a patient who refuses to inform relatives of a genetic risk. Genetic risk information can, for instance in the case of malignant hyperthermia, literally save lives. In this line of argument, some advance a "duty to know" next to the generally accepted "right to know." An underlying value in the discourse of the advocates of breaching the confidentiality of medical information is the solidarity within a community (standpoint A). The proponents of the view that medical confidentiality can never be breached underline such values as privacy and respect for autonomy (standpoint C).

A more moderate standpoint (B) takes the view that for overriding confidentiality, the consequences of every case should be balanced against some fixed conditions. In the case of breast and ovarian cancer, these conditions are not entirely met. The disorder is not highly preventable (except by prophylactic surgery) nor always curable. In addition to this, disclosure of the family risk information does not necessarily urge people to let themselves be tested.[15–17] Some people do not wish to clarify their genetic status and show a preference not to know. So the reasons to believe that disclosure of the family risk will prevent harm to a relative are limited.

Medical confidentiality acknowledges respect for the patient's personal physical and psychological integrity. It decreases a sense of shame and vulnerability. The promise of confidentiality also permits patients to trust, to have confidence that the information revealed will not disseminate further. In this way patients are encouraged to communicate honestly and forthrightly with their counselors. This bond of trust is vitally important in both the diagnostic process and in the treatment phase.[18]

Although there is a moral obligation for relatives to protect each other from harm and so to inform each other, this cannot be extrapolated to the health care professionals who are not in a professional relationship with the relatives.

REFERENCES

1. MIKI, Y., J. SWENSEN, D. SHATTUCK-EIDENS, P.A. FUTREAL, K. HARSHMAN, S. TAVTI-GIAN et al. 1994. A strong candidate for the breast and ovarian cancer susceptibility gene BRCA1. Science 266: 66–71.
2. WOOSTER, R., G. BIGNELL, J. LANCASTER, S. SWIFT, S. SEAL, J. MANGLON et al. 1995. Identification of the breast cancer susceptibility gene BRCA2. Nature 378: 789–792.
3. RIGO, A., 1994. Genetic Counseling in Vlaanderen: een empirisch-ethische benadering. In Het gebruik van genetische informatie, Federale Diensten voor Wetenschappelijke. E. GULDIX, J. STUY, K. JACOBS & A. RIGO, Eds.: 49–82. Technische en Culturele Aangelegenheden. Belgium.
4. WERTZ, D. & J.C. FLETCHER. 1990. International perspectives on voluntary versus mandatory screening and third party access to test results. In Genetic Screening for Newborns to DNA Typing. B.M. Knoppers & C.M. Laberge, Eds.: 243–257. Excerpta Medica International Congress Series 901. Amsterdam.
5. CHADWICK, R., M. LEVITT & D. SHICKLE. 1997. The Right to Know and the Right Not to Know. Aldershot. Avebury.
6. A REPORT OF A WORKING GROUP OF THE ROYAL COLLEGE OF PHYSICIANS OF LONDON COMMITTEES ON ETHICAL ISSUES IN MEDICINE AND CLINICAL GENETICS. 1991. Ethical Issues in Clinical Genetics. par. 4.7. The Royal College of Physicians. London.
7. KIELSTEIN, R. & H.M. SASS. 1992. Right to Know or Duty to Know? Prenatal Screening for Polycystic Renal Disease. J. Med. Philos. 17: 395–405.
8. EDGAR, H.S.H. 1991. The genome project and the legal right to medical confidentiality. In Legal and Ethical Issues Raised by the Human Genome Project. Mark A. Rothstein, Ed.: 197–221. Health Law and Policy Institute. University of Texas. Texas.

9. BODDINGTON, P. 1994. Confidentiality in genetic counselling. *In* Genetic counselling. Pratice and principles. A. Clarke, Ed.: 223–240. Routledge. London.

10. PRESIDENT'S COMMISSION FOR THE STUDY OF ETHICAL PROBLEMS IN MEDICINE AND BIOMEDICAL AND BEHAVIORAL RESEARCH. 1983. Screening and counseling for genetic conditions. U.S. Government Printing. Washington, D.C.

11. COMMITTEE ON ASSESSING GENETIC RISKS, L.B. ANDREWS, J.E. FULLARTON, N.A. HOLTZMAN & A.G. MOTULSKY. 1994. Assessing Genetic Risks. Implications for Health and Social Policy. National Academy Press. Washington, D.C. pp. 23 and 267.

12. THE DANISH COUNCIL OF ETHICS. 1993. Ethics and mapping the human genome. Protection of sensitive personal information and genetic testing in appointments. The Danish Council of Ethics. Copenhagen.

13. WIDMER, P. 1994. Human Rights Issues in Research on Medical Genetics. *In* Council of Europe. Ethics and Genetics. Strasbourg.

14. GEZONDHEIDSRAAD, Erfelijkheid: wetenschap en maatschapij. 1989. Over de mogelijkheden en grenzen van erfelijkheidsdiagnostiek en gentherapie. Gravenhage. Nederland. 99–109.

15. RICHARDS, M. 1997. It Runs in the Family: Lay Knowledge about Inheritance. *In* Culture, Kinship and Genes. Towards Cross-Cultural Genetics. A. Clarke & E. Parsons, Eds.: 187. Antony Rowe Ltd., Chippenham, Wiltshire, Great Britain.

16. BINEDELL, JULIA & JO R. SOLDAN. 1997. Nonparticipation in Huntington's Disease Predictive Testing: Reasons for Caution in Interpreting Findings. J. Genet. Counsel. **6**(4): 419–431.

17. PONDER, M. & J.M. GREEN. 1996. BRCA 1 testing: Some issues in moving from research to service. Psycho-Oncology **5**: 223–232.

18. SIEGLER, MARK. 1989. Confidentiality in Medicine—A Decrepit Concept. *In* Contemporary Issues in Bioethics. L.T. Beauchamp & LeRoy Walters, Eds.: 405–407. Wadsworth Publishing Company. Belmont, California.

Index of Contributors